Research and
Statistical Methods in
Communication Disorders

Research and Statistical Methods in Communication Disorders

David L. Maxwell, PhD

Professor of Communication Disorders
School of Communication Sciences and Disorders
Emerson College
Boston, Massachusetts

Eiki Satake, PhD

Associate Professor of Mathematics
School of Communication Sciences and Disorders
Emerson College
Boston, Massachusetts

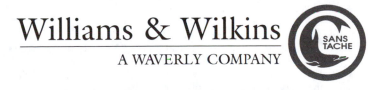

Williams & Wilkins

A WAVERLY COMPANY

BALTIMORE • PHILADELPHIA • LONDON • PARIS • BANGKOK
BUENOS AIRES • HONG KONG • MUNICH • SYDNEY • TOKYO • WROCLAW

Editor: Donna Balado
Managing Editor: Linda S. Napora
Marketing Manager: Christine Kushner
Production Coordinator: Raymond E. Reter
Copy Editors: Bonnie Montgomery and Kathy Gilbert
Designer: Dan Pfisterer
Illustration Planner: Lorraine Wrzosek
Cover Designer: Dan Pfisterer
Typesetter: Peirce Graphic Services, Stuart, Florida
Printer & Binder: Edwards Brothers, Inc., Ann Arbor, Michigan
Digitized Illustrations: Peirce Graphic Services, Stuart, Florida

Copyright © 1997 Williams & Wilkins

351 West Camden Street
Baltimore, Maryland 21201–2436 USA

Rose Tree Corporate Center
1400 North Providence Road
Building II, Suite 5025
Media, Pennsylvania 19063–2043 USA

Accurate indications, adverse reactions and dosage schedules for drugs are provided in this book, but it is possible that they may change. The reader is urged to review the package information data of the manufacturers of the medications mentioned.

Printed in the United States of America

Library of Congress Cataloging-in-Publication Data
Maxwell, David L.
    Research and statistical methods in communication disorders / David L. Maxwell, Eiki Satake.
      p. cm.
    Includes bibliographical references and index.
    ISBN 0-683-05655-7
    1. Communicative disorders—Research—Methodology. 2. Speech therapy—Research—Methodology. 3. Communicative disorders—Research—Statistical methods. I. Satake, Eiki. II. Title.
    [DNLM: 1. Communicative Disorders. 2. Research Design. 3. Statistics—methods. 4. Statistics—problems. WL 340.2 M465r 1997]
    RC423.M369 1997
    616.85′5′ 0072—dc21
    DNLM/DLC
    for Library of Congress   96-29698
                               CIP

The publishers have made every effort to trace the copyright holders for borrowed material. If they have inadvertently overlooked any, they will be pleased to make the necessary arrangements at the first opportunity.

To purchase additional copies of this book, call our customer service department at **(800) 638-0672** or fax orders to **(800) 447-8438.** For other book services, including chapter reprints and large quantity sales, ask for the Special Sales department.

Canadian customers should call **(800) 665-1148**, or fax **(800) 665-0103.** For all other calls originating outside of the United States, please call **(410) 528-4223** or fax us at **(410) 528-8550.**

Visit *Williams & Wilkins* on the Internet: http://www.wwilkins.com or contact our customer service department at **custserv@wwilkins.com**. Williams & Wilkins customer service representatives are available from 8:30 am to 6:00 pm, EST, Monday through Friday, for telephone access.

97 98 99 00 01
1 2 3 4 5 6 7 8 9 10

This book is dedicated to our parents:

Minnie Marie Maxwell & William Lowell Maxwell

and

Tsunehiro Satake & Nobue Satake

Preface

Philosophy and Goals

This text was written primarily for graduate students preparing for professional work in the field of communication disorders. The great majority of students will pursue clinical practice as opposed to research careers. Whatever their professional bent, however, all will benefit from a working knowledge of *both* the principles of research design and data analysis techniques, whether as intelligent consumers of scientific literature or actual producers of such literature. Scientific literacy is crucial for understanding research methodology as well as the statistical assumptions and techniques used for the analysis and interpretation of data. Without such literacy, it will be impossible to stay abreast of a rapidly flowing and ever-changing stream of information related to speech, language, and hearing disorders. The ability to assure quality in clinical care, to render valid diagnostic conclusions, and to discriminate factual information from fallacious reasoning is vital to the future success of communication disorders as a scientific discipline. Toward this end, an understanding of research and statistical methods helps to develop the kinds of analytic and critical thinking skills that can be "mind expanding" for ourselves personally and for the profession as a whole.

Within this book, the authors express the view that the term "science" is best conceived as a verb denoting certain systematic operations used in solving problems, making decisions, and communicating knowledge in a manner that can be objectively evaluated by others. As a noun, the concept of "science" can be intimidating if not shrouded in mystery. As a verb, it is understood to be merely a set of critical reasoning processes underlying strategies and tactics that culminate in an evolving body of facts, many of which are likely to change or be discarded as new facts are discovered. Ultimately, the authors' general goal is to help readers acquire or further hone the kinds of critical thinking and problem solving skills important in the search for "scientific truth" however conditional or temporary such truth might turn out to be.

Features and Approach of Textbook

- Makes clear the philosophical and logical foundations for scientific reasoning and hypothesis testing based on the principles of empiricism, operationism, causality, and probability theory.

- Provides an integration of research methods with core statistical concepts and techniques using clinically relevant examples.

- Provides a simplified schema for classifying nonexperimental and experimental research designs according to the purpose of the investigation and the degree to which control over research variables is desired or achieved.

- Demonstrates step-by-step calculations of commonly used statistical tests while taking an intuitive approach to fostering an appreciation of more complex statistical applications. Every effort has been made to present statistical concepts and applications in a fashion that can be readily comprehended even by students with no background in statistics and only minimal mathematical sophistication.

- Includes detailed outlines to guide students in reading and evaluating research articles and in writing various types of research proposals such as theses, dissertations, and grant applications.

- Discusses the criteria used by academic committees, professional organizations, government agencies, private foundations, and corporations in reviewing and funding research proposals.

- Provides information on presenting research findings at scholarly meetings or professional conferences.

- Provides a Research Article Questionnaire (see Chapter 9).

- Provides a Research Proposal Outline (see Chapter 9).

- Provides a wide array of fully developed problem exercises and demonstrations in Appendix A that are based on representative statistical applications used in actual investigations.

- Includes complete topic outlines at the beginning of each chapter and highlights key terms and concepts throughout the text.

- Provides a comprehensive glossary of research and statistical terminology at the end of the book.

- Provides self-learning review exercises at the end of each chapter to reinforce and consolidate learning. These exercises are arranged in the form of "completion frames" with answers provided in the margin of the page. The task for students is to supply the missing words or numerical computation. To facilitate learning and retention of the material, it is recommended that a **mask** be used to conceal the answers provided until you have formulated your own answers based on memory or by consulting material read previously in the chapter. A mask can be easily constructed from a piece of construction paper folded to the appropriate dimension, or a bookmark may be used.

Chapter Synopses

Chapter 1. Provides an overview of the origin and nature of different kinds of research questions, the general types of research approaches to problem solving, and the role of the scientific method in planning and evaluating research. Presents a cybernetic model of the reasoning processes used by scientists as elucidated in the various components of a research article.

Chapter 2. Provides an overview of the history, nature, and philosophy of scientific thinking, as such thought processes have evolved from the human quest to explain, predict, and control natural phenomena. Shows the linkage between logical reasoning, empiricism, and operationism as forces that have shaped modern scientific approaches to theory construction and hypothesis testing. Discusses some of the major reasons for scientific inquiry and the relevance of scientific problem-solving skills to clinical practice.

Chapter 3. Discusses the conceptual basis of set theory as an approach to exploring associative and causal relations among variables. Reviews the types of *variance* important in the statistical analysis of data sets and the relevance of such variance to testing research hypotheses. Discusses further the kinds of reasoning processes that provide the intuitive foundation for constructing theories, testing hypotheses, and evaluating the significance of statistical outcomes. Makes clear the concepts of validity and reliability, some types thereof, and the importance of carefully evaluating factors related to each of these types in the search for causal relations among variables.

Chapter 4. Discusses several important questions to raise in selecting and defining a research problem, including how questions originate. Emphasizes the significance of developing a well-founded rationale for a research question and gives factors to consider, including ethical considerations, in evaluating the feasibility of answering the question. Distinguishes among the various ways of defining a problem: i.e., as a research question, research hypothesis, or null hypothesis. Examines the statistical logic underlying null hypotheses and some alternative approaches based on Bayesian methods for testing "personal probabilities" or the use of small-N research designs.

Chapter 5. Expands and extends the discussion of concepts covered in earlier chapters to include a concise review of the eight major factors to consider as steps in planning and designing a research study prior to its implementation. These pertain to:

- Identifying a topic
- Conducting a literature review
- Stating a research problem
- Choosing a research design
- Selecting a sample of subjects
- Controlling the variables
- Specifying measurements
- Recording measurements

Chapter 6. Discusses different kinds of measurement scales and the type of data they yield. Presents the basic concepts underlying the application of various *descriptive statistics* in organizing, portraying, and analyzing data. Covers various measures of central tendency, variability, correlation, and regression.

Chapter 7. In preparation for a discussion of statistical inference in Chapter 8, introduces some of the elementary assumptions underlying mathematical models of probability and the rules for calculating the likelihood of various events. Shows an application of Bayes' theorem in reference to calculating the *sensitivity* and *specificity* of a diagnostic test.

Chapter 8. Presents the basic concepts of *inferential statistics* as reflected in parametric and nonparametric hypothesis testing. Covers the statistical theory underlying the notion of *sampling variability*. Discusses the Student t-test and its application to the one-sample and two-sample case along with nonparametric analogs suitable for testing comparable hypotheses. Introduces the intuitive basis of the analysis of variance (ANOVA) and its statistical relevance to multigroup designs and multivariate techniques. Discusses several complex statistical methods and the role of computer applications in the statistical analysis of data.

Chapter 9. Discusses reading and writing skills as expressions of critical thinking and reasoning processes. Outlines the criteria for evaluating a research article and writing a research proposal. Identifies major sources of funding. Notes the steps necessary in preparing proposals for theses and dissertations and the essential requirements for "well written" proposals, whatever purpose they might serve. Comments on the opportunities for professional presentations of research and the criteria used by scholarly organizations such as ASHA in evaluating the merit of such proposals for technical papers or poster sessions.

Acknowledgments

Special appreciation is given to: Professors Gene J. Brutten, for the years devoted to mentoring students, the first author among them, in the best traditions of science; and to Charles J. Klim, long standing teacher of research methods at Emerson College, who encouraged the writing of this book. In addition, words of thanks are owed to Danni Maxwell for her patience and support throughout the many months of this projects.

Both authors wish to express sincere appreciation to those people who have directly facilitated our work in writing this textbook. First, we are greatly indebted to the excellent editorial and publication design professionals at Williams & Wilkins, especially Ms. Linda Napora, Managing Editor, for her good advice and quality editorial standards relating to many publication details. We also wish to thank Ms. Heather Pimental, Ms. Meng-Fong Tan, Ms. Hiroko Ichikawa, Mr. Yoji Ichikawa, and Ms. Rachael Smith for their superb help in preparing many technical aspects of the manuscript involving word processing, computer graphical designs, and illustrations of statistical concepts and calculations. Also, we wish to express our gratitude to the many authors and journal editors who granted permission to use the data of published studies to illustrate various concepts as a part of problem exercises. Appreciation is likewise expressed to Ms. Sophia Belenky and Mr. David Daggett for their computer assitance during various stages of this project. We would also like to thank many faculty colleagues who offered valuable comments and suggestions. Finally, we wish to thank our many students, past, present and future, who inspired us to write this book.

David L. Maxwell
Eiki Satake
Boston, Massachusetts

Contents

Getting Started

The following is a true story out of the personal experience of the first author (D.L.M.) of this textbook. It attests to the fact that research problems are to be found everywhere, no matter how unsystematic our approach is to their solution. I think this story may have relevance to the student who is beginning to study the principles and applications of research—an often frustrating enterprise that also can be enjoyable and full of surprises.

At the end of the story, the co-author (E.S.) provides additional commentary.

In Search of the Wow Factor: a Research Odyssey

One muggy summer evening around midnight, I was awakened by a high-pitched oscillating noise. Through the bedroom window I saw brief flashes of lightening, and I could hear the distant roll of thunder. "Putting two and two together," I concluded it was about to rain, turned over, and tried to go back to sleep. Just as my conscious awareness began sliding into a pleasant state of somnolence, the shrill sound came back again, more piercing than before. As the sound continued, I opened my eyes and tried to focus half-awake sensory machinery on a possible cause. Looking toward the window, I realized that no lightening was now evident and I could no longer hear the rumble of thunder. Yet, not only did the oscillating noise continue, but it seemed louder and more eerie with each passing moment.

Unable to contain my agitation, I bounded from the bed with the unfortunate result of landing on the tail of my loyal sleeping companion, Tillie the cat. She let out a mournful shriek before making a fast exit into the adjoining hallway. Meanwhile, the high-pitched noise could no longer be heard. "Aha," I thought, it must have been Tillie making one of those feline sounds she is capable of composing—weird nocturnal arias that at one end of the scale evoke acoustic images of fingernails scraping a blackboard and, at the other end, sound like the hiss of an angry snake. Admittedly, the oscillating noise had not been quite like either of these, but then Tillie's vocal dynamics seem endlessly inventive.

Feeling remorseful about Tillie, but increasingly confident as to the validity of my hypothesis, I started back to bed. However, the mind set of a Sherlock Holmes is no guarantee of the same results. Soon, the noise was back, proving that for a hypothesis to be valid it must likewise be reliable. Determined to solve the problem, I turned on some lights and walked from the bedroom into the hall. Tillie was sitting at the far end of the corridor, her gaze transfixed on the ceiling. The noise seemed to be coming from a nearby smoke detector. Experience with other smoke detectors had taught me that, like cats, they are also capable of making funny little sounds but for a very different reason. Whereas cats are capable of producing a litany of strange noises when aroused, smoke alarms only seem to "chirp" as their batteries run down. As I stood contemplating the generality of this inference, the noise stopped once again.

Because it is common practice for researchers to acknowledge the assistance of others, I commended Tillie for helping to find what apparently was the cause of our mutual distress. But I was not at all sure that her hurt feelings were mollified by this late praise. After all, I had indicted her wrongly by inferring guilt on the basis of mere association when she had been no more than an innocent bystander. To add injury to insult, I had stepped on her tail.

This might have made a nice ending to the story, but there is more to tell. After replacing the smoke detector battery, I returned to bed hoping now for a good night's sleep. Who was it that said something about ". . . the best laid plans of . . . ?" Yes, the irascible sound was back invading my ears again! Emitting a few unpublishable expletives about the unreliability of even new batteries, I jumped from the bed, this time taking special care to avoid Tillie, ran into the hall, pulled open the cover to the smoke detector, and yanked out the @#%@@$^ battery. Yet, much to our dismay, not even this controlled experimental manipulation stilled the nuisance noise. It then occurred to me that perhaps the noise was not actually emanating from the smoke detector but from a source close by. I didn't want to tell Tillie that her earlier positive identification was perhaps false. She abhors making what we call, in the jargon of research, a type I error. Yet, neither did I want to dismiss the possible significance of such a strange if not ominous sound. To do so would put me in danger of making an even more serious mistake, a type II error.

What to do? I searched my memory for alternative hypotheses. I entered a metamorphic state of consciousness (some what akin to a dreamlike trance), and two rival hypotheses came to mind. The first involved the recent complaint of the next-door neighbors about a mockingbird roosting on their roof at night and keeping them awake. Although I was aware that such birds have a wide range of vocal dynamics, I knew they are best known for imitating the sounds of other birds—not for making the macabre noises in question. The second memory trace stirred up an alternative explanation that was much more daunting given the potential consequences.

I recalled that one summer evening at my cabin in Maine, I was awakened by a similar noise that turned out to be the hum of electrical circuits as they were disintegrating. During that event, the fuse box and some of the wiring in the walls of the cabin had burned up amidst a cloud of smoke as I waited anxiously for the fire department to arrive. The clarity of that particular memory also reminded me of Ben Franklin's well-worn adage: "An ounce of prevention is worth a pound of cure."

To make a long story short, I decided to call an appropriate research specialist—the fire department. The dispatcher at the station inquired politely as to whether or not I could smell any smoke. I replied "No" but went on to tell him of my experience in Maine. "Well," he said, sounding more than a little skeptical, "I guess we better investigate . . ."

Meanwhile, Tillie and I returned to the hall to search for additional evidence. The oscillating noise seemed even more high pitched and louder than before. Also, Tillie's agitation was clearly becoming more pronounced. She ran back and forth along the hallway, systematically investigating the ceiling, the walls, and the baseboard along the floor. Stopping abruptly at the corner of the bathroom door, her little nose twitched excitedly as though finding a new lead. Just then, the door bell rang and I hurried down the stairs to let in two burly fireman holding axes at their sides. "Where's the problem?" one of them mumbled, in a manner that suggested he was still half asleep or bored with his own question.

While directing the firemen to the upstairs hall, I was strangely comforted to hear the noise continuing, which, in the resonating chamber of the stairwell, seemed even more bizarre. Imagine the embarrassment if there had been no empirical evidence to support my claim. At the head of the stairs, the firemen stopped for a moment before focusing their gaze on the smoke alarm. Then one of them walked closer to the device, probing around inside its case with a screwdriver. "The batteries are gone," he said. "It can't be this." "How do we know for sure?" asked the second fireman. "Well, just think about it," replied the first. "All smoke detectors require batteries for their operation. This, being a smoke detector, likewise requires batteries to operate, does it not?" The second fireman scratched his head and asked, "Is that a question or an answer?" "You must learn to think deductively," replied the first fireman in an exasperated voice. "Meanwhile, maybe we should check the attic." "Why the attic?" asked the second fireman. "Because a bird or bat may be up there. Maybe even a squirrel or raccoon! To do your job right, you must not only think deductively but inductively as well."

Just then, the shrill noise stopped abruptly, followed by a moment of silence. Then I heard what sounded like another feline vocalization but this time more like a "wow!" than a simple "meow." "What's on the other side of this wall?" the first fireman asked. "Just the bathroom," I replied. "Lets check it out," said the second fireman, appearing more authoritative and confident. We walked back down the hall to enter the bathroom. Tillie was nowhere to be seen. Then I saw the tip of a fat and furry tail quite unlike the long and lean Abyssinian shape of Tillie's. Pulling back the shower curtain, we discovered the other family cat, Hallie, who was usually the more phlegmatic of the two. Yet, at that moment, crouched down and ready to pounce, her gaze was fixed raptly on what I and both firemen readily agreed was the biggest cricket we had ever seen. "Wow!" said Hallie. "Wow!" said the firemen. And I too said, "Wow!"

As they were leaving, one fireman stopped abruptly in the middle of the driveway. "What's the matter?" asked the other fireman. "Nothing, I guess," said the first in a rather tentative tone. He looked back toward the house with his head cocked slightly and his hand cupped to his ear. "For a moment there, I thought I heard a screech owl." "Naw," said the other fireman with a big grin on his face. "That was a mockingbird. You know," he said, ". . . speaking inductively, that bird can sound like almost anything!"

David Maxwell

Eiki's Reaction

David's account of his "research odyssey" may seem strange as a beginning to a serious book. Yet, the word "odyssey," typically associated with Homer's epic account of the long wandering of Greek soldiers after the battle of Troy, is certainly appropriate to describe the mental meandering of David, his cats, and the two firemen in search of the "Wow Factor." Still, an important question remains unanswered: "Is the 'Wow Factor' the means or end goal of science?" Like a lot of research questions, the answer to this one is quite complex. Some interesting comments on this matter can be found in the words of a fictional character named Donald Shimoda:

> The world is an exercise-book, the pages on which you do your sums. It is not reality although you are free to express reality there if you wish. You are also free to write nonsense, or lies, or to tear the pages. (Bach, p. 97)

Henceforth, our pledge to you, despite the well-known prevaricating reputations of some researchers and statisticians, is to do our best to tell no lies and to avoid writing nonsense. In return, we hope you will persist in reading rather than tearing the pages of our book as we all try to get as close to the truth as we can.

Eiki Satake

1. Basic Concepts of Research and Statistics

Origins of Research Questions

Types of Research

Quantitative Research

Qualitative Research

True Experimental Research

Quasi-Experimental Research

Nonexperimental Research

Clinical Research

Applied versus Basic Research

Planning and Evaluating Research

Scientific Method as a Research Plan

Structure of a Research Article

—*Abstract*

—*Introduction*

—*Method*

—*Results*

—*Discussion*

—*References*

Science as a Cybernetic System

ORIGINS OF RESEARCH QUESTIONS

Ultimately, every research investigation begins with a motivation to solve a particular problem. Sometimes, the solution may lie merely in achieving an improved description of the observable characteristics of certain objects and events, termed **phenomena**. For example, we might ask a **descriptive question** about the prevalence of particular phonologic errors observed in the speech of preschool children delayed in expressive language development. In so doing, we could set about to *classify* or *categorize* the frequency of certain errors according to the type of errors observed. Descriptive procedures are commonly used by clinicians to document the quality or quantity of observed attributes or behavioral characteristics, as typically represented in such nonexperimental approaches as interviews, case studies, or surveys.

On the other hand, we might wish to go beyond the static analysis of behavioral features by noting the manner in which their frequency of occurrence changes in relation to the varying characteristics of other phenomena. Phenomena that are observed to vary in this way are called **variables.** Thus, we might ask a **relationship question** pertaining to the degree to which certain classes or categories of phonologic errors relate to or change in association with other variables such as age, gender, ethnicity, cognitive level, auditory processing skills, etc. When the measure of one variable predicts the measure of a second variable, it can be said that the two variables are **correlated.** Although prediction is an important basis for examining the covariation of phenomena, it does not explain *why* a particular relationship may be found to exist.

A third type of question that can be asked is a **difference question.** Conceivably, this might entail comparisons of **between-group differences** in the prevalence of various phonologic errors or **within-group differences,** reflecting the prevalence of one specific

1

type of error versus another type. Although description and prediction are important first steps in understanding a phenomenon, asking and answering difference questions is generally recognized as the best means for deriving **causal explanations**—the major goal of science. This is because an understanding of the cause or causes of variation of a phenomenon is essential for establishing future conditions under which it might be influenced or controlled. Difference questions are particularly relevant to the goals of clinicians who wish to demonstrate the efficacy of their treatment procedures. By examining performance differences under one particular method as compared to alternative treatment strategies or to the absence of any such active manipulation, causal inferences can be made. Ideally, such an investigation would be designed to restrict the interpretation of differences only to those resulting from the systematic influence of the established treatment condition (**independent variable**) on the behavioral target affected by such manipulation (**dependent variable**).

TYPES OF RESEARCH

Quantitative Research

From the outset, it is important to recognize that scientific research is not a unitary approach to problem solving but includes a broad range of activities and methods that contribute toward the development or refinement of knowledge. In the field of communication disorders, perhaps the most common type of research involves the testing of relations presumed to exist among various processes of speech, language, and hearing.

Typically, **quantitative** measurements and methods of data analysis are used to compare a collection of individuals having a particular communication disorder (**experimental group**) with a normal group of speakers (**control group**). As we shall see in later chapters, comparative measures of averages and variances **between groups** are considered by many to be the *sine qua non* of valid research. Such an approach may be described as an **extensive research model** because it involves the collapse and subsequent analysis of numerous individual scores into unitary indices of group performance.

Although the majority of research studies in communication disorders and related behavioral sciences have been based on the extensive research model, there has been a shift in recent years to an increased use of **intensive approaches (N-of-1 designs),** which are particularly adaptable to studying changes in individuals over a relatively long time frame. Such methods should not be confused with the so-called **one shot case study** that is often subject to illusory retrospective interpretations that are, in addition, potentially biased, unreliable, and lacking in scientific value (Campbell and Stanley, 1966).

The essential criterion for any study is the **reliability** of findings as judged by replication. As discussed in Chapter 5, N-of-1 studies typically take the form of a series of baseline-treatment trials on the same subject. Differences between the baseline and treatment conditions are evaluated **within** each individual subject separately. Intensive designs are particularly applicable to many clinical studies in which generalizations about individual subjects rather than groups of subjects are sought. The "clinical situation" can provide a highly fertile source of research because human problems can be seen and intensively evaluated under controlled conditions apart from the ordinary circumstances and confounding influences of everyday life.

Qualitative Research

Some researchers hold that **qualitative** rather than quantitative methods are more appropriate for the study of human behavior. Such behavior is believed to involve a subject matter that is far more complex, dynamic, and less amenable to quantification than are the phenomena studied by biologists, chemists, and physicists (Filstead, 1970).

Qualitative research involves several types of data collection procedures that emphasize data collection in the **"natural setting"** such as in the home, school, community, etc. Such methods may involve surveys, focused in-depth interviews, direct observation, etc., all of which are designed to allow the investigator to "get close to the data." In his research of street corner culture, Liebow (1967) emphasized the importance of the investigator actually entering the experience of the individuals under study in order to adopt their perspective from the "inside."

A classic example of naturalistic research is embodied in the work of Piaget (1932), whose approach to the study of language development consisted primarily of observing and recording childrens' questions, reflections, and conversations. From such qualitative methods, he published a number of scientific papers concerning various stages of what he termed "egocentric" and "sociocentric" speech development that in turn stimulated much additional research of a similar kind.

Studies that seek to document the customs, social patterns, and rule-governed interactions of a culture or group of individuals are often called **ethnographic research studies.** The methods of such studies attempt to uncover the logic underlying such social rules as might operate, for example, in taking turns in conversations. The type of data emerging from ethnographic studies might also be evaluated in combination with other qualitative techniques. One such method, known as **content analysis,** could be used in the case of our example to observe and code the frequency of certain verbal and nonverbal behaviors during group conversations. Later, the frequencies of particular response patterns could be closely scrutinized and perhaps explained.

An often-cited strength of qualitative research orientations is that, unhampered by preconceived and rigidly structured quantitative techniques, they tend to foster the emergence of new concepts, explanations, and theories. In addition, such methods are said to allow for certain potentially significant *chance* observations that sometimes turn out to be more important than the hypothesis being tested. The term **serendipity** was first used by Cannon (1945) to describe the process of accidentally discovering scientifically valuable information while exploring some unrelated problem.

A classic example experiment frequently cited in support of serendipitous research is based on a study carried out at the Walter Reed Laboratories in the 1950s. In an investigation of avoidance conditioning paradigms that entailed the use of electric shock, Joseph Brady (1958) was frustrated by the inability to complete his experiments as planned because of the high mortality among the monkeys that were used as subjects. During subsequent autopsy investigations, it was discovered that the animals had been subjected to a certain type of negative reinforcement schedule that had apparently resulted in a high incidence of perforated stomach ulcers. Although far from the intent of the original research, Brady and his colleagues appeared to have accidentally stumbled onto an important link between psychological stress of a certain kind and physical disease. Despite such fortuitous observations that occasionally lead to new insights and ideas, these discoveries are best viewed as by-products of research rather than as a replacement for the kind of findings that evolve from more structured and well-planned research activities.

Although an advantage of qualitative research may be found in its flexibility, this type of research can also lead to floundering about from one trivial and time-consuming activity to the next with the potential of losing sight of the main research goal. Unless attention is focused carefully on central issues, it is possible that efforts to collect, organize, and interpret data will be rendered meaningless, as humorously depicted in Figure 1.1.

The Far Side by Gary Larson

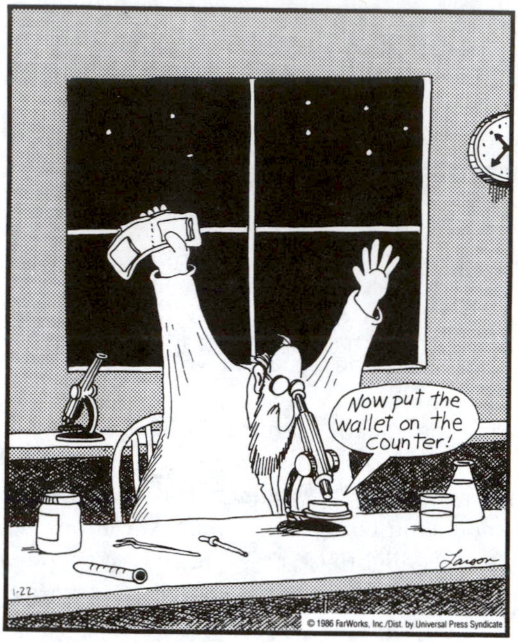

Working alone, Professor Dawson stumbles
into a bad section of the petri dish.

Figure 1.1. The perils of serendipity. The Far Side © 1986 Farworks, Inc. / Dist. by Universal Press Syndicate. Reprinted with permission. All rights reserved.

Another danger of qualitative research is that the interior world of the individuals or groups under study may be distorted by the mere presence of another outside observer or by whatever biases the researcher may impose based on his or her own subjective views.

When possible, practitioners of qualitative research are likely to eschew the use of preconceived measurements or data analysis techniques that could potentially influence or obfuscate the natural interaction of research subjects with their environment. When numbers are used, their primary purpose most often is to describe or represent the mere presence or absence of the quality under study rather than to quantify a specific attribute. Categories of behavior are compared, contrasted, and sorted in the search for meaningful patterns and relationships (Shaffir and Stebbins, 1991).

True Experimental Research

A large number of experimental methods are available for use in scientific research that seek to establish lawful relationships among variables. The use of all such methods go beyond efforts to observe and describe problems to their prediction and control.

True experimental designs can be distinguished from all others on the basis of three main factors. The first of these requirements is the **random assignment** of subjects to at least two or more groups. The second requirement is for some type of **active manipulation** to be performed. Third, one group of subjects **(experimental group)** is then compared with another nonmanipulated group **(control group).** When compared to other research methods, true experimental designs are the most effective in controlling for sources of variance extraneous to the causal relationships under study.

For many practical and ethical reasons, it is sometimes impossible for an investigator to assign subjects randomly to treatment groups or to indiscriminately apply a particular treatment to one group while withholding it from another. This is often the case in many clinical studies in which an insufficient numbers of appropriate subjects may preclude the use of randomization procedures. In addition, it could be argued that withholding a treatment from a target population or administering an alternative treatment with unknown effects rather than one with established benefits is unfair or perhaps illegal (Cook, Cox, and Mark, 1977).

Quasi-Experimental Research

Quasi-experimental research designs are generally selected when true experimentation is impractical or impossible to perform. Typically, subjects are assigned to groups on the basis of preexisting conditions or circumstances. Suppose you work in a hospital clinic where you treat many adult patients for hoarseness accompanied by vocal nodules. Following diagnosis, the availability of therapy is on a "first-come, first-served" basis so that many patients are on a waiting list for 3 months or more. Although the use of randomization procedures may not be possible, you still wish to draw some conclusions about the efficacy of your treatment program.

An alternative way to estimate your program's effectiveness would be to use a **constructed control group** suitable for comparison with a treated group of patients. The two groups would be matched on a number of variables prior to treatment; these variables would possibly include such factors as the degree of hoarseness, size of the nodules, duration of illness, occupation, age, sex, alcohol/tobacco consumption, etc. Such matching would be done to rule out as many extraneous variables as possible so that any subsequent positive between-group differences could be confidently attributed to your program.

As a means of coping with extraneous variables that might invalidate an experiment, quasi-experimental methods often necessitate the use of more control procedures that do true experiments. Consequently, they are considered to be less powerful and, as stated previously, are generally recommended only when true experimentation is not possible. Yet, some investigators believe that, if properly conducted, quasi-experimental designs can be as effective as true experiments (Rossi, Freeman, and Wright, 1979).

Both true experimental and quasi-experimental designs incorporate protocols that are aimed at establishing causal relations among variables. Although it is sometimes impossible in any research study to determine that an experimental manipulation has clearly produced an intended effect, designs of this type offer the greatest promise of producing unambiguous results.

Nonexperimental Research

One type of investigation in which causal relations definitely cannot be established is **nonexperimental research**. In such research, there is no attempt to achieve randomization, nor is any purposeful effort made to manipulate the variables under study. In such studies, many of which involve qualitative approaches of the type described previously, only correlational, as opposed to causal, relations can be evaluated.

Attempting to infer causal relations on the basis of the mere association between factors X, Y, or Z is risky. To illustrate why correlational designs are subject to ambiguity, consider the associative relations often found to exist between attention deficits, low IQ levels, and developmental language delays (Rutter, 1989). It might be argued that any one of these factors could give rise to the others. Alternatively, all three factors could be the common result of still another more generalized delay or abnormality in development.

Efforts to derive causative relations from correlational findings alone can lead to the kind of fallacious reasoning that is represented metaphorically in the "horse and cart" problem or by the "dog chasing its tail." Such tautological reasoning, sometimes described as **vicious circularity,** occurs when an answer is based on a question and a question on the answer. For example, one might ask, "Why do slow learners experience academic failure?" Answer: "Because of language-learning disabilities." Question: "But how do we know they are language-learning disabled?" Answer: "Because they exhibit academic failure."

Correlational studies are generally lacking in purposeful experimental manipulations that are external to or independent of the variables under study. For this reason, they are often called **ex post facto studies** because they search for past causes of a phenomenon that has already occurred. Efforts to derive causal relations in this manner can become hopelessly engulfed in the type of circular reasoning processes described above. As Dember and Jenkins (1970) succinctly noted, ". . . correlational designs are subject to an ambiguity of interpretation considerably greater than the normal uncertainty inherent in any research attempt" (p. 47).

Clinical Research

In evaluating and selecting a particular research design, it is important to bear in mind the purpose of the study. Particularly in the context of the clinical setting, problems are initially encountered in a qualitative form. It is often the case that numerical data are unavailable. Information must be collected from a variety of sources, including written questionnaires, client and family interviews, preexisting records, formal and informal test procedures, etc. Ultimately, the clinician must work from the grist of the historical and current information available about individual clients. By examining the possible relations among antecedent factors and current conditions, an effort is made to form both a tentative hypothesis about the cause(s) of the problem and an appropriate treatment plan.

The research-oriented clinician may collect data on a number of clients with similar problems under controlled conditions of testing or treatment. It is generally the case that a preliminary or **exploratory investigation** begins because of the apparent association between two or more variables. For example, the clinician may have noted during his or her work with children that weaknesses in phonologic encoding and word retrieval seem to go hand in hand. Subsequently, a formal research study may be performed, wherein a strong positive relationship is demonstrated based on the statistical calculation of **correlation coefficients** (see Chapter 6). The next step may be to sharpen the investigative focus through the use of a true experimental or quasi-experimental design in an effort to determine whether or not the observed relationship is associative or causal in nature. To accomplish this objective, special conditions must be established to determine the extent to which an active manipulation of one factor might cause a significant change in another. Given the hypothesis that phonologic encoding skills underlie word retrieval abilities, the investigator might set up an *antecedent* program designed to improve phonologic awareness in a randomly assigned experimental group and then systematically evaluate the *consequent* effects of such training against a randomly assigned control group (a true experiment). Alternatively, in the case of a quasi-experimental design, a comparison group matched on relevant variables might be used instead.

In choosing a particular research design, the investigator must weigh the design's relative advantages and disadvantages in view of the questions asked and the answers sought. Some designs are more appropriate at one stage of an investigation than another. Furthermore, the physical limitations imposed by certain experimental settings, the unavailability of suitable subjects and instrumentation or test materials, excessive costs, and the potential for ethical or legal violations are but some of the constraints that may influence the final selection of a specific research plan.

Applied versus Basic Research

Because the main orientation of the profession of communication disorders is to help clients solve practical problems, most scientific research in the field is directed toward solving **applied,** as opposed to **basic,** research problems; the latter involves the advancement of knowledge for its own sake. This is not to say that one type of research emphasis, applied versus basic, is better than the other. Indeed, much of the foundation of our clinical knowledge is enlightened and directed by advances in the study of "pure" or "normal" processes of speech, language, and hearing. For example, from the study of normal physiology of the inner ear, invaluable information has been gained leading to applications involving cochlea implantation. Through efforts to understand the molecular genetics of normal hearing, genetically transmitted hearing loss may be preventable in the future. Conversely, an understanding of the genetics of normal hearing may be gained by studying individuals with heritable hearing loss. Apropos to the value of studies involving what he called "accidents of nature," Pruzansky (1973) called attention to the eloquent statement written by the great physician William Harvey in 1657:

> Nature is nowhere accustomed more openly to display her mysteries than in cases where she shows tracings of her workings apart from the beaten path . . . For it has been found, in almost all things, that what they contain of useful or applicable nature is hardly perceived unless we are deprived of them, or they become deranged in some way.

In the opinion of the present authors, the applied versus basic research distinction is somewhat spurious to the actual work of scientists who, regardless of the problem, engage certain thinking and action processes designed to provide better and more representative solutions to problems. Such work proceeds by what is commonly called the **scientific method.**

PLANNING AND EVALUATING SCIENTIFIC RESEARCH

Scientific Method as a Research Plan

Science involves a systematic way of thinking and behaving to solve problems. Although the term "scientific method" is often used to describe an interconnected series of steps or organized activities that are uniformly followed by scientists in achieving their research goals, such a view can be erroneous or misleading. In reality, the so-called scientific method is better conceived as a *research plan,* often constituted of diverse approaches and techniques rather than a rigid set of step-wise procedures to be invariably followed by all investigators. According to Thomas (1929), the scientific method can be viewed simply as any set of procedures aimed at the control and measurement of the influence of one variable upon another while excluding extraneous influences.

As noted previously, perhaps the most practical way to conceptualize the scientific method is in terms of the origination and development of the research plan. Although there is no precise template or set of rules to follow, most research plans evolve based on the following factors:

1. Observation of a problem that leads to a question.
2. Development of a problem statement in the form of a testable hypothesis.
3. Use of appropriate methods for testing the hypothesis.
4. Statement and interpretation of results.
5. Discussion and evaluation of results.

Such thinking and acting processes that form the basis of scientific work are reflected in the prototypic structure of a research article, as outlined in Table 1.1.

Table 1.1.
Structure of a Research Article

Section	Includes
Abstract	• Concise summary of the research (approximately 100–150 words) that includes a description of the problem, the experimental procedurres, highlights of results, and a statement of implications
Introduction	• Review of relevant literature, theoretical foundations and rationale, and purpose statement/research questions or hypotheses
Method	• Design of study, subjects, and sampling techniques, controls used, apparatus or test materials, experimental procedures, logical basis for choice of statistics
Results	• Systematic presentation of relevant data, figures and tables, evaluation of data to point out significant/nonsignificant findings
Discussion	• Interpretation of the meaning and importance of findings, evaluation of hypotheses and their generality, implications for future studies
References	• Complete citations of the work of others

Structure of a Research Article

Abstract

Most research articles begin with an **abstract** or concise summary of the problem investigated, the methods used, highlights of the results and their statistical significance, and a concluding statement of implications. Key words are sometimes listed at the bottom of the abstract as cues to the specific topics covered. In essence, a good abstract provides a convenient yet accurate means of scanning the substance of the article as a whole.

Introduction

The **introduction** section of an article includes an historical overview of the theoretical foundations of the problem to be investigated that is usually based on the results of previous research. A review of relevant literature is akin to the process of scientific observation which, as noted previously, involves collecting, organizing, and interpreting available background information (data) related to the current problem. Such research forms the basis for developing a logical argument or **research rationale** that is used to justify the need for additional investigation.

The introductory section of an article most often reflects a thinking process called **deductive reasoning.** Based on a review of theoretical propositions and preexisting knowledge, the introduction should lead naturally to a statement of the current problem. The problem might be stated by denoting the **purpose** of the research or given as a **question.**

For example:

> The purpose of this study was to examine the relative frequency of different types of phonologic errors (omissions, substitutions, distortions) in the speech of children with verbal apraxia.

or

> What is the relative frequency of different types of phonologic errors (omissions, substitutions, distortions) in the speech of children with verbal apraxia?

A third type of problem statement based on theoretical reasoning, prior data, or both is called a **research hypothesis.** As a means of defining a research problem, the use of a formal hypothesis is typically reserved for predicting associative or causal relations among the variables under study. For example:

> Verbal apraxia in children is associated with (or causative of) a significantly higher frequency of substitutions than other types of phonologic errors involving omissions or distortions.

The manner in which the problem is stated in the introduction often provides some hint about the general type of statistics used in analyzing the data. Of the problem statements illustrated here, all three imply that measurements will be carried out to quantify the frequency of certain types of phonologic errors. In the case of the first two statements, the frequency measures will at least be totaled, averaged, converted to percentages, or **statistically described** in other ways. However, it is clear only in the case of the third statement, involving the research hypothesis, that sampling statistics also will be used to infer the **significance of difference** in the frequency of error types.

Method

Unfortunately, the method section of a research article is frequently given the least attention by the reader because, as the *structural blueprint* for the investigation, this section often contains many tedious details. Yet, the framework of the entire investigation either stands or falls based on the strength of its methodological foundation. Most scientific investigations include important methodological considerations that relate to selecting an appropriate (1) design for the question or hypothesis; (2) group or sample of subjects; (3) apparatus or test materials; (4) set of procedures for conducting the study; and (5) statistical analysis technique(s).

Selecting a Design. Choosing an appropriate design relates primarily to whether the intent of the investigator is to describe the characteristics and/or associative relations among variables or to arrive at causal explanations through the use of experimental strategies. If **descriptive methods** are chosen, the research chiefly will entail observing, recording, and perhaps measuring certain events, but no attempt will be made to manipulate the variables of interest. The basic tool of description is systematic observation of the phenomena under investigation. *Observations* of individual cases or groups in the clinical or natural setting, *surveys* of attitudes and opinions, *normative studies*, *prevalence and incidence studies*, and *evaluative studies* of policies and programs are examples of problems that usually call for nonexperimental research designs. As noted previously, descriptive methods are often important in categorizing or classifying variables according to their physical or psychological attributes; this is a preliminary step that leads toward more definitive studies of their causal relations.

When the researcher is primarily interested in explaining the effect of one variable, the independent variable, upon another, the dependent variable, he or she selects either experimental or quasi-experimental techniques. In the field of communication disorders, such **explanatory methods** are frequently used to test a hypothesis about a cause and effect relationship. Such methods are commonly employed in the search for explanations for the causes of specific disorders or to evaluate the efficacy of new diagnostic techniques or therapy procedures.

The defining feature of a true experiment versus a quasi-experiment is that the former requires random assignment of subjects to different treatment conditions, whereas the latter simply involves classifying subjects on the basis of a particular characteristic (e.g., normal hearing versus hearing impairment). Subsequently, the groups are compared on some dependent variable or performance measure. Quasi-experimental designs are weaker than true experiments because of the potential for preexisting subject differences and other extraneous variables to contaminate the results.

Selecting Subjects. Three major factors must be considered in selecting subjects for any investigation. First, the subjects should be appropriate to the goals of the study. If your intent is to study syntactical errors in Broca's aphasics, avoid the inclusion of Wernicke's aphasics or of other types of aphasic disorders in your sample. Ultimately, your goal is to assure the **internal validity** of your results, or the degree to which they can be directly attributed to the effect of a chosen independent variable as opposed to some unwanted extraneous variable. A **confounding effect** owing to selection can result if subject characteristics in one group differ from those in a comparison group. The old adage that "apples and oranges can't be compared" summarizes well this particular problem. In the subject section of the Methods portion of the research article, it is important to list the characteristics of all subject participants, including age, sex, intelligence, type of disorder if present, and any other relevant identifying information.

A second issue is the degree to which subjects in a study are representative of the population from which they were selected. This concern relates importantly to the establishment of **external validity** or the degree to which the results can be transferred to the population from which the sample was originally drawn. If a sample of subjects is not highly similar to the parent population, the study results will be of little or no value as they might apply to other cases under comparable conditions or circumstances. Although **random selection** of a sample of subjects does not assure that the sample will be **representative** of the population from which it was drawn, it is the best means available for accomplishing this goal.

A third issue in subject selection pertains to the number of subjects to be used. Decisions about the number of subjects (denoted by the letter **N**) to be used in an investigation are complex. From a pragmatic perspective, the investigator will include whatever number of subjects are appropriate and available given the particular aims of the experiment. As Sidman (1960) noted, the problem of generality cannot be disposed of simply by employing a large number of subjects. Nevertheless, it is also the case that, for purposes of detecting significant between-group differences when present, large samples lend greater power to a statistical test than do small samples. If the sample size is too small, there is a risk of failing to detect the real effect of an independent variable on a dependent variable—the main purpose of the experiment.

Apparatus and Materials. The apparatus used in presenting stimuli and recording responses, test materials, questionnaires, and related measurement tools must also be described. All identifying information, including the names of manufacturers, model numbers, publishers, calibration procedures for electrical or mechanical equipment, and evidence of the reliability and validity of such instruments, should likewise be included.

Procedures. It is necessary that the procedures used in conducting an experiment be precisely delineated. This is important for at least two reasons. First, research procedures reflect the plan for the actual steps to be followed in carrying out the investigation. As far as possible, the following issues should be clarified by describing (1) the manner in which the independent variable was administered; (2) the way the dependent variable was recorded; (3) the instructions given to subjects; and (4) the nature of the test environment.

A second and equally important reason for carefully documenting research procedures is to allow for replication by other investigators. For this to occur, the essential conditions of the original experiment must be reproducible. Unfortunately, in communication disorders and other behavioral fields, replication is not yet given sufficient emphasis as a part of the scientific method as it is in many of the physical sciences. Although replication experiments in several fields, including our own, do not appear to be highly esteemed, the ability to substantiate research findings through experimental replication ought to be an integral goal of all scientific studies irrespective of the nature of the problem. Perhaps greater value will be placed on such research by future investigators and the editors of professional journals as we are increasingly required to justify, through empirical means, the efficacy of our clinical programs.

Statistical Analysis. Typically, the types of statistical analyses used and their manner of application also are described under the Method section of a research article. The type of statistical methods selected will vary according to the purposes they are intended to serve but will essentially consist of one or more types of three major techniques. If the aim of the statistic is only to describe the features of a set of measurable observations, **descriptive statistics** will be used to *summarize, condense,* and *organize* such observations into a more convenient and interpretable form of data. Tables and graphic figures may be used to display the data in a "pictorial" manner. Such descriptive statistics are also used to derive what are called measures of central tendency **(averages),** and the way in which individual scores are dispersed around such averages **(variability).**

A second major type of statistic is based on investigative efforts to describe an apparent association between two or more sets of data. For example, one might wish to know the degree to which academic performance measures in children are related to various aspects of language expression or comprehension. Statistical tests of **correlation** may be used to describe the degree of relatedness between these or other sets of data. However, it is impossible to derive **causative relationships** on the basis of such comparisons alone.

A third type of statistical technique will go beyond the mere description of individual data sets or their associative relations to making inferences about the degree to which a particular sample of subjects is representative of the population from which it was drawn. In clinical science fields, such as communication disorders, **sampling** or **inferential statistics** commonly are used to study specific disorders or diseases in a relatively small number of individuals. Subsequently, by means of **inductive reasoning,** inferences about the general nature of such conditions in the population at large may be drawn. Most often, we do not investigate specific groups of aphasic individuals, individuals with a stutter, dysarthric individuals, hearing impaired individuals, or individuals with voice disorders for their own sake but to learn more generally about how to explain or modify such problems as found in similar persons from the same population.

Essentially, we want to know the extent to which a **"sample fact"** derived from a small sample of observations approximates a **"true fact"**—the fact that would have been obtained had we examined the entire population. By applying the techniques of statistical inference, we are able quantitatively to determine the degree of **confidence** that we can have in generalizing our findings to large groups or populations based on sample results for individuals believed to represent these populations. Such confidence is based on the tolerance for making certain kinds of **sampling errors** owing to chance factors beyond the investigator's control.

In addition to the need for determining, prior to initiating a study, what type of statistical procedures can best be used, the *risk tolerance* for sampling errors should likewise be decided beforehand if the results are to be fairly evaluated. Such risk is commonly preset at either a 1% (.01) or a 5% (.05) chance of error. Unfortunately, the practice of many investigators is to neglect stating the risk for error they are willing to tolerate prior to disclosing the results of their study. In our opinion, this practice is akin to waiting for the last bounce of the ball at the roulette wheel before finally placing bets.

Perhaps the best way to conceive of statistics is as an implicit logical reasoning system made explicit in quantitative terms. Its laws are neither absolute nor universal in the sense that a consequent event will always follow a given antecedent cause or condition. More accurately, the laws of statistics can be described only in terms of the **probability** for a particular event occurring a certain percentage of time under highly defined conditions and within specified confidence limits. Furthermore, although one may be able to predict with 95% confidence that some hypothetical number of cases similar to one's own will improve in response to treatment X under certain conditions, one still will be unable to forecast which particular cases might do so. Because statistical methods do not lead to invariant answers, they are best viewed as general guides rather than precise maps in the search for new knowledge and understanding.

Results

The main goal of the results section of a research article is to provide a straightforward presentation of the relevant data. Some research publications include not only a detailed explanation of the empirical data within this section but also a discussion of their theoretical implications. However, it is common practice within the results section to present and explain the data only in relation to the research hypotheses. *Interpretation* of findings should be avoided. The latter task is reserved for the discussion section of the research article.

Within the results section, a systemic presentation of the data should be included beginning with a precise summary of the evidence and then proceeding to a point-by-point report of each statistical analysis. Figures or graphs may be used to illustrate relevant research findings in pictorial form. Tables provide a convenient format for condensing data according to such average measures as the **mean** and measures of variability (the dispersion of scores around the mean) such as the **standard deviation**. Based on the comparison of such composite measures, which reflects differences in sets of scores *between* or *within* groups of subjects, statistical formulae can be used to calculate the **significance** of the results expressed as a probability value, or **P.** For example, the notation $P < .05$ would be interpreted to mean that you could expect your hypothesis to be true at least 95% of the time with a 5% chance of error (i.e., one chance in 20 of drawing the wrong conclusion).

As noted previously, a combination of descriptive and inferential methods, rather than a single statistical technique, usually are employed in the study of communication disorders. Although descriptive statistics permit observed variables to be specified in mathematical terms, it is only through the use of inferential statistics that generalizations are made from a selected sample of subjects to a larger population.

For reasons to be discussed more fully in Chapters 4 and 5, several researchers favor the use of intensive single subject or small-N designs over extensive large-N studies for some types of problems. Single-subject studies, sometimes called **applied behavior analyses,** are aimed at the precise analysis, control, or modification of behavior. Often, data description procedures are based on the mere visual inspection of results recorded in graphic form. Furthermore, as opposed to most group designs, single subject experimentation emphasizes *repeated measurements* of single subjects under controlled conditions.

Although there are many types of single subject designs, a common paradigm involves (1) establishing during a **baseline period** of recording an operant level of stable responding for a dependent variable prior to treatment; (2) introducing during a **treatment period** a single independent variable while recording any response changes in the dependent variable; (3) removing the independent variable during a **withdrawal period** while recording any response changes in the dependent variable (Figure 1.2). Although it is impossible to generalize results to a population based on one subject, the so-called

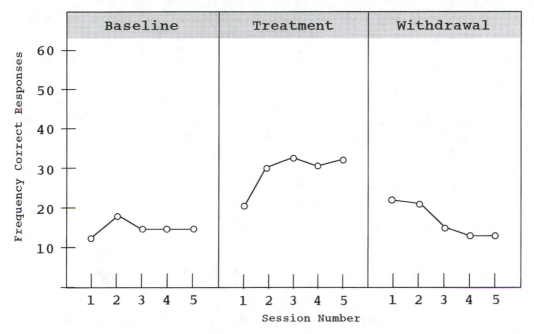

Figure 1.2. Basic paradigm for small-N designs.

small-N or N-of-1 designs may attempt to bolster the external validity of experimental findings by (1) describing the results from a number of individual subjects with similar characteristics (e.g., age, sex, IQ); (2) controlling sources of variability for each subject; and (3) demonstrating replicated findings with different subjects within the same experiment (Sidman, 1960).

Discussion

After objectively presenting and explaining the results of a study in relation to the hypotheses under test, the next step is to interpret the factual information in terms of the overall issues that served as the original impetus for the investigation. In essence, the task requires looking for meaningful patterns in the data to see how they might fit within the larger framework of knowledge—i.e., preexisting theories, conceptual models, and other research findings as reviewed in the introduction.

Whereas the form of scientific reasoning leading up to the results of an experiment was largely deductive in nature, the researcher is now required to inductively draw inferences *back* to the real world based on the specific data obtained. In more specific statistical terms, the degree to which the sample data can be generalized to the population from which it was drawn is carefully evaluated. This requires a rigorous analysis of the strengths and weaknesses of the current research design with respect to such matters as the effectiveness of the sampling procedures and the adequacy of experimental controls in dealing with the unwanted effects of extraneous variables.

In a figurative sense, the discussion section of a research article requires using data not only to look backward at "things as they have been" but also forward to how "things might be" in the future. Practical recommendations for improving various aspects of the methodology may be offered. Even new hypotheses may be advanced along with suggestions about the types of experiments needed for their testing. Thus, the discussion section of a study provides a mechanism for integrating inductive and deductive reasoning processes that together foster continuity of knowledge and new understanding.

References

All citations of previous studies must be listed in a reference list at the end of the research article. The references used need not be exhaustive but should reflect the work of previous investigations that are clearly related to the problem under investigation. The specific manner in which references should be cited within text and in the reference list is discussed in Chapter 9.

Science as a Cybernetic System

Thus far, we have argued that science can be conceived as systematic thinking and action processes that are well exemplified in the various sections of a scientific plan or research article. However, this is not to say that these same processes are necessarily straightforward or easily implemented as the casual reading of such an article otherwise might suggest. Rather than simply consisting of a few prescribed steps leading smoothly from point A to B, the gait of science is better viewed as often slow and halting, sometimes stumbling back and forth along a rocky path toward new facts or discoveries.

In many ways, the work of science is comparable to piloting a ship, adjusting its sails as needed as it tacks back and forth across the wind. Apropos to this analogy is the meaning of the term **cybernetics,** borrowed from the Greek word *cybernetica.* Plato used the latter word in the *Republic to* describe the skills acquired by sailors in charting the seas and steering ships (McGuigan, 1994). In his well-known book entitled *Cybernetics* (1948), Norman Weiner adopted this term to characterize the interactive components of communications systems and the theory of their control.

According to a biological model of a cybernetic system developed by McGuigan (1994) and adapted here for our purposes, the processing of information begins with a **source** as illustrated in Figure 1.3. Earlier, we noted that the source of information for researchers is found in systematized bodies of general knowledge that serve as a basis for deductive reasoning. Through deduction, we attempt to explain new facts or observations as they arise. Our explanations are based on cognitive structures of understanding as they exist in our brain (source). However, if an event cannot be accounted for on the basis of ex-

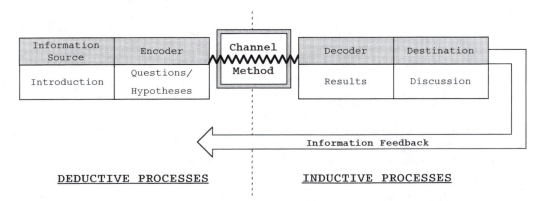

Figure 1.3. Comparison of a cybernetic information system with the scientific thinking processes and structure of a scientific article.

isting concepts or theories, perhaps because the event fails to conform with logic and reason, then the problem-solving tactics of science will need to be implemented. As noted previously, the process of articulating *conceptual gaps* in knowledge or understanding typically begins with a thorough review of the several dimensions of a problem as found in the introduction to a research article. Here, the evidence for the conceptual gap is distilled, organized, and focused in such a way as to suggest a compelling need for additional research.

In cybernetic terms, for a message to convey meaning, it must be **encoded** into a sequence of measurable events. Likewise, for a problem to be solvable, science demands that its various features first be specified (encoded) in an empirical manner that allows for the evaluation of hypothesized relationships among variables. In other words, to be useful, the message content of hypotheses must be stated in the form of predictions that can be statistically tested.

The "logistics" or methodological steps employed in the actual testing of a hypothesis is analogous to the purpose served by the communication **channel component** of a cybernetic system. In order for such a channel to transmit information reliably and accurately, it must be free of "noise" or any unwanted influences that might degrade the message. Similarly, researchers often speak of the need for a "clean" design. Such a design involves the use of a well-planned methodology uncluttered by the kinds of extraneous variables that often undermine the integrity of data. As in a cybernetic system, the ability to control interactions among variables is essential for sound results.

The next component comprising a cybernetic system is the unit used for **decoding** messages so that they can be understood. In a research plan, this is comparable to the function of appropriate statistical techniques used to analyze and record the results. Such techniques are applied in order to inform the researcher as to whether or not the findings can be confidently attributed to systematic and intentional effects of the experiment or merely to chance factors.

The final component of a cybernetic system is termed the **destination**. This is a pivotal control unit in the sense that the message is not only finally interpreted here but is then "fed back" to the source for collaborating or correcting information as required. A comparable interpretative operation is performed in the discussion section of a research article. The conceptual meaning of the specific results are not only evaluated but also related (fed back) to the original theoretical models and research hypotheses as outlined in the introduction. Through this process, inductive inferences are drawn that either confirm or fail to support theories and research hypotheses, adding or subtracting from their explanatory value.

Ultimately, research involves the judicious use of existing knowledge in conjunction with empirical data-gathering techniques that together advance understanding. In subsequent chapters, many of the basic skills involved in conceptualizing and solving problems will be reviewed while emphasizing the dynamic and integrative nature of the research process.

SELF-LEARNING REVIEW

phenomena

1. The observable characteristics of objects and events are called _____.

Descriptive
classify
categorize
variables

2. _____ methods are commonly used by clinicians to _____ or _____ phenomena.

3. Phenomena that are observed to vary are called _____.

variables
association

4. Relationship questions ask about the degree to which certain classes or categories of _____ change in _____ with other variables.

correlated

5. When the measure of one variable predicts the measure of a second variable, the variables are said to be _____.

relation

6. Answering questions pertaining to differences among phenomena is generally recognized as the best means of determining causal _____.

between
within

7. Two types of difference questions pertain to the search for _____-group and _____ -group differences.

control

8. Establishing the cause(s) of variation of a phenomenon is necessary for establishing the conditions for its future _____ .

independent
dependent

9. Studies involving difference questions tend to restrict the interpretation of group differences to the systematic influence of the treatment condition, called the _____ variable on the target of such manipulation, called the _____ variable.

extensive
groups
intensive
subject

10. The _____ research approach involves the study of _____ , whereas the _____ research approach is best adapted to the study of a single _____.

reliability
replication

11. The primary criterion for any study is the _____ of findings based on _____.

qualitative

12. A classic example of _____ research is embodied in the work of Piaget.

ethnographic

13. The study of customs, social patterns, and rule-governed interactions of a culture or group of individuals is termed _____ research.

14. _____ analysis is a qualitative research technique that allows for communication messages to be coded and classified based on frequency of occurrence.

Content

15. An approach to research that factors in the worth of accidental discoveries is based on _____.

serendipity

16. True experimental designs can be distinguished from all others on the basis of two major factors: (1) random _____ of subjects to at least two groups and (2) some type of active _____ to be performed on an experimental group of subjects who are then compared with a _____ group.

assignment
manipulation
control

17. _____ -experimental designs are generally selected when true experimentation is unfeasible or impossible to perform.

Quasi

18. With the exception of _____ , quasi-experiments are like _____ experiments.

randomization
true

19. As opposed to a randomized control group, a _____ group generally requires careful _____ of subjects in order to control for the _____ influence of extraneous variables.

constructed
matching
confounding

20. Nonexperimental research makes no effort to achieve _____ in the assignment of subjects to groups, nor are _____ procedures used in an effort to achieve _____ between groups.

randomization
matching
equivalence

21. Instead of using a randomized control group and actively manipulating an independent variable, many nonexperimental studies rely on _____ interpretations of preexisting data or observations.

ex post facto

22. Vicious _____ occurs when an answer is based on a question and a question on the answer.

circularity

23. A correlation _____ is used to express the degree of association between two variables.

coefficient

24. The _____ method entails certain _____ and _____ processes designed to produce better and more representative solutions to problems.

scientific
thinking
action

25. The introductory section of a research article can be seen as the structural _____ for the investigation.

blueprint

internal
external
generalizable

26. The degree to which the results of an experiment are directly attributable to the influence of an independent variable pertains to their _____ validity; _____ validity concerns the degree to which the results are _____.

Descriptive
Inferential
sample
population

27. _____ statistics are used to summarize, condense, and organize data. _____ statistics are used to draw inductive inferences from a _____ to a _____.

sample
true

28. A _____ fact is derived from a sample of observations. A _____ fact would require that we examine the entire population.

probability
confidence

29. Statistics are concerned with determining the _____ of certain observations or events within specified _____ limits.

presenting
explaining
hypotheses
Interpretation

30. The results section of a research article is generally restricted to _____ and _____ data in relation to the research _____. _____ of data is usually reserved for the discussion section.

N-of-one
descriptive
inferential

31. ___-___-___ designs typically rely on the use of _____ rather than _____ statistics.

cybernetic
research article

32. The thinking and action processes of science can be viewed as a _____ system with a number of interactive components for transmitting information accurately and efficiently. The systemization of such information is reflected in the various sections of a _____ _____.

2. History and Philosophy of Science

History of Scientific Thought	**Science and Empiricism**
Nature of Scientific Thought	**Language of Science**
Scientific versus Nonscientific Knowledge	**Reasons for Scientific Inquiry**
Logic of Science	**Clinical Relevance of Science**
Metamorphism	

Since the time of its rudimentary beginnings, from a substrate of related disciplines including education, medicine, and psychology, the profession of communication disorders has made remarkable strides in developing a fund of knowledge firmly grounded in scientific research. The substance and relevance of our current clinical endeavors owe much to a preexisting scientific ethos that values critical thinking and objectivity in evaluating the reliability and validity of evidence and a willingness to change our theories and approaches to problems as new facts emerge. Faith in the worth of science and a commitment to its philosophy of thought and method of action have long been established.

HISTORY OF SCIENTIFIC THOUGHT

Scientific thought began with the earliest humans whose brains had developed sufficiently to convert and elaborate raw sensory experience from a state of primitive wonderment into coherent and organized perceptions of experience. From that time onward, our evolution has been characterized by a continuous unfolding of increasingly complex mental capacities out of a quest to **explain, predict,** and **control** cause-effect relationships existing among multitudinous variables. Perhaps what we learned that was most important to the advancement of science was the way to control our environment and one another through language and the gradual emergence of powerful communication technologies.

In early history, the perceived causes for natural phenomena were attributed to the work of **deities.** For the Babylonians, the Bull of Heaven brought drought; the great bird Imdugud caused rain. Yet, the will of these spirits could be mediated or altered through prayer, sacrificial offerings, and related rituals. Eventually, modified forms of these early doctrines evolved into the major tenets of the world religions. These religions promulgated the belief that the superstructures of knowledge were largely impenetrable.

With the advent of numerical systems, humans began to refine their observations into quantifiable measurements. Efforts to explain the relation between causes and effects were increasingly cast as mathematical formulations of order and coherence. The secrets of the Gods began to be encoded into sets of empirical definitions unified by a system of higher definitions called **theories.** Such theories provided for humankind a systematic structure for thought in guiding the processes of inquiry as new facts were organized into larger units of useful knowledge.

Ancient evidence of relatively abstract theoretical thinking is found in the calculations of areas and volumes recorded on Egyptian papyrus and Babylonian tablets dating from 2000 BC. About the same time, the Chinese were beginning to formulate the first written hypotheses about the elemental composition of matter, which appeared in the *Shu-ching,* or Canonical Book of Records. With the advent of written language, the record of the **causal relations** between objects and events **(variables)** forming the structure of the world was removed from the heavens and placed in human repositories of knowledge called libraries. From these budding scientific efforts, ingenious **constructs** have emerged spanning all fields of human knowledge, allowing us to observe, investigate, and apprehend the relations between variables within the framework of particular sets of propositions **(theoretical structures).**

NATURE OF SCIENTIFIC THOUGHT

The work that entails the search for the answers to certain questions is called **science** and the tools of such work consist of systematically applied research and statistical methods. In the preface of this book, the authors expressed their conviction that, for pragmatic reasons, the term science is best viewed as a **verb** rather than a noun. This viewpoint is consistent with Kerlinger's (1964) notion of science as an *activity* that people do in the pursuit of **valid** and **reliable** answers to questions. Although such activity often culminates in new knowledge, science is best seen as the means to this end. As we shall see, the "means" involves **hypothesis testing** under systematic, controlled, and empirical conditions. According to Dewey (1922), the actual distinction between the **"means"** and **"ends"** of science often is arbitrary because both involve a series of actions with the means simply occurring at an earlier stage.

SCIENTIFIC VERSUS NONSCIENTIFIC KNOWLEDGE

Science is but one means of obtaining knowledge of the world. An understanding of one's experience can also be gained through subjective or personal analysis, intuition, or spiritual or religious convictions, or it can be based on what are perceived to be the omniscient pronouncements of certain authority figures. But science, unlike such alternative approaches to knowledge, deals in **temporary hypotheses** of cause and effect relations. Events in the universe are interconnected and causally determined by natural factors under certain conditions of observation and measurement. Such causal relations may change under different conditions of time or space.

As made clear by modern statistical theory, nature's laws are not forged as rigid truths but exist as expressions of **probability,** having a degree of **error** that is inherent in nature itself. Unlike most dogma, the language of science involves statements of probability, under certain conditions or proscribed limits, not statements of absolute certainty.

LOGIC OF SCIENCE

The rational character of science is manifested in two major types of logical reasoning processes: **deduction** and **induction.** Deductive logic begins with a general premise or law, assumed to be true, which is then used to explain a specific observation or behavioral occurrence. Conversely, induction involves a form of reasoning wherein a general theory or set of laws is ultimately derived from specific observations or individual cases. In actual practice, inductive reasoning **(inferences based on particulars)** is the initial starting point for most research activity from which a more general understanding or theory may be derived. Once formulated, the theory may be used to deduce or predict specific aspects of other phenomena to which its tenets might be generalized.

Although logical reasoning is an important tool in scientific thinking, it does not necessarily assure or provide correct answers to problems. Essentially, logic is first and foremost concerned with the **form** or degree of agreement between certain stated premises rather than the inherent truth of statements such as, "All men are mortal. Socrates is a man. Thus, Socrates is mortal." If the original premise (all men are mortal) is faulty, the edifice of the entire logical structure will crumble.

METAMORPHISM

According to Pirsig (1974), the word "logic" stems from the Greek root word "logos," referring to the sum total of a human being's rational understanding of the world. He goes on to suggest that there is another level of understanding, recognized by the ancient Greeks, called "mythos" that transcends "logos" as a kind of overall complex mental structure. Mythos is an older form of knowledge, consisting of the accumulated historic and prehistoric myths and legends of culture. The notion of the mythos is embedded in the pledge given in a court of law ". . . to tell the whole truth and nothing but the truth, so help me God." Mythos is the quality that is sought after and found in our common experience.

Perhaps the best science, like fine art, is grounded in metamorphic schema that intuitively appear correct or true. Many believe that the qualities of such schema actually exist as symbolic images in the "mind's eye" prior to their empirical expression through a particular medium. The specific method selected provides the basis for revealing in a systematic way that which is already known. According to literary lore, Milton conceived "Paradise Lost" as a unitary whole before writing this classic work. Similarly, Mozart is reported to have heard whole symphonies in his head prior to their actual composition. Einstein, who noted that the creative mind is informed and directed by a state "akin to a religious conviction," envisioned the Special Theory of Relativity, the photoelectric effect, and other conceptual schema that rocked the basic tenets of existing scientific theory years before his ideas were actually validated by empirical research methods.

As an avenue to knowledge, the idea of metamorphism is similar to what Boulding (1978) called "literary knowledge," or the knowledge that comes from the imagination as created by an abstracting process whereby symbolic realities are formed. From such cognitive structures, theories are formed that stimulate the major activities of empirical science—observation, description, and testing.

SCIENCE AND EMPIRICISM

Whereas logical reasoning and metamorphic understanding are important in the framework of the philosophy of science, perhaps a more significant requirement guiding actual scientific research is based on the **doctrine of empiricism:** "nothing can be said to exist until it is actually *observed* to exist to some degree." Empiricism insists that the elements of the problem under investigation be observed, tested, or measured rather than left to the realm of hypothetical argument or subjective opinion. Strict reliance on logic or common sense is an untrustworthy means of gaining knowledge, and metamorphism may be a lofty cognitive attribute unattainable by most scientists who must pursue knowledge using more pedestrian or "pick and shovel" methods. According to the doctrine of empiricism, the ultimate arbiter of an issue ought to be either direct or indirect observation of the phenomenon itself (Lundber et al., 1968).

Without the "seeing is believing" requirement of empiricism, one's approach to knowledge would have to be based largely on folklore, mysticism, speculation, hearsay, or unverified authoritarian pronouncements.

LANGUAGE OF SCIENCE

Despite the major premise of empiricism that "seeing is believing," the idea that "truth is within the eye of the beholder" must also be borne in mind. Different individuals may behold different things through the lens of their unique personal experiences. Perhaps for this reason, Francis Bacon (1561–1626) warned scientists in 1620 to beware of four illusory idols that certain biased perspectives can impose on the reasoning process, leading to erroneous ways of "seeing." These included:

1. Idols of the Tribe: Errors inherent in the beliefs of culture or humankind in general.
2. Idols of the Cave: Errors inherent in the beliefs of a particular individual owing to private prejudices or idiosyncratic personality factors.
3. Idols of the Marketplace: Errors arising from misleading messages or systems of thought.
4. Idols of the Theater: Errors resulting from the influence of mere words over our minds.

Because of these potential pitfalls in discerning the true nature of phenomena, Bacon advocated systematizing and improving the precision of observation methods in all sciences, including those concerned with the study of human behavior.

The notion of empiricism eventually spurred the development of new requirements in the language of science. The terms and definitions applied to objects and events would include only **objective language** descriptions. As much as possible, objective language communicates an observation according to the physical attributes of the phenomenon observed. On the other hand, the focus of **speculative language** is on what are largely the unobservable or private perceptions of an individual.

The new emphasis on objectivity in scientific work led the renowned physicist P. W. Bridgeman in 1927 to introduce a movement called **operationism,** which emphasized the importance of defining the quantitative meaning of theoretical terms in accordance with the conditions of their measurement. This movement had a profound influence on not only developments in the physical sciences but the behavioral sciences as well. In order to sharpen the level of scientific discourse, the abstract and often vague meaning of various concepts began to be specified as measurable values. Concepts deliberately reconstructed in this way for scientific use are called **constructs.** The factors that constructs describe that are capable of assuming different values are called **variables.** For research purposes, variables are typically **defined operationally** according to the manner in which they are assigned, manipulated, or measured. In addition, a variable can be defined according to whether or not it is considered to be the antecedent cause **(independent variable)** or consequent effect **(dependent variable)** under the experimental conditions. The conjectured relationship among such variables is usually stated in the form of a tentative **research hypothesis** formulated to be tested or evaluated under controlled circumstances termed **conditions.**

REASONS FOR SCIENTIFIC INQUIRY

Most scientific investigations begin with a problem caused by an obstacle to understanding. Such an obstacle leads to what is often a **compelling motivation** to describe, predict, or control behavior or circumstances. Although such motivation is a necessary ingredient of any problem solving activity, it is not sufficient for the work of science. According to Kerlinger (1964), the majority of scientific research involves: "systematic, controlled, empirical and critical investigation of natural phenomena guided by theory and hypotheses about the presumed relations among such phenomena" (p. 10).

Like Kerlinger, many scientists believe that the primary reason for conducting research is to investigate hypotheses in relation to the tenets of particular theories. Such theories contain a number of statements or hypotheses about presumed relationships among classes of variables.

Three major criteria can be used in assessing the ultimate worth of any theory. First, and most important, a theory must be **empirical,** i.e., one must generate hypotheses that are amenable to operational definition, objective testing, and evaluation. Unless a theory contains hypotheses that can be disproved, it has little or no scientific worth. Psychoanalytic theories of stuttering that attribute etiologic significance to repressed needs, stemming from immature sexual impulses and other unconscious urges along Freudian lines, are examples of the type for which scientific corroboration is largely lacking and is extremely difficult to achieve (Bloodstein, 1987). A second criterion for assessing the value of a theory is its relative **parsimony** in explaining the known facts about a phenomenon. A parsimonious theory of stuttering would be one that could consistently explain the known and newly emerging facts about its origin, development, and maintenance with the fewest contradictions. A third characteristic of a "good" theory is to be found in its **heuristic quality.** Is the theory fruitful in stimulating new and creative research endeavors, or does it "die on the vine" as a passing fad?

Some scientists believe that there are several important justifications for research beyond testing and evaluating theories. Indeed, advocates of strict behaviorism in the mode of B. F. Skinner believe that the tactics of hypothesis testing may blind investigators to significant bodies of knowledge that lie outside the narrow range of one's theoretical biases and problem solving. This particular philosophy is perhaps best summed up by the advice of Skinner: "When you run into something interesting, drop everything else and study it" (1956).

Sidman (1960) offered several reasons for research beyond theory testing and evaluation. These included research to:

- Try out new methods or techniques
- Indulge or satisfy curiosity
- Demonstrate a new behavioral phenomenon
- Deepen understanding of the conditions influencing a behavioral phenomenon

These research rationales are especially applicable to the clinical environment wherein the needs of diverse individuals must be addressed, often by means of an **eclectic approach,** emphasizing flexibility and innovation in behavioral management.

Applying and evaluating the efficacy of certain treatment procedures is the primary concern of most "clinical situations," not formal theory testing. Nevertheless, it is often the case that theories and hypotheses operate either implicitly or explicitly in guiding diagnosis and therapeutic intervention. Furthermore, data may be collected and conclusions drawn that support existing theoretic frameworks or ultimately are translated into new theories and hypotheses suitable for empirical testing. As clinicians, we ought to remember that the richest substrate of our science is to be found in the problems we treat.

CLINICAL RELEVANCE OF SCIENCE

Students who aspire to careers in various clinical fields often ask, "Why study research and statistical methods when my goal is to help people—not to study them?" Whereas this expression of human concern is admirable, such an interest does not conflict with the use of scientific approaches in the realm of diagnosis and therapy. Many years ago, the recognition of this fact by the eminent physician Harvey Cushing led him to proclaim that he had two main questions about any patient. First he asked, "What can I learn from this person?", and second, "How can I be of help?" By the order of his questions, Cushing wished to make clear that clinical effectiveness is maximized through critical thinking and the application of problem-solving skills.

The need for critical thinking and problem-solving skills among speech-language pathologists and audiologists is steadily increasing with the ever-expanding body of diverse yet highly specialized information. The basis of knowledge for the field of human communication disorders is related importantly to developments in such overlapping professions as education, psychology, rehabilitation, and medicine, each having a host of subspecialties. The quality of our own work depends in large measure on the ability to evaluate and use relevant information as it emerges, regardless of the source. To do so, we must be **scientifically literate**—i.e., be able to read professional literature not merely in terms of its content but also with respect to possible shortcomings in the design and conduct of a particular study or in the methods of data analysis. Scientific literacy will help us in deciding whether or not certain research findings are plausible and clinically relevant based on reliable and valid evidence rather than hope, faith, or the pronouncements of authority figures. Unless a study is properly designed and the data appropriately analyzed, the results are invalidated no matter how important the original investigative goals.

In addition to improving our ability to evaluate a constantly expanding body of research literature, scientific thinking and research skills also assist us in designing better clinical programs and in assessing their reliability and validity. Support and reimbursement for health and human services is increasingly dependent on the ability of providers to demonstrate the **efficacy** of their professional services. If the field of communication disorders is to continue to be respected and supported by state and federal regulatory agencies and other third-party fiscal agencies that set standards and policies for health care delivery, the profession must demonstrate **accountability.** This will have to be done by empirically documenting the utility of our clinical programs and their relevance to the individuals we serve.

Regardless of the clinical role you might play in the future, keep in mind that you will augment your professional effectiveness by thinking and behaving as a **clinical scientist.** To perform well in any work setting, it will be necessary for you to:

- Identify problems
- Develop hypotheses about the causal relations among variables
- Formulate suitable methods of treatment
- Collect and evaluate data relevant to treatment outcomes

In other words, you will be using the same thinking and behavior processes that characterize the so-called **scientific method** as it might be applied to almost any problem-solving endeavor.

Remember also that research involves scientific thoughts and actions that have immediate relevance to clinical as well as experimental problems. In addition to expanding our knowledge base, research provides the practical means of achieving quality outcomes in our everyday professional activities. As we shall see, the types of research that can be done are quite varied, ranging from simple to highly complex designs, depending on the nature of the questions raised and the answers sought.

SELF-LEARNING REVIEW

1. Scientific thinking grew out of early human efforts to _____, _____, and _____ causal relationships.

explain
predict
control

2. Initially, the perceived causes of natural phenomena were attributed to _____ forces or spiritual _____.

animistic
deities

3. With the advent of the numerical system, presumed causes of certain effects began to be formulated in _____ terms. _____ definitions were unified into a system of higher-order definitions called _____.

quantifiable or
mathematical
Empirical
theories

4. Theories offered explanations of the _____ relations between observed objects and events termed _____.

causal
variables

5. Through various _____ propositions or frameworks, we apprehend the _____ between variables.

theoretical
relations

6. In essence, _____ entails the systematic search for _____ and _____ answers to questions.

science
valid
reliable

7. Important tools of science include _____ and _____ methods.

research
statistical

8. Because science involves dynamic thought processes translated into systematic research activity, the term science is better viewed as a _____ rather than a _____.

verb
noun

9. Dewey believed that the distinction between the _____ and the _____ of science is arbitrary because they are simply different stages of the same process.

means
ends

10. The "means" of science, which involves _____ testing, is carried out under controlled _____ or circumstances.

hypothesis
conditions

11. A central tenet of science is that events in the universe are _____ and _____ determined.

interconnected
causally

12. Nature's _____ are not viewed as rigid truths but express a _____ for a certain outcome having a degree of inherent _____ .

laws
probability
error

13. _____ reasoning processes attest to the rational character of science. Deriving general laws or rules, based on observations of specific cases involves _____ reasoning. On the

Logical
inductive

deduction

other hand, _____ entails the use of a general premise believed to be true in order to explain a specific observation.

form
content

14. Logic is first and foremost concerned with the _____ of propositions rather than their _____ .

empiricism

15. The edict of _____ states that "nothing can be said to exist until it is observed to exist to some degree."

objective
speculative

16. Empiricism spurred new requirements in the language of science requiring _____ as opposed to _____ descriptions of objects and events.

operationism
concepts
constructs

17. This movement, called _____ , required that _____ be intentionally reconstructed as _____ for scientific use.

Variables

18. _____ are the factors that constructs describe that are capable of assuming different values.

operationally

19. Variables may be defined _____ according to the manner in which they are assigned, manipulated, or measured.

independent
dependent

20. Antecedent causes are defined as _____ variables, whereas those viewed as the consequent effects are called _____ variables.

hypothesis
controlled

21. A conjectural statement as to the relationship between the dependent and independent variables is called a research _____ , formulated to be tested under _____ conditions.

Case Example

Interest in the study of communication disorders has existed for a very long time. Notation of the existence of speech disorders, such as stuttering, is found in the writings of ancient Greece. For example, there is the well-known legend of Demosthenes who is reported to have reduced his stuttering by holding pebbles in his mouth while speaking. One possible explanation of this purported therapeutic effect is that the pebbles served to distract Demosthenes from his fears and apprehensions as he spoke with

cause

the Gods. The role that fear may play in the _____ or development of stuttering symptoms has been and continues to be a subject of widespread debate in the literature.

concept

As a _____ , fear is too general to be of much use in explaining the role of emotion in stuttering. Thus, theories of stuttering have refined the abstract meaning of this concept into the

_____ of anxiety as an aggravating or associated feature of the behavior. Many theories agree that, unlike fear, anxiety is not a natural response to immediate danger but is instead a learned reaction to impending or anticipated threat evoked by stimulus objects or situations.

As noted earlier, constructs that are capable of assuming different values, which can vary in amount or degree, are termed _____. In the case of stuttering, the variable of anxiety has been considered by some theorists to be a learned reaction to certain conditions or stimuli. For example, Wischner (1950; 1952) attempted to reformulate earlier concepts about the role of anxiety in stuttering according to the _____ of a scientifically based theory of learning. Within the framework of his theory, two types of conditioned stimuli were _____ to evoke anxiety and consequent stuttering behavior. One class of these, involving nonverbal stimuli, was said to evoke situational anxiety (e.g., anxiety in response to certain people or speaking circumstances). A second class of verbal stimuli evoked what Wischner termed "word anxiety." Both types of stimuli, through the intervening variable of learned anxiety, could serve as what Wischner termed "current instigators" of stuttering and maladaptive avoidance patterns. The original instigator of such learned anxiety reactions was _____ to lie in some type of actual pain-producing stimulation of the past.

Because anxiety itself cannot be directly observed, its influence must be inferred based on _____ defined stimulus-response variables. To support his theory, Wischner (1952) marshaled evidence pertaining to the so-called expectancy effect in stuttering, which he equated with anxiety. For Wischner, equating expectancy and anxiety seemed meaningful given his review of numerous investigations in which a high agreement was found between stutterers' predictions of their stuttering and its subsequent occurrence. Such findings prevailed for the ability of stutterers to reliably predict actual frequencies of stuttering on specific words and during various kinds of speaking situations or _____. In these studies, systematic variations in levels of predicted stuttering, during the silent reading of words or under different speaking conditions, served as _____ variables for theorizing about the causal relation of expectancy (anxiety) to stuttering. The influence of such antecedent predictions of stuttering on the _____ variable of observed stuttering was inferred. This _____ inference was based largely on statistically _____ associations found between predicted and actual stuttering moments.

Despite the reliable _____ [associations] found to exist between occurrences of expected stuttering and actual stuttering, the truth of a theorized causative relation between two or more variables, such as expectancy and anxiety, cannot be demon-

construct

variables

propositions or hypotheses

hypothesized

hypothesized

operationally

conditions

independent

dependent
causal
reliable

associations

construct
validity

validity

hypotheses or
explanations

strated merely on the basis of their observed correlation. Ultimately, the question of the truth of any theoretical _____
pertains to its inherent _____. In this respect, there is some
evidence that reliable predictions of stuttering may occur in the
absence of detectable changes in emotional arousal (Baumgartner
and Brutten, 1983; Bloodstein, 1974). Furthermore, the ability to
predict stuttering moments reliably may depend, at least in part,
on abnormalities in the tone and postural adjustments of speech
muscles that have been shown to precede stuttering in some studies. Rather than being artifacts of an anxiety reaction, such
"preparatory adjustments" may simply represent early components of a moment of stuttering that signal or inform the speaker
about impending speech difficulty. Thus, the _____ of
Wischner's theory can be challenged by contradictory data as well
as alternative _____ that deserve further testing.

3. Encountering Problems and Their Causal Relations

PROBLEM SETS

Each day, we encounter a host of problems in our personal and professional lives that require resolution. Not all of these problems are suitable for formal research, yet each presents us with an opportunity to observe, describe, and interpret the phenomenal features of various objects and events. Such phenomena constitute the elements of our conscious awareness. Human senses are remarkably specialized for organizing data into perceptual schema, or **data sets.** A data set is a well-defined aggregate of characteristics that serve to categorize or classify experience. In neurologic terms, there is evidence that the human brain automatically organizes and interprets sensory phenomena within modules or networks where images of the world are represented and stored in the records of memory.

In the common vernacular, it could be said that a data set is actually a "mind set" that influences the schema or frame of reference used in deriving meaning from sensory experience. An apt example of this property of mind can be found in a well-known figure-ground problem. When one is shown the picture illustrated in Figure 3.1a, what one sees, whether a white vase against a dark background or two dark faces in profile against a white background, is a result of reference to internal models (Gregory, 1968).

Sometimes the ambiguity of a problem may be so great as to render it almost unsolvable. Such is the case in one of the "picture puzzles" devised by K. M. Dallenback (1951). When asked to name the animal shown in Figure 3.1b, it is impossible for most people to do so. But when told to look for a white animal with black ears and a black muzzle, people typically see the abstract image of a cow. Moreover, once the figure has been perceived

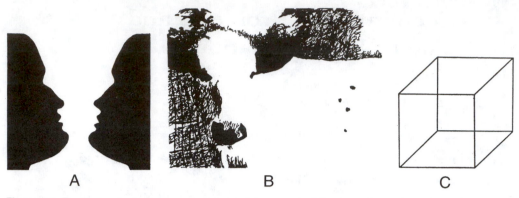

Figure 3.1. The human brain "makes sense" out of data sets by referring to internal representations of external phenomena. As these picture puzzles illustrate, our frame of reference may change substantially when given new information (see text).

as a cow, it is very difficult to perceive the image of the animal in a new or different way. Here, as elsewhere, the mind set that we apply to a particular problem may **bias** the outcome.

Despite the remarkable ability of the brain to *reliably* discern the features of specific objects and events according to a particular perspective, this does not exclude the possibility that different points of view may exist having equal or greater *validity.* Fortunately, most people have the ability to change or even reverse their subjective impressions when exposed to alternative suggestions or interpretations. A good example of this latter ability is found in the differing schema or frames of reference that the brain may use in perceiving the lines of a cube, as shown in Figure 3.1c. The drawing is a modified version of an earlier illustration by C. A. Necker, who discovered in 1832 that crystals seemed to change their spatial orientation as he peered at them through the lens of a microscope. Although some people may find it difficult to see Necker's cube in more than one orientation, it is possible for most to do so when instructed to view it from above or below, switching back and forth from one perspective to the other.

All of the examples cited above illustrate the tendency of people to adopt a particular set in response to a problem based on the brain's natural propensity to create order out of chaos. According to Kerlinger (1964), the "set idea" is fundamental to human thinking and problem solving. The tendency to group objects and events into categories or classes of phenomena that can be labeled or named is preliminary to the study of the rules governing their respective relations and functions. In this respect, Singer (1959) quotes Descartes, who noted that the proof for such rules " . . . embraces at once all the objects to which these are devoted and a great many more besides."

Associative Relations Among Sets

Although set theory is often used in describing various phenomena in mathematical terms, sets can also help more generally in conceptualizing many different kinds of problems and the relations among them. A useful means for the purpose of illustrating sets and their relations are **Venn diagrams**. As shown in Figure 3.2, such diagrams can be used to represent all members belonging to a **population** such as, for example, the American Speech-Language-Hearing-Association (ASHA). Individual subsets of this population (speech-language pathologists and audiologists) can also be represented, as may be their area of professional intersection (e.g., members certified in both specialties). Three, four, or even

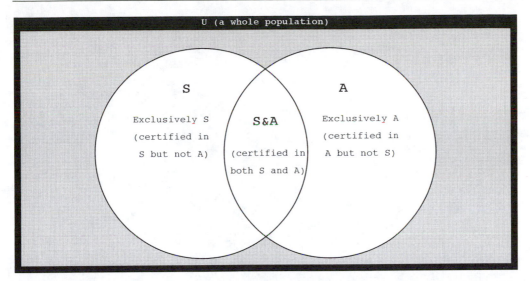

Figure 3.2. Venn diagram for a population and subsets, in which **U** represents a universal set of all speech-language pathologists and audiologists (certified or uncertified); **S** represents a subset of all certified speech-language pathologists; and **A** represents a subset of all certified audiologists.

more subsets could be specified according to such factors as membership in more narrowly defined subspecialties as aphasia or fluency disorders, work setting, etc.

Ultimately, the goal of science in problem solving is to go beyond the mere description and categorization of sets of objects and events to a determination of the manner in which they are related to one another. Set relations can be specified in at least two ways. First, through the **method of association,** it is possible to describe the correspondence **(correlation)** between two or more sets of objects or events. This can be done by arranging pairs of observations according to the relative magnitude of one or the other factor.

Let us assume we have observed that many children with language impairments later evidence a high prevalence of reading disabilities. In order to evaluate this relationship further, we might wish to compare language development test scores obtained by such children on standardized tests in kindergarten with their performance on tests of reading achievement upon entering the second grade. Hypothetically, the following two sets of standard scores might be obtained for a sample of six children:

Language Ability	Reading Achievement
82	77
80	84
75	79
70	78
67	59
52	55

These sets of sample scores, with each pair ordered first according to the factor of language ability, describe the overall relation of such ability to subsequent reading competence. Our ability to visualize this relation can be further aided by graphing the two sets of scores on X and Y axes, as in Figure 3.3. Here, the existing correlation between the two sets of scores can be more readily seen: for the majority of the children evaluated, higher language scores (X) tend to be associated with higher reading scores (Y).

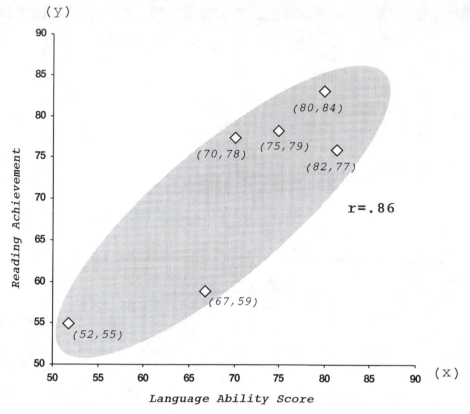

Figure 3.3. Relationship of reading achievement to language ability.

In statistical terms, the relation between these two sets of scores can be expressed as a **coefficient of correlation**. Such coefficients can be used to denote a range of relations in which +1 expresses a perfect positive correlation and −1 a perfect negative correlation. In reality, a correlation indicative of either perfect **covariance** (+1) or a perfect inverse relation (−1) is highly improbable.

Typically, coefficients range from 0 to 1 in either the positive or negative direction. A common test used for calculating the degree of relation between two sets of scores is the **product-moment coefficient of correlation (r).** For the set of scores displayed previously, $r = .86$.

Causal Relations Among Sets

The second major means and ultimate goal of most problem-solving activities is to go beyond mere description of the associations between objects and events to a study of their cause and effect relations. Essentially, the idea underlying the concept of causality is that one event is the *consequence* of another known or knowable event that can be specified. Although an association between one or more data sets may suggest that they tend to covary or vary inversely in their relative direction or degree of expression, we cannot conclude, on this basis alone, that one such factor is the cause of the other.

In the previous chapter, the notion that expectancy of stuttering causes stuttering was challenged on the basis of alternative explanations hypothetically involving the influence of a **third variable.** In addition, deriving conclusions about causality based on correlation is typically hampered by the so-called **directionality problem.** More specifically, it is often difficult, if not impossible, to say whether variable X (expectancy or anxiety) causes variable Y (e.g., stuttering) or vice versa. Both the third variable and directionality problem are examples of how plausible **alternative** or **rival hypotheses** lend credence to what is perhaps the most-often cited dictum of research practice: "Correlation does not imply causation."

In the field of communication disorders, we attempt to understand and treat what are generally recognized as the behavioral products of a **complex system.** Speech-language-hearing is the result of vast neural linkages among sensory end organs and motor end plates coordinated by higher order association areas within the brain. Theories regarding the linguistic rules that govern a myriad of interactions occurring within this system are as yet incomplete and unproved. Indeed, the sheer number of associations among its variables may be so complex that no single theory could ever account for all of their causal relations. Nevertheless, the history of science suggests that the challenge of solving complex problems more often stimulates rather than dampens the interest and motivation of researchers as they seek to determine how one event gives rise or brings about definite changes in the next.

Previously, it was noted that although a correlation may suggest the existence of some type of relationship between two or more data sets, it is impossible to conclude on this basis alone that factor X influences or changes factor Y. By what means, then, can causality be determined? According to the logic expounded in the writings of John Stuart Mill (1806–1873), causality can be inferred, all else being equal, only when factor Y occurs in the presence of factor X and does not occur in the absence of factor X. Mill's **"method of difference"** does not exclude other possible causes of Y. However, when such other influences are absent or under control (all things being equal), X is inferred as *sufficient* to cause Y. Mill's premise is the touchstone for most modern research hypothesis testing procedures in which at least two effects are typically examined: the first when preceded by the presumed cause and the other when the presumed cause is absent.

CAUSALITY AND VARIANCE

The subject matter of most scientific research is the study of relations among objects and events that are capable of assuming different values. Such phenomena are called **variables.** More specifically, researchers are interested in answering questions pertaining to **differences** in a dependent variable (hypothesized effect) that *has* and *has not* been preceded by an independent variable (hypothesized cause). The quantitative evaluation of such differences relates to what statisticians call **variance** (the extent to which scores differ from each other).

The testing of research hypotheses usually entails the comparison of variances of different types. The three major types of variance are (1) population and sample variance; (2) systematic variance; and (3) error variance. Each type is discussed more fully below.

Population and Sample Variance

Researchers and statisticians use the term **population** to describe an all-inclusive data set about which they wish to draw a conclusion or causal inference. Typically, the term encompasses a large collection of animate or inanimate objects or events that share common attributes. In the field of communication disorders, a population might include all certified members of ASHA, all patients with whom they work, all patient files, all treatment facilities, etc.

A population will include at least one common characteristic, but more can be defined as desired. For example, all certified members of ASHA would include all those holding the Certificate of Clinical Competence in the specialty Speech-Language Pathology or the specialty Audiology. However, another population could be defined as only those who hold dual certification in both specialties. Should we decide to count all members belonging to one or the other of these populations, the resulting number would be referred to as a **parameter.** A parameter is a number or measured characteristic derived from the entire population.

A **sample** is a subset of a population ideally drawn in such a way that each member of the population has an equal chance of being selected. Thus drawn, such a sample is said to be **representative** of the larger population. In the example above, a sample could be drawn from the entire pool of certified members of ASHA or from the smaller population of members who hold both certifications. A **statistic** is a number derived from counting or measuring sample observations that have been drawn from a population of numbers.

Statistical methods allow researchers to make inferences about the characteristics of a population on the basis of information obtained from the sample. If the population consists of a finite number of observations, and provided that it is both possible and practical to count or measure each member of the data set, then variance for a particular population attribute can be measured.

Conceivably, one might wish to determine the mean age for the entire population and then calculate the variance of each member from such an average measure. Although such a task might be accomplished, to do so would be a tedious and highly laborious undertaking, particularly for an organization with more than 80,000 members.

A more feasible approach to this goal would be to draw a random sample to use as an estimate of the mean and variance of the **target population.** A target population can be defined as the population for which the investigator wishes to generalize. In so doing, the investigator must expect a certain degree of **sampling error,** which is the difference between the measures collected for a randomly selected sample and the population it is believed to represent. More specifically, sampling error can be defined as the expected amount of variance owing to chance alone rather than to systematic influences. The methods and statistical problems associated with sampling procedures are discussed more fully in Chapter 5.

Systematic Variance

Known causes of variation in an experiment are termed **systematic variance** or **between-group variance.** Variance of this kind is usually reflected in systematic differences between the scores of two groups resulting from the *assignment* or *active manipulation* of independent variables by the experimenter. In the typical experiment, the variance between at least two groups is examined. If we wish to examine the influence of different amounts of a particular independent variable on the dependent variable, one means of doing so is assigning individuals possessing different levels of the independent variable to two or more groups. For example, suppose that we wish to investigate systematic variations in stuttering severity in relation to different levels of anxiety.

One way to accomplish this would be to divide subjects into two groups consisting of "low anxious" and "high anxious" individuals based on their scores obtained on an anxiety questionnaire such as the Speech Situation Checklist (Brutten, 1975). Between-group variance on measures of stuttering severity, such as those found on the Stuttering Severity Instrument (Riley, 1986), could then be examined. A frequent difficulty surrounding the interpretation of between-group differences based on assignment stems from the directionality problem discussed previously. With respect to the study just discussed, we would be unable to determine whether or not any hypothetical between-group differences in stuttering severity resulted from or were a cause of the predictor variable (anxiety).

In order to avoid or diminish such "cart before the horse" dilemmas in making causal inferences, many investigators tend to favor a design strategy that allows for the active manipulation of independent variables when possible. Designs that involve the active and systematic manipulation of one or more independent variables are called **controlled experimental studies.** Such experiments allow for a more direct determination of causal relations than do methods that are based solely on the between-group assignment of independent variables according to preexisting subject characteristics. For instance, several studies have explored the relationship between anxiety and stuttering by varying (manipulating) the difficulty of reading tasks or speaking situations while recording changes in autonomic arousal. In the majority of these experiments, no consistent relationship between changes in such anxiety measures as palmar sweating, galvanic skin response, heart rate, or pulse volume and the frequency of stuttering behavior was found (Bloodstein, 1987).

Some independent variables, such as those involving relatively stable physical or psychological characteristics, are not subject to active experimental manipulation. Examples of such **organismic variables** might include age, sex, height, weight, auditory and visual acuity, motor skills, intelligence, memory, and health status. By and large, such intrinsic subject characteristics would be impossible or impractical to alter in human investigations, and their influence on dependent variables can be better controlled or investigated through group assignment.

Error Variance

Effective problem solving involves not only the determination of systemic relations among variables but the degree to which random fluctuations in measured observations occur as a result of unidentified and uncontrolled circumstances. In the opening pages of *Moby Dick*, Herman Melville set out to explore the often-hidden and disorderly forces in nature by stating, "The classification of the constituents of chaos, nothing less here is essayed."

Whether and to what extent randomness actually exists in the universe is a continuing debate among scientists. As noted earlier, a primary tenet of science is that the relations among objects and events are causally determined by lawful and orderly processes that are subject to discovery. Given this mind set, the idea that some element of chaos is to be found within the workings of all biological and physical systems is difficult to accept. Nonetheless, researchers are aware that relatively small unsystematic changes in variables owing to random fluctuations of unknown factors commonly exist in experiments. Influences that cannot be held constant from subject to subject and that do not systematically favor any one particular treatment over another are random sources of error.

One way to think about error variance is that it is the amount of variation that still remains after all known sources of systematic variance have been eliminated (Kerlinger, 1964). Conceptually, tests of the significance of difference between groups, such as the F test, can be defined as the ratio of systematic variance to error variance, or

$$F = \frac{V_b}{V_e}$$

The larger the denominator (error variance) in relation to the numerator (systematic variance), the less likely it would have been that the independent variable produced a true between-group difference. The relationship of systematic variance to error variance is depicted in Figure 3.4.

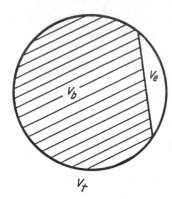

Figure 3.4. Total variance constituted of sources of variation between groups, owing to (1) systematic influences (V_b) and (2) unknown causes of uncontrolled influences (V_e). As V_e increases, the between-group variance attributable to systematic influences (shaded area) decreases.

Sources of systematic variance tend to produce a directional effect in a set of scores, i.e., either a measurable increase or a decrease is caused. However, sources of error variance can cause scores to fluctuate in a willy-nilly fashion, going sometimes up and sometimes down. As noted previously, such residual variance is typically ascribed to random or **chance** factors.

One possible source of error variance are **errors in sampling.** One should remember that such deviations are normally expected and are not due to mistakes on the part of the experimenter. To illustrate the nature of such errors more clearly, suppose that we know that the true mean intelligence quotient for the population of certified ASHA members is 110. Next, assume that we decide to repeatedly draw 20 random samples, each consisting of 100 individuals from the ASHA population, and calculate the mean scores of intelligence for each sample. Based on the averages thus calculated, we would expect to find about half of the sample means falling above the true population mean and the other half below. In either case, the grand average of the sample means would be expected to approximate the population mean, as would the individual averages. Furthermore, with progressive increments in sample size, small individual differences in intelligence would eventually even out, thereby diminishing the variation among the sample scores.

A second source of uncontrolled variation of the dependent variable can arise from **errors of measurement.** Suppose you wish to compare the voice initiation times of stutterers as compared to normal speakers. A means of doing so might entail using a stop watch to measure the two groups' response latencies in vocalizing the schwa vowel in response to a defined visual or auditory cue that signals the onset of vocalization. In such a study, an important question to raise is to what degree efforts to measure response latency accurately reflect subject performance. Are there inconsistencies related to errors within the experimenter in starting and stopping the watch? Other errors in measurement might result from instability in the measuring devices themselves.

A third class of error variance can result from **fluctuations in the conditions of testing.** Imagine that different experimenters are collecting data on different subjects, who stutter as noted previously. Variations in scoring *between* experimenters as well as *within* experimenters could account for chance errors of measurement. Other sources of variation in the test conditions such as distracting noises, unwanted interruptions, changes in temperature or lighting, or alterations in the appearance of the test environment are additional examples of uncontrolled variations that might unduly influence the outcome of an experiment.

In later chapters, statistical procedures will be described that allow us to evaluate the relative influence of systematic variance versus error variance in accounting for the results of an experiment. This evaluation is of great importance for two reasons:

First, significant differences observed between the measured values of two or more groups or treatment conditions can result as the consequence of random sources of error.

Second, the converse is also possible: the failure to find significant differences can likewise result from random sources of error.

Calculating Major Sources of Variance

Two major sources of variance must be calculated in any experiment. As noted previously, the first of these are the effects of systematic influences that contribute to between-group variance. The second source involves **within-group variance,** consisting primarily of error variance plus variations owing to differences within individual subjects that constitute the group. According to strict definition, error variance is a random phenomenon that is beyond the control of the experimenter. However, **secondary influences** involving individual differences among subjects within a group can be controlled to some degree.

Because the main goal of any experiment is to demonstrate that the assignment or manipulation of an independent variable influences the dependent variable, it is desirable that the subjects within a group be as closely alike as possible. The importance of this principle can be readily understood in relation to important issues as might be involved in assessing the efficacy of our diagnostic or treatment procedures. Given such hypothetical within-group group differences resulting from individual variations in cognitive level, degree of motivation, severity of problem, etc., how could valid answers to these or other significant questions ever be obtained? The difficulty in doing so is the reason that secondary sources of variance must be reduced as much as possible. Because it is often difficult to separate sources of error variance from secondary variance, they are considered jointly in statistical calculations.

SEARCHING FOR TRUTH VERSUS PROBABLE CAUSE

Deductive Reasoning: Problem Making

In Chapter 1, we identified two kinds of cognitive processes that are used in deriving or inferring causal relations. The first of these, deductive reasoning, is used in the conclusive derivation of truth provided that the premises leading to the conclusion are also true. Deductive reasoning is usually based on a triad of propositions called a **syllogism**—a kind of top-down mode of problem solving introduced by Aristotle. The initial syllogistic premise is usually quite broad, encompassing all of the attributes of a phenomenon that you might wish to describe, whereas the second premise is more narrowly defined. The third statement is the conclusion (proof) derived from a combination of premises one and two.

Deductive reasoning can be illustrated in abstract form by the following syllogism: *If all phenomenon that have property* X *also have property* Y *(premise one), and if a given phenomenon* Z *has property* X *(premise two), then it follows that* Z *also has property* Y *(conclusion).*

In more concrete and relevant terms, we might develop the following syllogism: *If all children born with a cleft of the hard palate also have a cleft of the soft palate (premise one), and if Bobby has a cleft of the hard palate (premise two), then it follows that Bobby also has a cleft of the soft palate (conclusion).*

As a form of reasoning that proceeds from broad interpretative statements to extrapolating about a particular set of observations, deductive logic is most suited to what might be termed **problem making-**the mental activities emanating from a general theory or explanatory model that in turn leads to a hypothesis about a specific behavior or expected outcome. In this sense, the application of deductive logic is future oriented toward drawing conclusions from a set of **a priori generalizations** believed to be true and, therefore, indisputable. If the general theory is correct, then the postulates derived from it should also be true. However, as the philosopher David Hume (1711–1776) so aptly noted, the past is not necessarily a predictor of the future. More specifically, it can be said that neither the postulates nor conclusions derived from a finite set of data can be assumed to be permanently true. Indeed, perhaps the only truism in nature is "things are subject to change."

Inductive Reasoning: Problem Solving

A second major type of reasoning based on inductive logic forms the basis for what might be called **problem solving.** Whereas deductive reasoning argues for the truth of a particular statement beginning with a general theory, the cornerstone of scientific reasoning is based on **inductive inferences** empirically derived from actual experiments. The universal application **(generality)** of a theory can be supported only as long as the data derived from testing its hypotheses in specific experimental instances or conditions are consistent with it. A theory is disproved or weakened to the degree that generalizations based on its component hypotheses are contradicted by data.

In reality, most scientists hold that the actual truth of a theory can never be unequivocally proved or disproved. This is because of the so-called **inductive gap,** or the gap between *existing knowledge* and *predictive knowledge* (Figure 3.5). The foundation of existing knowledge is based on the data of past experiments. Predictive knowledge rests on the relative likelihood or **probability** of obtaining certain results in future experiments. As the consequence of the inductive gap, inductive inferences yield empirical data that are logi-

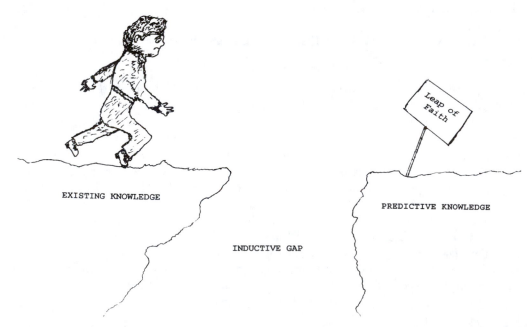

Figure 3.5. An inductive gap lies between *existing knowledge* (based on the past) and *predictive knowledge* (estimates of probable outcomes).

cally **inconclusive.** Although we use past experience to guide our behavior and decision making, it is no guarantee of future results.

Because all assertions about the future carry with them the possibility of error, no matter how small, such assertions must be stated as **probability estimates,** reflecting relative degrees of certainty as compared to uncertainty. In statistical terms, such probability is a ratio that reflects long-run percentages for the generality of certain observed results. For example, using various kinds of statistical tests, we might wish to derive an **inductive inference** about the general effectiveness of some treatment procedure, **a posteriori,** given the results observed from its use with a specific number of cases.

Let us suppose that the proportion of 10 cases responding favorably to therapy was found to be 8. Does this mean that we might reasonable expect 80% of the population of all highly similar subjects to show such positive gains? Keeping in mind that the true probability for successful treatment can be expressed as the ratio of successes to the total number of cases **in the long run,** we must say no. To conclude otherwise would require establishing a long-run percentage in an infinitely large number of cases-an obvious mathematical impossibility. Furthermore, even slight variations in subject characteristics, treatment variables, recording techniques, and certain chance fluctuations resulting from the passage of time can contribute toward the inductive gap.

The best we can do in resolving such a gap is to estimate the true probability based on our sample observations. Thus, whereas our estimated success rate is 80%, the true probability of successful treatment may be as low as 65% or as high as 95% or could reflect a range of other hypothetical values. Such a range of values, within which the true probability might fall, is termed an **interval probability estimate.** This estimate and its conceptual basis provides the major foundation for much of modern statistical theory and its methods involving **confidence interval testing.**

Gaining Confidence: Statistical Testing

A common goal of many clinical research studies is to estimate the degree of certainty **(level of confidence)** with which one particular treatment has a greater probability of success than another. Suppose we found in one group that 8 out of 10 cases (80%) were successfully treated with Method A. In a similar group, only 6 out of 10 cases achieved success in response to Method B. What we wish to know is whether or not the between-group difference in the percentage of successful outcomes resulted merely from random fluctuations or reflected a **significant difference** in the probability of an efficacious result.

Using suitable statistical techniques for calculating probabilities, it could be shown that such a large difference between the two percentages might have resulted from chance factors in only 1 out of 20 studies of a similar kind (see Chapter 8). More specifically, an **odds ratio against chance** of 19 to 1 translates into a probability termed the .05 level of significance. All else being equal, this means that we can be 95% confident that Method A has a significantly higher probability for a successful outcome than Method B. Had the odds against chance been 99 to 1, the difference would have reached the .01 level of significance, resulting in our being 99% confident in the validity of the findings.

Confidence interval testing, although somewhat arbitrary, typically entails the use of either the .05 or .01 level of significance depending on the degree of confidence that one wishes to have in concluding that one observation truly differs from another. In considering the probability that an inductive inference will result in a true conclusion, it is important to understand that the meaning and interpretation of a *statistically significant effect* may not be necessarily considered the same as a *clinically significant effect.* For example, a gain of only 0.2 IQ points for a sample size of 10,000 may be just as statistically significant as a gain of 10 IQ points for a sample size of 4 (Streiner, 1986). Yet, from a clinical perspective, the former outcome might reasonably be viewed as trivial when compared to the latter. The point we wish to make is that statistics have meaning only in relation to the uses to which they are put and the contexts in which they are interpreted.

VALIDITY AND RELIABILITY

The main goal of scientific research is to draw valid and reliable conclusion about causal relations among variables based on empirical observations, measurement instruments, and test procedures. The terms validity and reliability have broad or specific applications depending on the purpose(s) they are intended to serve.

Drawing Valid Conclusions

As a concept, the notion of validity commonly pertains to making correct or well-founded arguments based on deductive reasoning. Nevertheless, as noted previously, a "good argument" does not necessarily establish its truth unless all of the premises that comprise the argument are likewise true. For scientific purposes, the criteria for establishing validity extend beyond deductive reasoning to inductively inferring the **relative truth** of an observation based on its operational definition and empirical measurement.

Again, we have intentionally highlighted the words "relative truth" to underscore the difficulties in actually assessing and measuring the validity of a phenomenon. This is because one's concept of validity may change depending on the purposes of the experiment and the measurements or procedures used. Whereas a scale in a supermarket may be deemed acceptable for weighing fruits or vegetables, its perceived validity would no doubt sharply decline as a device for establishing the weight of precious metals or gemstones. Similarly, an audiometric test may be deemed clinically useful and appropriate as a general "screening" test for hearing loss, yet judged deficient for diagnosing the specific type of loss. The use of the norms and values of a particular test to evaluate the language abilities of one group of children from a particular educational, linguistic, and socioeconomic background may be entirely appropriate provided that such children are representative of the population for whom the test was developed. The same test may be deemed invalid for children who do not share the same level of attainment or cultural upbringing.

The degree to which a particular measure actually assesses what it was intended and designed for pertains to its **content validity,** sometimes called **face validity.** Content validity refers to the **representativeness** or sampling adequacy of a measure or procedure. Content validity is dependent on the degree to which clinicians or researchers agree that a measuring instrument is adequate for sampling or representing the characteristics of a phenomenon.

Thus, a particular measure of language competence ought to adequately represent the linguistic skills and behaviors it is *generally presumed* to evaluate in order to possess content validity. Despite the lack of such validity, a measure or procedure may still be able to predict some other variable or performance outcome. A test such as the previous example of one designed to assess language competence may fail to represent certain subcultures of sample cases and yet still accurately predict academic success or failure. Thus, **predictive validity** of tests or procedures may exist independent of their content validity. Essentially, the extent to which a measure or procedure is judged valid depends on its demonstrated usefulness in achieving the specific aims of an investigation (Nunnally, 1978).

Thus far, we have discussed the meaning of the term validity in reference to measurement instruments or procedures. Other meanings of the term pertain to the overall validity of an investigation. Four types of validity pertain to the accuracy of the conclusions or inferences made on the basis of scientific research, namely, (1) internal validity; (2) external validity; (3) statistical validity; and (4) construct (theoretical) validity.

Internal Validity

Internal validity refers to the extent that causal inferences are justified based on observed changes in a dependent variable in response to systematic variations in an independent variable. Shaughnessy and Zechmeister (1994) identified three important conditions that must be established for making valid causal inferences. The first of these involves the *co-variation of events*. More specifically, this principle states that a change in one variable should be accompanied by a corresponding change in another variable. Second, a *time-order relationship* should be demonstrated so that the presumed cause should occur before the presumed effect. Third, causality can be demonstrated only when *other possible causes have been ruled out*.

In order for a conclusion to be drawn with confidence, *alternative plausible causes* involving extraneous variables must be eliminated or controlled. Failure to do so could result in a **confounding effect** as a result of two variables being allowed to vary simultaneously. For example, if you wished to evaluate the comparative effectiveness of two therapy programs for treating aphasia, you could avoid the potential confounding effect of age on performance by matching subjects on this variable prior to their group assignment.

Threats to Internal Validity

The purpose of most experimental-type studies is to establish conditions that allow an investigator to conclude with confidence that an observed *effect* is the consequence of a particular *cause*. Consistent with this goal, various research designs are selected to maximize the intended systematic influence of the independent variable on the dependent while controlling or eliminating extraneous influences that might otherwise invalidate conclusions by allowing for alternative explanations.

Several extraneous factors have been identified (Campbell and Stanley, 1966; Cook and Campbell, 1979) which, if not controlled, can produced unwanted changes (**confounding effects**) in a dependent variable unrelated to the influence of the independent variable. Among these are the following:

- **History:** The influence of change-producing external events, tangential to the purposes of an experiment, that intervene between two observations or measurements (e.g., between a pretest and a posttest). *Example: We wish to determine the effect of completing a research and statistical methods course on graduate students' attitudes about the importance of such content to their future day-to-day work as clinicians. Attitudes are pretested at the beginning of the course and posttested upon completion. In the interim, the coordinator of graduate studies circulates a memorandum with study tips for students preparing for comprehensive examinations, many of whom are presently enrolled in our course. The memorandum states, among other things, that the " . . . ability to critically evaluate research literature will be emphasized and necessary in order to satisfy the academic standards of the program."*

- **Maturation:** Internal biological or psychologic changes within subjects that may occur over a span of time, resulting in performance variations unrelated to the treatment of interest. *Example: At the beginning of the school year, you decide to evaluate the efficacy of an articulation training program for a group of first grade students who have yet to acquire correct production of the /s/ phoneme. You pretest the children in September before commencing treatment* *and provide therapy until June of the following year, when you posttest their performance. Happily, for most, a significant reduction in the severity of frontal lisping has occurred. Perhaps coincidentally, because of the full eruption of their central incisors, the dental appearance of many of these children has likewise greatly improved!*

- **Testing:** The facilitative influence of previous testing on performance measures, accruing as the result of familiarity, practice, or learning with repeated exposure to the same or similar test. *Example: There is evidence that people tend to score better on IQ measures merely as the result of repeated testing (Anastasi, 1988). Some measures of verbal ability, such as the Peabody Picture Vocabulary Test, have addressed the potential for such a **"practice effect"** by developing two standardized forms of this particular instrument. Of course, there also is the familiar refrain of students proclaiming to their instructors after taking the first test of the semester, "Now that I know what to expect, I'll do better the second time around."*

- **Instrumentation:** Changes in the accuracy or precision of measuring devices or human observations. *Examples: The calibration of an audiometer is altered or an electrical short in the wiring of a headphone produces intermittent static noise during an experiment. The audiologist conducting the experiment develops an ear infection accompanied by tinnitus (ringing sensations) that is likely to interfere with his or her own accuracy in judging and recording subject responses during speech discrimination testing.*

- **Statistical Regression:** In the nineteenth century, Francis Galton observed from hereditary studies of nature that the characteristics of phenomena not only evolve but end up clustering in such a way as to be more similar than dissimilar. Statistically, this is reflected in the tendency for extreme scores in a data set, on repeated testing, to move toward the average score of the distribution. *Example: A researcher wishes to examine voice onset times in two groups of childhood stutterers who differ in stuttering severity. Subjects whose severity scores are atypical of their average level of disfluency may be inappropriately delegated to one group or the other. Greater regression is likely for subjects whose scores are the most extreme. Given a large number of such subjects, resulting comparisons between the two groups would be inappropriate because the groups tend to be more alike than initially believed.*

- **Experimental Mortality:** We prefer to call this extraneous variable **differential attrition** because subjects may terminate their participation in an experiment for reasons other than that implied by the more ominous term. Hopefully, when the loss of subjects occurs, as often happens, especially in the course of lengthy experiments, it will be for reasons related to ordinary living circumstances (e.g., job changes, family or school demands, moving from the area, temporary illness, etc.). Whatever the reason, the differential loss of subjects from comparison groups can seriously impair an experiment. *Example: Suppose you wish to study the speed and accuracy of sentence comprehension in two groups of subjects, one group during a quiet condition and the other under a condition of ambient noise. You know or suspect that a subject's performance may be related differentially to such extraneous factors as age, intelligence, motivation, attention, etc. As a means of controlling these extraneous variables, you may attempt to distribute their effects equivalently in the two groups through random assignment or try to control for such influences through careful matching of groups on all important factors so that they differ only with respect to the independent variable. Despite your best efforts to achieve control, subjects drop out from one group in significant numbers, invalidating the assumption of group equivalency. The resulting imbalance is reflected not only in a disproportionate number of subjects constituting the comparison groups, but in the loss of control over important variables that are likely to differentially impact group performance.*

- **Selection Bias:** Preexisting factors may preclude or interfere with the establishment of equivalent groups, so it cannot be assumed that the operative influences or treatments in an experiment differ systematically only with respect to the independent variable. *Example: You wish to determine the effectiveness of a parent counseling program in facilitating the language acquisition of preschool children judged to be mildly delayed on standardized language tests. You ask for volunteers and divide children into two groups based on their parents' participation or lack thereof. Some months later, posttesting reveals that the children whose parents participated in the counseling program made significant gains in language development, whereas the children of the nonparticipating parents did not. Can you conclude that parent counseling was effective in achieving the intended goals? You cannot.*

One major problem relates to the volunteer status of the parent participants who may have been more highly motivated to provide direct assistance to their children despite the counseling program. Furthermore, the children of the parent volunteers may have come from cultural or socioeconomic backgrounds in which greater emphasis is placed on developing the same type of verbal skills as those measured by the testing procedures.

All of the factors described can individually or interactively threaten the internal validity of an experiment. Some experimental designs better control or, through randomization, distribute in a chance fashion the potential for such extraneous variables to prevent or weaken the interpretation of results. For reasons noted previously, true experimental designs offer more effective control over threats to internal validity than quasi-experimental designs. Pre-experimental designs are by far the weakest of all in controlling for pitfalls that can invalidate an experiment. Such designs, particularly one-group studies, should only be undertaken when nothing better can be done and the essential goal is to explore or describe new phenomena rather than to explain their causes (see Chapter 5).

Whereas true experiments are effective at eliminating most, if not all, threats to their internal validity, some pitfalls are sometimes difficult, if not impossible, to avoid no matter how well the study is planned. Such threats often are due to inherent biases within the experimenter or subjects of an investigation rather than to structural faults in the research design.

Rosenthal (1966) has documented several sources of observer bias that have come to be known as **experimenter effects.** Such bias often exists in the form of expectations about what the results of an investigation *ought to be* that can lead an experimenter, perhaps unknowingly, to treat subjects differently in certain respects or to favor a particular outcome. An even earlier awareness of this phenomenon is contained in the story of Clever Hans, the horse who was believed to be able to understand words, spell, and perform arithmetic in response to his trainer's instructions. What first were considered remarkable abilities were later discovered to represent conditioned responses to subtle movements and related cues unintentionally provided by the trainer.

The practical implication of this story is represented in the problems resulting from labeling school children as "cognitively impaired," "learning disabled," "conduct disordered," etc. Research has demonstrated quite clearly that such labels can mold teachers' expectations in ways that influence their evaluation of student performance (Rosenthal and Jacobson, 1968).

Another source of bias can stem merely from **subject awareness** of having been selected to participate in a study. Changes in performance, found to occur when subjects believe that they have attracted the attention or have been "singled out" by a significant other(s), have come to be known as the **Hawthorne Effect.** This phenomenon is named after a production plant of the Western Electric Company, where the effect was first observed in a study of worker productivity in response to changes (increases or decreases) in illumination. Improvements in productivity seemed to be related to subjects' awareness of their participation in the experiment independent of the type of manipulation employed. Although the reasons for the effect are no doubt complex, it is believed that the action of an independent variable can alter the behavior of subjects based on how they perceive that the experimenter might expect or hope they will behave (Franke and Kaul, 1978). In such cases, subjects' presumptions about the intended effect of an independent variable may turn out to be quite different than the effect actually intended by the experimenter.

In estimating the internal validity of a research study, Cook and Campbell (1979) have emphasized the importance of:

> . . . a deductive process in which the investigator has to systematically think through how each of the internal validity threats may have influenced the data . . . the researcher has to be his or her own best critic, trenchantly examining all of the threats he or she can imagine (pp. 55–56).

Whereas the need for careful reflection in evaluating data is undeniable, it is more important to consider how threats to internal validity can be eliminated or controlled in planning and designing an experiment from the outset. As in the case of caring for one's own health, weak or ill-conceived research plans are better treated prospectively than lamented posthumously.

External Validity

External validity pertains to the generalizability of results from a specific study sample of cases to one or more populations, settings, treatment variables, or measurement variables (Campbell and Stanley, 1966). In addressing the problem of external validity, we are asking about the usefulness of our findings to the world beyond the narrow domain of our own investigation. It is possible for data to be internally valid but lack external validity. For example, we know that it is often possible to achieve marked reductions in stuttering behavior within the clinic or laboratory but also difficult to generalize these same results to other speaking conditions. The same could be said for many other types of cases and treatment programs in the field of communication disorders. A common argument for the use of inclusion models of therapy intervention, as commonly practiced in many school systems, is that such programs are purported to foster improved functioning in more "real life situations" than can be provided in relatively "artificial settings" as the therapy room. Yet, a study's prospects of replication are of major concern in matters pertaining to its external validity. If a study cannot be replicated, it has little or no scientific value regardless of the internal validity of its results.

In most investigations, the researcher is faced with balancing the often conflicting or competitive demands for external and internal validity. Efforts to achieve relevancy can result in the loss of experimental control over important variables. On the other hand, gains in control can reduce the meaning of the results as they might otherwise apply to the outside world.

Threats to External Validity

It will be recalled that external validity refers to the generalizability of experimental data. When one asks about the external validity of a particular study, the question pertains to the limits of how far the results can be extended beyond the confines of a particular study to other persons, settings, or circumstances. Just as the factors that jeopardize internal validity must be weighed, threats to the generality of research findings require careful evaluation. Three main types of factors may operate to restrict external invalidity.

Measurement restrictions are those in which the measure selected to represent a dependent variable is not truly representative of the phenomenon that the experimenter wants to assess. Imagine an experimental study of stutterers designed to explore the level of anxiety associated with speaking in the presence of photographs of certain individuals. The investigator selects galvanic skin response or palmar sweating as the measure of anxiety to be recorded at predetermined times during the experiment. The question is whether or not the degree of physiologic (autonomic) arousal is the variable that was actually of interest to the investigator. After the experiment, a problem arises should he or she decide to the contrary. For example, it might be decided that the more intriguing issue pertains to the nature of the threats posed by the photographs as *consciously perceived* by the speaker. In this case, cognitive measures of apprehension or rating scales of avoidance about speaking engendered by the photographs may have proved more useful in examining the "real" question of interest. Before initiating an experiment, it is important to determine the degree to which a selected measure is appropriate for its intended use and thus capable of producing relevant (generalizable) results.

Treatment restrictions, involving the selection of an independent variable that is unsuitable for generalizing results, can also limit the external validity of an experiment. In our example above, it could be argued that the use of photographs to examine speech-related anxiety is an *artificial research arrangement* having little or no relevance to actual speaking situations—i.e., individuals typically speak to other people directly rather than having imaginary conversations in response to their photographs. Based on this line of reasoning, the investigator might alter the experiment by substituting actual listeners in place of photographs in an effort to create testing conditions more like "real-life" speaking circumstances. While admitting that the generality of results could be improved by such an alteration, critics might still contend that any testing arrangement involving experimental research is artificial to the degree that it departs from naturally occurring circumstances or ordinary experience. Although such a conclusion is technically correct, the internal validity of some research studies simply cannot be evaluated short of the controls and constancy imposed by the structure of a laboratory experiment. The investigator is generally faced with alternative choices that require perspicacious judgment in weighing threats to external validity against internal validity. As the risks to external validity increase because of the artificiality of a treatment or setting, the influence of extraneous variables mitigating against internal validity often decreases. The reverse is also found.

Sample restrictions that might adversely affect the external validity of an experiment pose still another concern that relates to **representativeness** of the subjects used. More specifically, a question that must be raised pertains to the degree that a sample of subjects truly reflects the behaviors, physical and mental attributes, socioeconomic status, motivation, level of skill, etc. as the target population to whom we wish to extrapolate our findings. If a sample of subjects is not representative, there is no justification for inductively inferring the meaning of an experiment beyond the immediate results. Indeed, citing philosopher David Hume (1711–1776), Campbell and Stanley (1966) noted that there is in fact no logical basis for ever making generalizations beyond the limits of a particular study in absolute terms. This is because the precise characteristics of subjects, conditions, or circumstances surrounding the time and place of an original experiment can never be fully duplicated. The best a researcher can do is to make the best guesses possible about what pitfalls might undermine the generality of an experiment. A reasonable safeguard is to clearly identify the specific population characteristics of the population for which generalization is desired prior to an experiment. Having done so, the next step is to implement sampling procedures that are estimated to yield a subject pool most like the population of interest.

Statistical Conclusion Validity

A third type of validity in a scientific study, **statistical conclusion validity,** pertains to the relative truth upon which its statistical conclusions are based. In most investigations, statistical methods are used for collecting, organizing, analyzing, and interpreting the results of a study in a mathematical form. A characteristic of such data that usually interests the researcher is its variability. More specially, a major concern is the degree to which data are indicative of intended systematic influences as opposed to uncontrolled chance factors. Based on the available information, an educated guess in the form of a hypothesis is formulated as to the likely outcomes (statistical findings) of the experiment.

In the vernacular of statistics, hypotheses are generally formulated in the *null* form. A **null hypothesis** is one formulated for the specific goal of statistical significance testing, thereby permitting generalization from a sample of cases to the population from which such cases were drawn. Briefly defined, the word *null* means "no difference" and generally refers to a predicted finding of no significant differences between or within groups of subjects or treatment conditions.

Associated with null hypotheses are probability estimates for making certain types of statistical inference errors (sampling errors): **type I or type II errors.** A type I error involves rejecting a particular null hypothesis when it is true. For example, there is a chance of erroneously concluding that treatment A is significantly better than treatment B when it is not. On the other hand, one might make a **type II error** (retaining a null hypothesis when it is false) by erroneously concluding that a particular treatment is no more effective than another.

As noted previously, the researcher typically selects an acceptable risk for error in the form of a significance level—i.e., ($p = .05$ or $p = .01$) prior to initiating an experiment. For a finding to be regarded as "significant," the odds for making an inferential error must be quite small: no greater than 5% of the time in the case of the first probability value noted above. In the case of the second value, an inferential error would be expected only 1% of the time.

Remember that statistical significance testing involves *estimating* the odds for a systematic influence controlled by the experimenter against the *expected amount* of deviation in the measures of interest owing to chance alone. As a part of null hypothesis testing, errors of inference can and do occur. The nature of such errors and their statistical relevance for formulating and testing null hypotheses is discussed more fully in Chapters 4 and 8.

Construct Validity

The final type of validity that we wish to discuss pertains to the notion of the truth of a construct or theory. **Construct validity** (theoretical validity) is perhaps the most abstract and difficult type of validity to establish because it requires establishing not only the content and predictive validity of a particular measurement tool or procedure but also the extent to which the obtained results converge with those found in other investigations of the same phenomenon.

For example, it was noted earlier that numerous researchers have attempted to study anxiety in stutterers as a characteristic feature of the behavior (see Chapter 2). It was also pointed out that the inconclusive nature of the research findings may be the result of employing widely differing methods that measure unrelated things. Physiologic measures of autonomic arousal like galvanic skin response or palmar sweating may tap into aspects of anxiety that are quite distinct from other indicators based on anxiety questionnaires, expectancy, or certain behavioral observations. Because of discrepancies among the results of several pertinent experiments, the role of anxiety and its theoretical importance in reference to various aspects of stuttering behavior can be said to lack **construct validity.** Construct validity can only be established based on the evidence accumulated from several studies performed by different researchers employing the same operational definitions or criterion measures of anxiety.

Statistical methods have been developed that allow for the analysis and summary of the results of independent experiments. In the future, such a sophisticated group of statistical procedures, called **meta-analysis,** will no doubt play a critical role in helping to validate the theoretical constructs that serve as a basis for explaining and managing problems in numerous professional fields, including communication disorders (see Chapter 8).

Drawing Reliable Conclusions

In addition to striving for valid research findings relevant to the underlying phenomena under investigation, researchers also wish to assure reliability in a set of data. Although the concepts of validity and reliability are closely related, they are by no means identical. One's observations or measurement techniques may be highly precise and consistent, illustrating so-called **test-retest reliability,** but lack validity. A case in point is a poorly calibrated audiometer that *reliably* produces erroneous results in the measurement of hearing acuity. Thus, whereas validity is dependent on the attainment of reliable measures or procedures, the reverse is not true.

As with validity, there are different meanings and applications of the term *reliability*. In the most general sense of the concept, reliability implies dependability, as in the case of a reliable person or piece of equipment that can be counted on to consistently supply some need. Yet, the idea of reliability carries with it the possibility of something being erratic or prone to errors even though such errors may be infrequent. Thus, the reliability of a measuring instrument, procedure, or person is best viewed in relative rather than absolute terms.

From the viewpoint of a researcher, important aspects of reliability that must be assessed in any experiment relate to the *stability* and *accuracy* of the measures or procedures employed (Kerlinger, 1973). The factor of stability reflects the extent to which the observations or results obtained in an investigation are consistent across time. More specifically, the measures reflecting the characteristics of a dependent variable ought to yield results that are identical or highly similar regardless of when a particular data set is obtained. The one exception to this rule would involve changes in a dependent variable that could be accounted for on the basis of systematic influences while ruling out the effect of chance or random fluctuations.

Another concern pertaining to the reliability of experimental measures or procedures relates to their *accuracy* in accomplishing the intended goal of the investigation. If a device designed to assess the acoustic features of hypernasality in cleft palate speakers should inadvertently measure hyponasality as well, it could hardly be called a trustworthy or reliable measure. As a general rule, concern about the accuracy of a measure or procedure should take precedence over issues pertaining to its stability. If a measure can be said to be accurate, it is likely that it will also yield results that are stable across time.

Researchers often are interested in quantifying the degree of error associated with a measure or procedure in accurately assessing a **true score.** A true score is one that would result as the consequence of repeated sampling over a very long series of trials under ideal conditions using a perfect test instrument. Such a score, representing perfect consistency in one's observations or measurement procedures, would be expressed mathematically as a value of one (1.0). This value, indicative of the greatest degree of reliability, is an idealized number that is generally believed to be unattainable. However, it is reasonable to believe that no measurement instruments or recording procedures are perfect in all respects. Furthermore, random fluctuations associated with extraneous circumstances beyond the experimenter's control appear to be characteristic of all phenomena. Based on these considerations, reliability can be defined as the *extent to which departures from a true score reflect random errors in measurement.*

The actual statistical calculation of reliability is usually accomplished by means of a correlational technique, resulting in a reliability coefficient. Such a value typically falls between 0 and 1.

In addition to concerns related to the internal stability and accuracy of one's measuring instruments, workers in clinical fields often are interested in assessing the reliability of professional individuals in administering diagnostic tests or treatment programs. Two types of *observer reliability* are typically of interest in any clinical study or research investigation. The first of these, termed **intraobserver reliability,** is the degree of internal consistency of an individual observer with her or himself in administering proscribed experimental procedures (independent variables) and in measuring or judging certain empirical phenomena (dependent variables) under the same conditions but at different times. Fluctuations within the observer, such as those resulting from extraneous distracters or changes in one's mental or physical state, can impair intraobserver reliability that is related to the stability of judgment.

Another form of reliability that is of equal or greater importance to assess in most clinical studies or experiments is concerned with the accuracy rather than the stability of judgment. This is termed **interobserver reliability** and is calculated as the degree or proportion of agreement between two or more observers. A relatively simple and useful method for measuring agreement between two observers in making judgments about behaviors that are assigned to one category or another is based on the kappa formula developed by Cohen (1977). The method has relevance to many clinical situations in which clinicians might wish to measure their agreement in diagnosing a particular disorder based on judgments of the *presence* or *absence* of abnormality. Such dichotomous results can be expressed as either "normal" or "abnormal" outcomes in leading to a diagnosis.

Imagine that two clinicians independently evaluate 100 children suspected of stuttering and render judgments about the normality or abnormality of disfluent speech using the same diagnostic criteria. Hypothetic data based on their observations can be cast in the form of a 2 × 2 contingency table (Table 3.1). Based on the results shown, we can proceed to illustrate the calculation of kappa (κ), defined as the agreement beyond chance divided by the amount of agreement *possible* beyond chance, such that:

$$\kappa = \frac{o - c}{1 - c}$$

where o = the observed agreement, and c = the chance agreement. Calculate o through the following formula:

o = (# of "normality agreements") + (# of "abnormality agreements")/the grand total
= (18 + 60)/100
= 78/100 (.78) or 78% = o

The calculation of the chance agreement is next accomplished by the following steps:

Table 3.1.
Observed Agreement on Judging Disfluent Children as "Normal" or "Abnormal"

| | Clinician B | | |
Clinician A	Abnormal	Normal	Subtotal
Abnormal	18	12	30
Normal	10	60	70
Subtotal	28	72	100

1. Calculate how many observations the clinicians may agree are abnormal by chance, determined by multiplying the number each found abnormal and then dividing by the grand total of 100 observations:

$$(30 \times 28)/100 = 8.4.$$

2. Calculate how many observations the two may agree are normal by chance, determined by multiplying the number each found normal and dividing by the grand total of 100 observations:

$$(70 \times 72)/100 = 50.4.$$

3. Add the two numbers found in the first two steps and divide by 100 to obtain the proportion of chance agreement:

$$(8.4 + 50.4)/100 = 0.588 \text{ or } 58.8\% = c.$$

Given that the observed agreement (o) is 78%, or 0.78, the agreement beyond chance (o-c) is 0.78–0.588 = 0.192, representing the numerator of k.

The potential agreement beyond chance is 100% minus the chance agreement of 58.8%, or $1 - .588 = .412$, the denominator of k. Thus, in our example, k = 0.192/0.412 = 0.47, or 47%.

For a two-category system of the type described above, chance would dictate that the observers would agree .25 or 25% of the time. Thus, based on the results of our hypothetic example in which a kappa of 47% was found, we can conclude that the extent of agreement between our two clinicians well exceeded chance expectations.

The kappa formula represents a convenient and straight-forward method for calculating the degree of reliability based on probability theory. Other more complex statistical procedures such as tests of correlation are available for determining the accuracy and stability of observations; some of these will be discussed in subsequent chapters. Meanwhile, remember that with respect to measurement considerations in research, the concept of reliability relates to the need for assessing errors resulting from inaccurate or unstable recording devices, including our own eyes and ears as they too may be used for such purposes.

SELF-LEARNING REVIEW

Data

1. _____ sets may be described as perceptual schema that serve to categorize or classify experience.

bias

2. The way we perceive a particular problem may _____ the outcome.

3. The ability of the brain to _____ discern specific objects

reliably

and events does not exclude other points of view from having

validity

equal or greater _____.

Venn

4. _____ diagrams are useful in illustrating the

associative

_____ relations among data sets. Typically, a population

subsets

can be divided into a number of individual _____ of data.

association
correlation

5. The method of _____ is used to describe the correspon-

coefficient

dence or _____ between data sets. The result can be ex-

correlation

pressed as a _____ of _____.

6. Determining causality based on correlation is typically unwar-

third

ranted because of the potential influence of a _____ vari-

directionality

able and the _____ problem.

correlation

7. A well-known dictum of research practice is that

causation

"_____ does not imply _____."

8. According to Mill's "method of difference," causality can be

presence

inferred only where factor Y occurs in the _____ of factor

absence

X and does not occur in the _____ of factor X.

difference

9. Asking and answering _____ questions is the chief

causal

means of determining _____ relations.

10. The quantitative evaluation of differences between two con-

variance

ditions relates to what statisticians call _____.

11. Essentially, causal research asks questions pertaining to dif-

variable

ferences in a dependent _____ that has and has not been

independent

preceded by an _____ variable.

causal

12. An all-inconclusive data set about which _____ infer-

population

ences are drawn is called a _____.

parameter

13. A number descriptive of a population is called a _____.

statistics

Numbers descriptive of samples are called _____.

14. The extent to which a variable changes in response to an ex-

systematic

perimental manipulation is called _____ variance. Change

owing to unknown or uncontrolled variables is termed
_____ variance.

error

15. _____ variables are those that are relatively
_____ and typically not subject to experimental
_____.

Organismic
stable
manipulation

16. After all known sources of _____ variance have been
eliminated, what remains is _____ variance.

systematic
error

17. Mathematically, the total variance in an experiment can be
expressed as an F ratio, where F = _____.

$$\frac{V_b}{V_e}$$

18. Whereas _____ -group variance is attributable to systematic influences, _____-group variance consists primarily
of _____ variance plus secondary influences including
_____ differences.

between
within
error
individual

19. Deductive reasoning is essentially based on a triad of propositions called a _____.

syllogism

20. Deductive logic is best suited for _____ making that
begins with set of _____ generalizations believed to be true.

problem
a priori

21. Problem solving, the cornerstone of scientific reasoning, is
based on _____ inferences.

inductive

22. Intervening between existing knowledge and predictive
knowledge is the _____ _____.

inductive gap

23. Because of the possibility of error, scientific assertions involve probability statements reflecting _____ degrees of certainty as compared to uncertainty.

relative

24. Inductive inferences are generally made _____ -after
data collection.

a posteriori

25. The best a researcher can do in resolving the inductive gap is
to _____ the true probability of an observation based on
_____ interval testing.

estimate
confidence

26. Statistical testing of the _____ of _____ involves
calculating an _____ _____ against chance.

significance
difference
odds ratio

27. Interpreting the results of statistical testing typically entails
the use of either the _____ or _____ level of significance depending on the degree of _____ desired in the test
results.

.05
.01
confidence

relative

28. In scientific terms, the concept of validity pertains to establishing the _____ truth of an observation.

Content
intended or designed

29. _____ validity refers to the extent that a particular measure actually does measure what it was _____ to assess.

validity

30. A measure may predict a particular outcome independent of its _____.

validity
dependent
independent

31. Internal _____ refers to the extent that causal inferences are justified based on changes in a _____ variable in response to the systematic influence of an _____ variable.

extraneous
controlled
confounding

32. Internal validity can be undermined when _____ variables are not eliminated or _____. Failure to do so could result in a _____ effect.

internally
external

33. It is possible for a study to be _____ valid but lack _____ validity so that the results cannot be generalized.

confounding

34. Unwanted changes in a dependent variable unrelated to the influence of the independent variable are called _____ effects.

history

35. A study may be invalidated as a result of change-producing external events occurring between a pretest and a posttest. Such changes are attributed to _____.

human
instrumentation

36. Changes in the accuracy or precision of measuring devices or _____ observations are attributed to _____.

test

37. A threat to internal validity as a result of familiarity, practice, or learning can occur with repeated exposure to the same or similar _____.

regression

38. The tendency for extreme scores in a distribution to move toward the average score is called statistical _____ .

attrition
differentially

39. Another name for experimental mortality is differential _____. This threat to internal validity may _____ impact group performance.

Hawthorne

40. A bias that stems merely from subject awareness of having been selected for an experiment is called the _____ effect.

experimenter

41. Sources of observer bias that result in treating subjects differently in certain respects or that favor a particular outcome are called _____ effects.

42. Three types of factors that can threaten the external validity of an experiment include _____ , _____ , and _____ restrictions.

measurement
treatment
sample

43. Selecting an independent variable that is unsuitable for generalizing results is an example of a _____ restriction.

treatment

44. _____ restrictions occur when the measure selected to represent the dependent variable is not representative of the phenomenon that the experimenter wants to assess.

Measurement

45. _____ restrictions relate to the representativeness of the subjects used in an experiment.

Sample

46. Associated with null hypothesis testing is the possibility of making _____ _____ and _____ _____ errors. The first type of error entails _____ the null when it is true, whereas the second error involves _____ to reject the null when it is _____ .

type I
type II
rejecting
failing
false

47. _____ validity can only be established based on the accumulated evidence of several studies. A sophisticated group of statistical procedures developed for this purpose is based on _____ -analysis.

Construct
meta

48. The test-retest _____ of a measure may be established, but the measure may still lack _____ .

reliability
validity

49. _____ reliability pertains to establishing the degree of _____ consistency of an individual observer. _____ reliability pertains to establishing the degree or proportion of agreement between two or more observers beyond that expected from _____ alone.

Intraobserver
internal
Interobserver
chance

50. A statistic that calculates the reliability between two observers in terms of their degree of agreement beyond chance is called _____ .

kappa

4. Selecting and Defining Problems

SELECTING A RESEARCH PROBLEM

A common concern among students beginning to think seriously about the importance of research and its potential relevance to their future careers is how to select and define a problem in a way that is amenable to systematic investigation. Certainly, we are all accustomed to asking routine questions in subjective terms that generally produce opinionated or nonscientific answers. For example, we might ask about therapy techniques that could prove useful in "motivating a client," "improving rapport," or facilitating "family intervention." Helpful colleagues may offer advice or opinions based on their own professional experience. Although many concerns of this type are quite appropriate for informal discussion and might eventually qualify as fertile areas for research, they lack the objective criteria necessary for framing a specific research question or hypothesis. Nevertheless, prior to asking a "researchable question" and developing a suitable research design for answering it, one must select a problem for study that one wishes to understand.

Before taking one or more courses in research and statistical methods, it is understandable why students might complain of difficulties in comprehending scientific concepts and investigative processes that underlie existing fields of knowledge. Although unfamiliarity with the methods of science can certainly impede the selection of cogent problems for research, even experienced investigators commonly encounter such difficulty. Indeed, as Hoover (1976) noted, "The hardest problem in scientific thinking occurs at the beginning of the investigation. Once you have solved it, other steps will fall into place." (p. 42)

Significant Questions Lead to Significant Answers

From the outset, the primary concern in forming a research question ought to be with the likely significance of the answer. Trivial questions generally culminate in inconsequential results. As summed up by Henri Poincaré,

> There is a hierarchy of facts; some have no reach; they teach us nothing but themselves . . .
> There are, on the other hand, facts of great yield; each of them teaches us a new law . . . it is to
> these that the scientist should devote himself. (p. 554)

Although this is a lofty goal, many of the routine tasks that become ritualized in our everyday professional lives fail to stimulate the kind of creative questions that advance a field
of knowledge. Nevertheless, only when faced with challenging tasks that demand solution
is the imagination taxed (Merton, 1959).

Previously, it was noted that questions aimed at solving some problem are typically focused on achieving at least one of three levels of understanding. At the simplest level, researchers ask **"who"** or **"what"** questions that are answered through the use of various descriptive techniques designed to categorize or classify the attributes of a particular
phenomenon. Often, the intended goal of such questions is to develop taxonomies of various types or subtypes of communication disorders, such as stuttering, aphasia, cleft lip and
palate, and hearing loss. Such knowledge is important in setting up mutually exclusive diagnostic criteria for identifying such disorders according to clusters of certain signs and
symptoms. This is often the main goal and chief value of descriptive research techniques.

At the next level of complexity, **"where"** questions might be raised pertaining to the
direction of associated changes in one variable (e.g., an attribute of a disorder) in relation
to another. If both variables move in the same direction, they may be positively related.
On the other hand, if they move in opposite directions, they may be negatively related.

Characterizing the various features of variables and their relationship to others is frequently an essential requisite to asking **"why"** questions geared toward discerning causal
relations among variables-the highest level of understanding. In answering such questions,
inferential statistics are often used to examine the significance of the difference between
two or more variables, and an effort is made to explain the basis for any such differences.

As Merton (1959) pointed out, merely asking a question does not constitute a problem. The formulation of a problem actually consists of a three-part process involving (1)
originating a question; (2) developing a rationale or statement of its importance; and (3)
determining the feasibility for answering it.

Origination of a Question

Most questions arise after one encounters a problem that needs to be solved. Such questions arise in the context of clinical practice; in interacting with one's professional peers;
through attending professional conferences and workshops; and by reading and critiquing
research articles.

For obvious reasons, researchers normally wish to identify interesting questions as opposed to dull or trivial concerns. Nevertheless, it would be a mistake to believe that, in order to be worthy of investigation, the subject matter must have revolutionary significance.
As clinicians, we are constantly faced with asking many questions in the search for the
kinds of *practical answers* that will allow us to better understand, predict, and interpret the
results of testing procedures and treatment programs. Few would deny the importance of
answering questions such as:

- Is this person's speech-language-hearing functioning within the normal range?
- Given the presence of certain signs or symptoms of abnormality, are they indicative of a particular disorder or disease process?
- How reliable or valid are the available diagnostic tests or strategies used for determining the
  specific nature of the problem?

- What etiologic factors are associated with an increased likelihood for the particular disorder or disease in question?
- How might the problem be modified through treatment?
- What intervention procedures can be expected to result in the best functional outcomes in cases of this kind?
- How can problems of this nature be prevented or their adverse consequences diminished?

These are a few of several questions that can arise from clinical efforts to solve practical problems. Although some of these may be answered through mechanisms other than highly formalized research designs, the knowledge of how to ask good questions and develop and apply scientific methods will likely improve the validity of our clinical observations and conclusions.

Important unresolved questions can also emerge from classroom discussions of research literature and the critical reading and evaluation of such literature. The American-Speech-Language-Hearing Association publishes several journals that contain research studies and scholarly articles related to important scientific issues. These include the *Journal of Speech and Hearing Research*; *Language, Speech, and Hearing Services in Schools*; *American Journal of Speech-Language Pathology: A Journal of Clinical Practice*; the *American Journal of Audiology: A Journal of Clinical Practice*; *ASHA Reports*; and *Asha*. One indicator of ASHA's commitment to scholarly publication is the increasing number of pages published annually in its journals that has occurred over the past several decades (Figure 4.1). Oc-

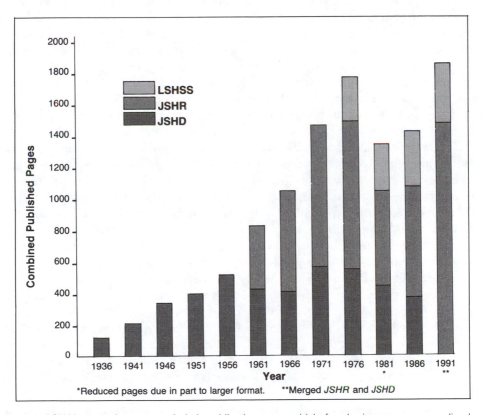

Figure 4.1. ASHA's commitment to scholarly publications as a vehicle for sharing an ever-expanding body of knowledge.

casionally, a Task Force on Research is appointed by ASHA (1989) to review and prioritize issues as a national research agenda.

Although each of ASHA's journals has a distinctive focus, some being more research oriented than others, all of them typically contain research reports that not only summarize the findings of a specific investigation but also provide an overview of other important studies relevant to the topic area. Moreover, such articles frequently contain a discussion of unresolved issues and research problems that warrant further investigation.

Journal publications of research articles that are useful and relevant to the interests of speech-language pathologists and audiologists are too numerous to list. A partial listing, including those published by related disciplines or specialty journals that have an interdisciplinary focus, can be found in Appendix D.

In a field as diverse as communication disorders, it is understandable why students may have difficulty in identifying a specific research question of interest to them. However, with minimal prompting, most can identify a broad issue or topic of concern (e.g., the diagnosis of stuttering in young children; the surgical treatment of cleft palate speech; the recovery of language in aphasic disorders; the role of language in learning disabilities; etc.). Having described the overall character of a problem, the search for a particular research topic can begin in earnest.

Specific topics pertaining to current research trends, existing controversies, and critical areas for future inquiry are often identified in special sections or issues of professional journals, monographs, and "state of the art" reports. The published proceedings of research conferences provide additional insight about current trends and potential areas of inquiry. Moreover, the policies and priorities for various research projects along with guidelines for submitting research proposals and requests for funding are published by various branches of government, foundations, and corporations. Two publications of the U.S. government, the *Federal Register* and the National Institute of Health's *NIH Guide for Grants and Contracts*, announce scientific research initiatives on a regular basis. The National Institute on Deafness and Other Communication Disorders (NIDCD) is one of the major branches of NIH that supports biomedical and behavioral research and research training in normal and disordered processes of hearing, language, speech, and voice.

Despite the availability of such resources as noted, formulating a significant research question that is both personally interesting and relevant to current professional concerns can be a formidable task. Whereas journal articles and related literature generally provide rich sources of research ideas, wandering aimlessly through such material can be a frustrating and time-consuming experience. Fortunately, help is available in the form of cumulative abstracts and computerized data base services that allow for efficient searches of research literature. Through the use of library reference tools such as the monthly publication *Psychological Abstracts*, concise summaries of research studies appearing in more than 1,000 national and international periodicals can be accessed. Many of these abstracts pertain to communication disorders and can be located by the use of the author or subject index. Another highly useful directory for students who are considering a research topic about which there may be little published information is *Dissertation Abstracts International*. Locating a dissertation related to your research interest can be of great help because it is likely to provide a more comprehensive literature review and related bibliographic information than that available in most journal articles. A handy reference that lists all periodicals and the sources in which they are indexed is *Ulrich's International Periodical Directory*.

A good means of avoiding the rather tedious work of searching through the "hard copy" summaries of articles volume by volume is the use of one or more of the computerized data base services listed in Table 4.1. With the entry of **keywords** that represent the

Table 4.1.
Popular Library Reference Indexes

ERIC (Educational Resources Information Center)
This broad data base can be used with either key words from its Thesaurus or for on-line key word searches. In addition to providing a good source for searching many journal articles pertaining to children, this index typically reports on educationally relevant papers read at conventions that are not yet published in professional journals.

PsychLIT
One can search for both journal articles and book chapters on psychological topics using this data base.

SSCI (Social Sciences Citation Index)
Indexes journal articles related to studies in the social sciences and related fields.

MEDLINE
One whose topic is of a medical nature can search this index, which includes the majority of citations found in Cumulated Index Medicus.

Table 4.2.
Literature Annotation Chart

Author/Date	Source	Subjects/Age	Design	Variables	Results
Pratt et al., 1993	*JSHR, 36,* p. 1063	Six preschool hearing-impaired children (3:4–5:5 yrs)	Single subject Multiple baselines Multiple levels Changing criterion	Indep. var.: IBM speech viewer Depend var.: vowel accuracy	Treatment effect demonstrated for at least one of three vowels in five subjects

essence of your subject (e.g., Parkinson's disease, dysarthria, speaking rate), the computer can quickly scan the titles and abstracts of articles in its memory and identify intersecting terms. A systematic approach to retrieving bibliographic information "on-line" is to begin the search process for articles published in the current year and work backward as far as necessary, given your particular retrieval goals.

The reference sections of recent articles will likely include references to other important studies related to the topic of interest. One way to identify an *important* research study is by noting the frequency of its citation in other investigations. After identifying the titles and authors of such studies, abstracts of those expected to prove most relevant to your own questions or information needs can be printed as desired in addition to any other bibliographic information that you might wish to place on file for future reference. A literature review chart such as the one shown in Table 4.2 can be a useful device for summarizing the results of your search in a cogent and informative manner.

Most libraries in colleges and universities have resources for conducting such searches in one-half hour or less. Reference librarians can be of assistance in "honing in" on references pertinent to your topic and in teaching you to use the most efficient searching techniques.

Rationale for a Question

We noted previously that merely asking a question falls short of developing a researchable problem. Ultimately, one must ponder the significance of the question asked. Anybody who has played the game "Ten questions" is aware of the importance of asking not just any question but one that is most likely to yield the answer sought. Behind any such question is a **rationale** or underlying reason for asking the question in the first place. According to Merton (1959), "The requirement of a rationale curbs the flow of scientifically trivial questions and enlarges the share of consequential ones." (p. xix)

The fact of modern human existence is that we must deal with a vast amount of information. Choosing what to attend to and for what reason is necessary for the achievement of relevant and meaningful goals. Perhaps the best way to clarify the rationale for a particular question is to explain the thinking processes behind the research. As such, a rationale is best viewed as " . . . an explanation built around a research problem" (Van Wagenen, 1991).

We noted in Chapter 1 that the rationale for a study ought to evolve naturally in the introduction section of a research paper as a consequence of establishing what is known about a problem and what remains unanswered. In considering the rationale for a potential research study, some important issues to address include the following:

- Will the answer to the question help to confirm, refute, or extend previous research findings?
- Will the answer to the question provide new information of current clinical significance or scientific importance to the profession?
- Will the answer to the question possibly advance the development of theory and research directions in the future?

As noted by Sidman (1960), the reasons for a question are many and ultimately reflect the subjective views of the investigator(s) about the kind of data needed by a scientific discipline. Judging the potential importance of data or the merit of what one chooses to study must rest on personal conviction and the opinions of one's colleagues. Furthermore, the history of science suggests that perceptions about the significance of certain questions can change as the result of professional trends, policy initiatives, or funding opportunities.

Feasibility of Answering a Question

What we undertake in research also ought to be guided by the available means of accomplishing the intended task. Although the specific details of a research investigation may be ill-defined initially, there ought to be at least some tentative basis upon which to predict its successful accomplishment.

The first issue in determining the feasibility of a study is whether or not the question or hypothesis is stated in a testable form. For this determination, the constructs of an investigation and the variables selected to represent them must be defined in operational terms. Unless the dependent and independent variables can be clearly specified in accord with the empirical means of their observation and measurement, the **criterion of testability** cannot be met. Connotative or theoretical definitions fall short of satisfying this requirement. For example, some years ago it was suggested that developmental stuttering may result because of delayed myelination of critical neural pathways that underlie speech production. The testability of such a proposition would depend upon the precise specification of how and under what conditions both the dependent variable (stuttering) and the independent variable (delayed myelination) would be measured. Perhaps because of difficulties involved in such specification, the theory has yet to be taken seriously as a credible etiologic explanation. Although a question that is *potentially testable* in the future may prove to have value, the better question is one that is *presently testable*.

Additional factors to consider in assessing the feasibility of answering a particular question relate to certain **methodological constraints**. Suppose an investigation is planned to assess hemispheric activation in autistic children in response to acoustic signals of various kinds, using Functional Magnetic Resonance Imaging (FMRI). Obviously, *availability of appropriate equipment and subjects* will be necessary to achieve the goals of such a research project.

Other possible methodological constraints on answering research questions relate to the inherent *difficulty of the project* or to *time limitations*. In considering topics for theses or dissertations, students should weigh carefully their ability to execute the necessary experimental procedures and to do so successfully within an acceptable time frame-hopefully, to use a common adage, "before reaching retirement age."

Ethical Issues

Ethical issues may also hamper the feasibility of answering certain research questions. In 1974, the National Research Act was established, creating the National Commission for The Protection of Human Subjects of Biomedical and Behavioral Research. In order to qualify for research funds awarded by federal agencies, all investigators and their institutions must comply with established regulations specifically designed to protect the rights and welfare of human subjects. To do so, research institutions are required to set up **Institutional Review Boards (IRBs)** with the charge of reviewing research proposals to determine their compliance with existing regulations. Such a board, sometimes called a Human Studies Committee, typically consists of at least five members that include scientists and nonscientists (e.g., clergy, lawyers, nurses, social workers, etc.).

Most colleges and universities have established IRB committees charged with protecting the rights and safety of research subjects. At many institutions, research proposals may be reviewed by an appropriate committee at the departmental level before being referred to the IRB. Graduate students, like faculty and other research personnel on contract, who are planning to complete research on human subjects, must first submit a detailed research plan or protocol for review that describes the background, significance, purpose, and methods of the project as well as all risks/benefits to participants and the means of obtaining their informed consent. If a prospective research subject is not of legal age or deemed incompetent to make a judgment as to the risks and benefits of participating, the informed consent must be obtained from a parent or legal guardian. IRB committees have the power to approve, disapprove, or require revision of a research plan as they see fit. An outline of the procedures for preparing human investigation protocols used at our own institution is shown in Table 4.3.

Two issues that are of major concern in the deliberations of an IRB committee are the so-called **risk/benefit ratio** and the means of obtaining **informed consent** by making clear any physical or mental risk to potential participants and those participants' rights prior to, during, and after the research investigation. Any research study entails some degree of risk if only for minor apprehension, boredom, fatigue, inconvenience, etc. Risks that do not exceed those normally encountered in daily life or as a result of routine tests and examination procedures are typically classified as **"minimal risks"** by an IRB, in which case certain requirements may be waived. When the probability of discomfort or possible harm is judged to be greater than "minimal," the IRB will likely designate subjects as being **"at risk."** In that case, the potential for harm or injury must be weighed against the possible benefits of serving as a subject in the investigation. The resulting balance is termed the risk/benefit ratio.

In some investigations, the IRB might determine that even high levels of risk are tolerable if the magnitude of the probable short- or long-term benefits is judged to be substantially greater. For example, in the medical field, patients commonly are asked to participate in testing the therapeutic benefits of new drugs with known side effects that might

Table 4.3.

Procedures for Preparing Human Investigation Protocols

In accordancce with the Emerson College Graduate Policy Manual, Section 14.0, all studies involving human subjects must be approved by the Division's and the College's Institutional Review Borads (IRB). Approval by the Division and College Committees is required even if your protocol has been approved by the agency through which you plan to recruit subjects . . . Protocols should be approximately 5 pages in length and should conform to the following outline:

A. RESEARCH PLAN
- 1. Name of investigator(s)
- 2. Title of project
- 3. Background and significance of study
- 4. Specific aims
- 5. Study design
  - a. Subjects
  - b. Measures
  - c. Procedures
  - d. Confidentiality (procedures for insuring of subjects' names and records, including location and consent forms).
  - e. Financial compensation (to families, subjects, or others).
- 6. Risks and benefits
  - a. Include risks to and potential benefits, if any, to the subject, his or her family, and/or society, as well as an analysis of risk/benefit ratio.
  - b. Justification of study.

B. CONSENT FORM
The following information should be included in simple nontechnical terms, and it should be written in first person, i.e., "I understand that I am being asked to participate . . ."
- 1. Title
- 2. Purpose of study and why individual is being asked to to participate.
- 3. Brief description of study procedures, especially what the subjects will be asked to do, how long it will take, and other information important from the subject's perspective.
- 4. Risks and benefits, including all risks and discomforts that may be associated with the procedures. Benefits should be stated clearly with distinction between personal and societal benefits expected to be derived from the study.
- 5. Subject's rights, including a statement of subject's/family's right to ask questions of the investigator and withdraw from the study if desired.
- 6. Statement of compensation where applicable
- 7. Confidentiality statement
- 8. The name of responsible investigator and contact phone number.

---

eventually improve the quality of the patients' lives as well as those of others with similar problems. The investigation of experimental surgical procedures for the treatment of communication disorders associated with spastic dysphonia, hypernasality, or hearing loss might be equally justifiable despite the risks from anesthesia or other complications.

In evaluating risks and potential benefits, the IRB can render a judgment only after carefully evaluating as many pros and cons as possible and recognizing that individual subjects may perceive risks and benefits quite differently given their unique needs and expectations. From an ethical perspective, it is incumbent on researchers to reduce the degree of potential harm or discomfort associated with an investigation as much as possible while remaining consistent with the intended goals.

Ethical research practice requires that subjects be informed in writing about the general goals, specific procedures, and significance of the study; the risks of harm or discomfort; the benefits, including remuneration, if any; the plans for disseminating the findings; and the measures, such as various data-coding procedures, used to safeguard confidentiality or preserve the anonymity of participants. It is also important to describe the duration of the intended study and to make clear that participation is a voluntary act that can be terminated at any time without negative consequences.

Some investigators, particularly in the behavioral sciences, have argued that full disclosure of the purpose of an experiment can bias subject responses, thus distorting the outcome. Milgram (1977) has been particularly outspoken in this regard, suggesting that investigators ought to neutralize the term "deception," replacing it with more appropriate [sic] descriptors such as "masking" or "technical illusion." The authors of this text are well aware of the evidence showing that a subject's preexisting knowledge or expectations of the goals of an experiment may introduce an unwanted extraneous influence. Nevertheless, in our opinion, this is no excuse for misleading subjects by supplying them with misinformation. As an alternative to such deceptive practices, subjects might be told that certain information about the treatments or conditions to be used in a study will not be disclosed until after the experiment. Provided that they agree to participate under such circumstances, it is still the responsibility of the experimenter to inform them of any associated risks. In our view, studies that require the abandonment of ethical principles cannot be justified on any grounds.

DEFINING A RESEARCH PROBLEM

Once one has selected a problem that one believes to be amenable to solution, the next step is to define the problem's parameters very clearly, in the form of either a testable research question or a hypothesis.

Research Questions

When the goal of a study is to merely describe the characteristics of one or more variables, without regard to possible relationships existing among them, a question is better used to frame the problem than a hypothesis. Suppose the purpose of your study is to establish the order of phoneme acquisition in children. You might decide, as Olmsted (1971) did, to consider a phoneme acquired when it is produced correctly in spontaneous speech by more than half the children in your sample at any one age level.

In such a study, the research purpose might be stated in the form of specific questions, such as the following: (1) What sounds of English speech are acquired first?; (2) What sounds are acquired last?; and (3) In what position (initial, medial, final) are sounds first acquired? Questions of this nature are generally used to explore new problem areas or in the early phases of scientific research when knowledge about the characteristics of the variables under study is limited. In such cases, there is typically no attempt to manipulate variables but merely to identify or describe them more fully by means of what Maxwell (1970) termed "straight-forward fact-finding types of studies."

Research Hypotheses

A research hypothesis is an explicit statement about what will be studied along with a prediction of the outcome. Although hypotheses are unnecessary for studies that are essentially limited to describing the behavioral or physical attributes of variables, they are needed for testing relationships or differences among such variables. In the previous example, a hypothesis could be stated in the following way:

> There is a positive relationship between the age of children and the acquisition of sounds in the final positions of words—i.e., increments in age are associated with corresponding changes in the frequency of correct sound productions in the final position.

In addition to expressing associative relationships of this kind, a hypothesis often involves a statement or prediction of differences. Again, using the previous example, a hypothesis might be formulated as follows:

> There are age differences in the frequency of sounds used correctly in the final position of words—i.e., the frequency of sounds used correctly in the final position will be greater in five-year-old children than in four-year-old children and greater in four-year-old children than in three-year-old children.

As a statement of the relations among variables, research hypotheses emanate directly from a theory under test.

Null Hypotheses

For statistical purposes, hypotheses are generally stated in the null form. That is, our hypothesis might be that there is **no significant** relationship between childrens' ages and the production of consonants in certain word positions or that children of different ages do not differ **significantly** in their use of final position sounds. Having stated a proposition in the null form, we then apply statistical tests to determine if the null hypothesis can be **rejected.** By rejecting the null hypothesis, we conclude that whatever relationships or differences observed among the measured variables of the study are indeed significant (owing to systematic influences instead of chance).

Many students who are unfamiliar with the use of the null hypothesis in statistical inference testing initially complain that the notion seems cumbersome, if not illogical. To them it appears that a "straw man" has been set up with the sole purpose of knocking him down. In essence, this is indeed the principle underlying null hypothesis testing. Whereas our original research hypothesis, as stated before, implies that two or more sampled groups (e.g., three-, four-, and five-year-old children) represent different populations, the null hypothesis says that they all must be considered representative of the same population until proved otherwise. In fact, there is a kind of inversion of logic surrounding null hypothesis testing because the usual purpose of research is not to determine that some difference in, for example, the mean scores between two groups is the result of chance. Instead, the goal of research usually is to prove the alternative proposition (research hypothesis) that the observed differences can be validly attributed to systematic influences within the experiment rather than to random fluctuations.

Statistical Logic of Null Hypotheses

The general logic underlying a null hypothesis (H_0) comes from evaluating its probable truth against the research hypothesis (H_1). This is made possible through statistical significance testing, which permits generalization from a sample of cases to the population from which such cases were drawn. The procedures employed in testing hypotheses in a prototypic experimental study are shown in Figure 4.2.

To simplify matters, assume that we wish to investigate the influence of phonologic training in kindergarten on students' reading ability in the first grade. In setting up such an experiment, the first step would be to randomly select a sample of subjects from a population and randomly assign them to two groups designated as X and Y. Group X (the treatment group) will receive phonologic training, whereas group Y (the control group) will receive no training. Two situations or treatment outcomes are possible as the result of statistical testing of the differences between mean scores: either the null hypothesis or its logical alternative, the research hypothesis, will be supported. Our null hypothesis, as a *statement of equality*, might be stated as:

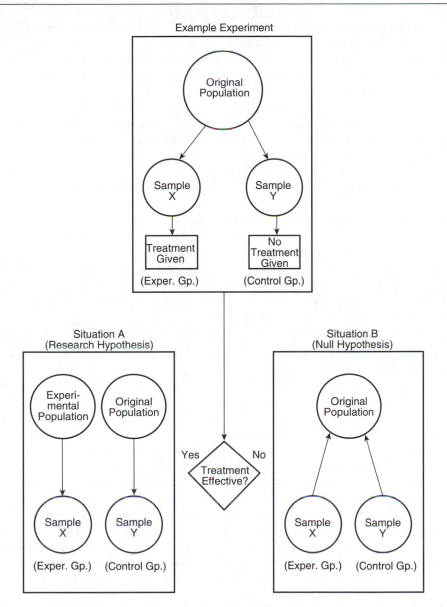

Figure 4.2. Relating the research hypothesis and the null hypothesis to the experimental results.

There is no difference in the reading ability of those first graders who receive phonologic train-ing in kindergarten and those who do not, or

$$\mu_X = \mu_Y \text{ (mean X is equal to mean Y)}$$

The logical alternative to that prediction would be expressed as the research hypothesis, which is a statement of statistical difference:

$$\mu_X \neq \mu_Y \text{ (mean X is not equal to mean Y)}$$

The first step in the decision-making process of a research study is to test the null hy-pothesis. Because the null hypothesis is the hypothesis of *no statistical difference*, if it is rejected, the alternative research hypothesis is supported. Thus, referring again to Figure 4.2, if phonologic training has not been found effective, then Situation B best represents the outcome wherein X is no different from Y. Alternatively, if Situation A prevails (the treatment was effective), then the research hypothesis may be supported on the basis of finding a significant difference.

Keeping in mind that a research hypothesis is a prediction derived from a theory, there are cases in which a researcher might want to explicitly predict the *direction* of an expected difference. Using our previous example, the research hypothesis in Situation A could have been expressed as $\mu_X > \mu_Y$, indicating that the mean of the treatment group is predicted to be greater than for the control group. In such a case, the implied null would read: $\mu_X \leq \mu_Y$, indicating that the mean of the treatment group is expected to be less than or equal to the control group.

In actual practice, null hypotheses are typically not stated explicitly in journal articles and related research reports unless they are predicting the direction of the differences. However, learning to formulate clear and concise hypotheses as a means of clarifying the purposes of an investigation is a valuable aid to inexperienced researchers such as students. Perhaps for this reason, the formal statement of null hypotheses is frequently required in theses, dissertations, and related academic projects designed to teach students how to conceptualize and investigate research problems.

Whether the null hypothesis is formally stated or simply implied, it must be formulated in a manner that allows for its rejection given certain probability estimates that are based on the results of statistical testing. As noted in Chapter 3, associated with null hypotheses are probability estimates for making certain types of statistical inference errors (sampling errors): either a **type I (alpha)** or **type II (beta) error** is possible. A type I error involves *rejecting a null hypothesis when it is true*. In such a case, one might conclude, for example, that Treatment A is significantly better than Treatment B when it is not. A type I error results in a **false positive conclusion.** On the other hand, one might instead make a type II error by *failing to reject a false null hypothesis*. In this case, it might be erroneously concluded that a particular treatment is no more effective than another. A type II error results in a **false negative conclusion.**

As noted in Chapter 3, researchers generally select an acceptable risk for error in the form of a **significance level** prior to an experiment. In the behavioral sciences, the conventional level of probability set by the researcher as the basis for rejecting the null hypothesis is either $p < .05$ or $p < .01$. Thus, for a finding to reach **significance** (the basis for rejecting the null), the odds for making an inferential error must be quite small. However, the tolerance for making an error is greater when the significance level is set at 5% (one time in 20 cases) than at 1% (one time in 100 cases).

A rejected null hypothesis indicates that the research results are significant leading to the acceptance of the research hypothesis. However, the failure to find a statistically significant result does not necessarily prove the null hypothesis to be true. All that can be said is that the accumulated data are as yet insufficient, casting doubt on the validity of the null hypothesis. Thus, the meaning of the term **"nonsignficant"** should be interpreted as "not yet proved" or "inconclusive." The failure to find significance can result because of many reasons, including a poorly designed study, experimenter mistakes, instrument failure or insensitivity, sampling errors, insufficient subjects, etc. In such cases, the best one can do is to live with the null hypothesis until it is otherwise proved invalid.

Conceptual Basis of Null Hypotheses

Science is concerned with discovering and documenting the "true nature" of objects and events in the real world and their lawful determination. In order to accomplish this, scientists have developed a philosophy that is aimed at divesting themselves from certain human limitations (e.g., prejudicial attitudes, personal preferences or beliefs, moralistic attitudes, emotions, etc.) that might otherwise bias the outcome of their work. Shaughnessy and Zechmeister (1994) have summarized well the attitude of most scientists:

> More than anything else, scientists are skeptical. Not only do they want to "see it before believing it," but they are likely to want to see it again, and again . . . people make mistakes. (p. 19)

The skepticism of scientists is reflected in their use of the null hypothesis that contends, in effect, that nothing exists until proved to exist based on certain statistically defined levels of confidence. Some investigators have drawn analogies between null hypothesis testing and the legal system as it exists in the United States (Browner, Newman, Cummings, and Hulley, 1988). A major assumption in a court of law is that the accused is innocent until proved guilty. A prosecuting attorney must marshal evidence to prove that the accused is indeed "guilty beyond a reasonable doubt" prior to rejecting the null hypothesis of "not guilty." However, in deciding a case, it is possible for a jury to make one of two errors: an innocent defendant may be wrongly convicted (type I error), or a guilty defendant may not be convicted (type II error). These two errors are related. By increasing the likelihood of a guilty conviction, more innocent people will suffer the consequences (more type I errors). On the other hand, should the legal system render more lenient judgments, there is a greater likelihood that the guilty will go free (more type II errors).

According to the laws of the United States, it is better to allow a guilty person to go free than to falsely convict an innocent person. In statistical testing, the relative seriousness of one type of error over the other is a subject for debate. Purely on statistical grounds, it could be argued that the research error of missing the presence of a significant treatment effect is less serious than concluding incorrectly that one is present. The logic behind this preference might be based on the possibility of finding a truly significant treatment effect in future studies that are perhaps better designed.

Certainly, from a clinical perspective, there are potential negative consequences associated with both kinds of errors. On the one hand, a false positive identification, involving an incorrect diagnosis and/or unnecessary treatment, might also result in unwarranted anxiety, expense, or stigmatization. On the other hand, a false negative identification, associated with the failure to diagnose and provide appropriate treatment for a disorder or disease, could likewise result in deleterious consequences. Of course, the best policy is to make every reasonable effort to reduce the potential for both type I and type II errors whenever possible. This can best be done through carefully designed experiments and the use of appropriate sampling procedures, including using an adequate number of subjects.

Case for Personal Probabilities in Hypothesis Testing

Despite the best intentions of researchers to suspend their personal beliefs in favor of adopting objective attitudes in selecting and defining research problems, seldom does one begin an experiment without at least some tentative preconceived ideas about the possible outcomes. Prior information about a problem is often available to a researcher from many sources, including theoretical knowledge, familiarity with the sample, documentation in the research literature, and subjective opinions of one's own or other colleagues. Given this understanding, it is a fallacy to believe that a state of "mindlessness" is attainable or even desirable in the conduct of research. According to Hayes (1973):

> The scientist does not operate in a vacuum . . . the experimenter has some initial ideas about
> how credible each of the hypotheses is . . . there are prior beliefs . . . that make some of the pos-
> sibilities for a true situation a better bet than others . . . (pp. 347–348)

The foregoing remarks by Hayes are in accord with the philosophy and methods of an alternative approach to null hypothesis testing based on directly determining the degree to
which a prior belief fits with the actual facts of a subsequent observation. The **Bayesian
method,** as it has come to be known, has existed longer than inferential statistics and null
hypothesis testing, yet its applications and relevance to many research problems remain
controversial.

First described by an English clergyman by the name of Thomas Bayes in 1763, the
Bayesian method provides a mathematical basis for expressing one's beliefs in the language
of probability prior to collecting data. Such a statement, called the **prior probability,** is
akin to the research hypothesis discussed previously, with the additional requirement of
including a numerical or quantitative estimate or "bet" reflecting the *degree of belief* about
a predicted result. The next step is to derive a **data probability** based on the sample of *data
actually collected*. The data probability can be regarded as the conditional credibility of a
particular view pending the calculation of a **posterior probability.** The latter probability,
reflecting the updated credibility of an original opinion or viewpoint, is derived from a
mathematical combination of the prior and data probabilities. The statistical basis of
Bayes' theorem (rule), the formula that describes the relation among these three sets of
probabilities, is further discussed and illustrated in Chapter 7.

Advocates of null hypothesis testing, based on the tenets of inferential statistics, as
originally expounded by Sir Ronald Fisher and developed further by Neyman and Pearson
in the early part of this century, have sometimes criticized if not denounced Bayesian methods. Such critics contend that subjective probabilities for a particular event may vary widely
among different individuals. The rejoinder to this concern is that no statistical method, including null hypothesis testing, is free of the influence of prior opinion. Evidence of this fact
can be found in the prior views of researchers that influence their choices in selecting and
defining problems for study; in decisions about sampling procedures and the number of subjects to study; and in the determination of a particular significance level (e.g., .05 or .01).

Bayesian statisticians contend that the ability of their methods to take into account
individual differences in the opinions of clinicians and researchers and to assess changes
in probabilities as new information evolves ought to be seen as a strength rather than a
weakness. In contrast to inferential statistics, that tend to treat and evaluate each new
sample as if it were the first drawn from a particular population, Bayesian methods rou-
tinely incorporate within the analysis information from *previous* samples.

As noted above, a clinician or researcher using Bayesian methods starts with an initial statement, tests its conditional credibility, and then revises the prior view in a straightforward manner as new data continue to be collected. It could be contended that its methods are more in keeping with the natural thought processes that underlay the making and
testing of actual research hypotheses than null hypothesis testing that " . . . gives only a
superficial appearance of objectivity." (Good, 1950). Furthermore, as Carver (1983)
noted, perhaps inferential statistical testing has become more popular than Bayesian
methods because the former has successfully advanced the illusion that a scientific decision can be made only if based on the results of a statistical calculation. More specifically,
the convention is to say that a result can be considered scientifically meaningful only if it
leads to the rejection of a null hypothesis at what often appears to be one of two *arbitrarily* decided significance levels (e.g., .05 or .01 level).

There are at least two problems in viewing these probability values as the defining goals for scientific research. First, as we have already noted, a scientifically important and statistically significant result are not one and the same. Virtually any study can yield a significant result at one of the conventional significance levels if it is replicated numerous times or if enough subjects are used. This can occur even though the actual difference in the size of the mean scores between two variables is minuscule. Unfortunately, it is the practice of many journal editors to accept articles for publication that fail to include measures of central tendency and deviation, reporting instead only the results of statistical testing that cannot be generalized to other experiments that have samples of different sizes.

The second point to bear in mind in evaluating the scientific importance of data is expressed in the following admonishment by Melton (1962), who said, "To insist upon the .05 level or .01 level is . . . to talk about the science of business, not the business of science" (p. 137). Obviously, there must be some basis available for judging the scientific importance of data, but Bayesian statisticians would argue against discounting a finding as trivial simply because it falls below some preordained probability value. For example, instead of arbitrarily pronouncing a probability value that falls short of the .05 mark as "no difference," the finding would be reported relying on what Morrison & Henkel (1970) called " . . . the application of imagination, common sense, informed judgment, and appropriate remaining research methods to achieve the scope, form, process, and purpose of scientific [not necessarily statistical] inference" (p. 311).

A major strength of Bayesian methods is that they permit the comparison of the prior opinions of one or more clinicians or researchers in relation to their own and each other's posterior distributions of data collected over time. Thus, such methods are capable of yielding a wealth of longitudinal information that can be useful in resolving many uncertainties pertaining to the diagnosis and treatment of communication disorders. The authors of this text have argued that Bayesian methods are particularly relevant to research efforts aimed toward achieving consensus definitions of such disorders as stuttering, and at improving the likelihood of their diagnosis given a particular symptom complex (Maxwell and Satake, 1994). The same principles apply to numerous other poorly understood and ill-defined communication disorders. Perhaps the greatest strength of Bayesian statistics is that such methods allow for the translation of an intuitive, yet often ill-formed, understanding of a problem into the kind of decision-making machinery that treats knowledge as cumulative and subject to continuous change.

In the 1960s, there began a **paradigm shift** in the field of radio broadcasting that involved an understanding that FM radio transmissions offered a number of transmission advantages over AM. The reasons for this type of a shift in "looking at the world" in scientific fields are complex and will not be reviewed here (see Kuhn, 1970). Nevertheless, it is possible that Bayesian statistics and other probabilistic methods will result in a similar paradigm shift in the future with far-reaching consequences in deciding the "significance" of scientific findings. Probabilistic models of decision making have already begun to replace long-standing mechanistic philosophies and practices in such fields as medicine (Bursztajn, Feinbloom, Hann, and Brodsky, 1990). Such methods can teach us that uncertainties in life are not only a part of life but can be incorporated advantageously into our scientific schema and clinical approaches to problems. Although these views reflect the subjective opinions of the authors, we believe they are worth stating.

Case Against Hypothesis Testing

Several researchers have argued that hypothesis testing, whatever its nature or statistical methods, is an often-misguided and counter-productive approach to developing a true science of behavior. For example, Sidman (1960) cautions not " . . . to fall into the error of insisting that all experimentation must derive from the testing of hypotheses. Such experimental activities can result in the piling up of trivia upon trivia" (p. 4). Sidman further advises the student to remember that which is most important in any experiment is a question that leads in the end to **good data** that owes allegiance to no particular hypothesis or theory.

According to Bakan (1966), it is often the case that by the time a researcher, intent on proving a particular theory, finally gets to the stage of hypothesis testing, most of the important work has already been done. In a similar vein, Mishler (1983) offered a counter view to the common notion of exemplary scientific research as an enterprise involving " . . . the elimination of plausible rival hypotheses to the preferred explicit hypothesis in any particular study" (p. 10). Instead, he proposed that the goal of behavioral science ought to be simply specifying the conditions under which lawful relationships of the form $Y = f(X)$ can be found and demonstrated.

There is a school of behavioral science that holds that the determination of causal relations among variables, of the type described by Mishler, can best proceed when the main goal is to improve **observation, prediction,** and **control** of behavior rather than to uncover or explain through hypothesis testing the factors that underlay its occurrence. The doctrine of this school has come to be known as **behaviorism,** and its methods are termed the **experimental analysis of behavior** or **applied behavioral analysis.** The defining feature of this approach is the emphasis it places on measuring the *effects* of manipulating aspects of the *observable behavior* of individuals.

The philosophic perspectives of behaviorism are rooted in a long effort among American psychologists to develop a science of learning, which began with William James (1890), who wrote at length "on the great law of habit." John Watson (1924) concluded that the *conditioned response* was the "fundamental unit of habit" and E. L. Thorndike (1938) later posited the "law of effect" to explain the influence of reward and punishment on behavior. The name of B. F. Skinner is most associated with the chief experimental method of behaviorism—**operant (instrumental) conditioning.** Although Skinner was influenced to some degree by Pavlovian principles of classical conditioning, his ideas incorporated to a much greater degree the principles of trial-and-error learning and response reinforcement as mechanisms for shaping behavior. The so-called operant approach emphasized that behavior is best explained through the use of *controlled conditions* that demonstrate its *controlling variables*. Hypothesis testing, inferential statistics, and the use of control subjects were all eschewed in favor of single-subject or small-N designs for controlling and monitoring the experimental situation. Skinner (1956) briefly summarized the essential steps of the operant paradigm as follows: "establish the behavior in which you are interested, submit the organism to a particular treatment, and look again at the behavior." As noted in Chapter 1, these three phases are commonly referred to as **baseline, conditioning,** and **withdrawal.**

The philosophic premises and experimental methods of behaviorism, particularly as reflected in operant conditioning, have been a subject of continuing controversy. The *Journal of Experimental Analysis of Behavior* was established in 1958 largely because of the refusal of other journals to accept small-N research studies for publication. As interest in the new field of **behavior modification** expanded, new journals and books began to appear that played an important role in developing applications that were therapeutically and educationally focused on a variety of human problems. The *Journal of Applied Behavioral Analysis*, first published in 1967, was devoted to human research in behavior modification and behavior therapy. New experimental methodologies and designs emphasizing small-N or single-subject research came into being and flourished throughout the 1970s (Krasner, 1971; Baer, 1975; Kazdin, 1978). The influence of these new developments also greatly impacted the field of communication disorders.

In support of the research strategies underlying the experimental analysis of behavior, Eysenck (1983) argued that its methods are likely to prove clinically more relevant and beneficial in the long run than therapies predicated on nebulous hypotheses or unfounded theories. Some researchers have countered by arguing against the generalizability of the data of small-N or N-of-1 designs.

As we shall see in later chapters, obtaining generality of findings is a common problem in all studies regardless of the sample size. In the case of null hypothesis testing, we never can be absolutely sure that the two sampled groups to be compared on some variable actually represent the *same* population. Because the variability of individual subject characteristics is unknown, the best we can do is to use the known variability in the sampled groups to *estimate* the unknown variability in the "assumed common population" (Carver, 1983). We must keep in mind that inferential statistics and null hypothesis testing are predicated on the use of average scores that reflect the "typical," "usual," "normal," "most representative," etc. performance measures for comparing *groups* of subjects, not *individual* subjects. More specifically, although it might be said that the group as a whole responded in a certain way to a particular treatment, the performance of individual subjects is typically not taken into account. In order to generalize the effect of a particular treatment from one individual to another, the **systematic replication** of a research study would be required—i.e., (a) similar participant(s) would need to be evaluated, ideally by different researchers in different test settings.

SELF-LEARNING REVIEW

descriptive
categorize
classify

1. "Who" or "what" questions are answered through the use of various _____ techniques designed to _____ or _____ phenomena.

diagnostic criteria

2. Developing taxonomies of various communication disorders is important in setting up mutually exclusive _____ _____ .

question
rationale
feasibility

3. The formulation of a problem consists of (1) originating a _____ ; (2) developing a _____ ; and (3) determining the _____ of finding the answer.

interpret
understand
predict

4. Asking and answering clinical questions allow us to better _____ , _____ , and _____ the results of testing procedures and treatment programs.

Federal Register
NIH

NIDCD, or
National Institute on
Deafness and other
Communicative
Disorders

5. Two publications of the federal government that summarize scientific research initiatives on a regular basis are the _____ _____ and the _____ Guidelines for Grants and Contracts.

6. A major branch of NIH that supports research and research training in the field of communication disorders is the _____ .

frequency
citations

7. One way to identify an *important* research study is by noting the _____ of its _____ by other researchers.

trivial
consequential

8. According to Merton, the importance of a research rationale is that it " . . . curbs the flow of scientifically _____ questions and enlarges the share of _____ ones."

introduction

9. The rationale for a study ought to evolve naturally in the _____ section of a paper.

question
hypothesis
testable

10. The first issue to settle in determining the feasibility of a study is whether or not the _____ or _____ is stated in a _____ form.

protection
IRB or Institutional
Review Board
compliance

11. In 1974, the National Research Act established a commission for the _____ of human subjects. Institutions are now required to set up an _____ to determine the _____ of research proposals with existing regulations.

risk/benefits
informed consent

12. Two issues of major concern in the deliberations of an IRB Committee pertains to the _____ / _____ ratio and the means of obtaining _____ _____ .

13. Once you have selected a problem, the next step is to define its parameters, in either the form of a _____ _____ or a _____ .

research question
hypothesis

14. Having stated a hypothesis in the _____ form, we then apply a statistical test to determine if it can be _____ .

null
rejected

15. Mathematically speaking, shortened expressions of the null hypothesis and its alternative, the research hypothesis, are _____ and _____ , respectively.

$\mu_1 = \mu_2$
$\mu_1 \neq \mu_2$

16. If the mean of the treatment group was predicted to be greater than that of the control group, the research hypothesis would have been expressed as _____ . Alternatively, given the opposite prediction, it would have been read as _____ .

$\mu_1 > \mu_2$
$\mu_1 < \mu_2$

17. Whether the null hypothesis is stated formally or is simply implied, it must be formulated as to allow for its _____ given the results of _____ _____ .

rejection
statistical testing

18. Concluding that Treatment A is better than Treatment B when it is not is an example of a _____ error. Concluding that Treatment A is no better than Treatment B when in fact it is results in a _____ error.

type I
type II

19. A _____ error results in a _____ _____ conclusion, whereas a _____ error results in a _____ _____ conclusion.

type I
false positive
type II
false negative

20. Other names for type I and type II errors are _____ and _____ errors, respectively.

alpha
beta

21. When a finding reaches significance, the null hypothesis can be _____ , typically at either p = _____ or p = _____ significance level. The significance level that one selects should be decided _____ an experiment.

rejected
$< .05$
$< .01$
before

22. The meaning of the term "nonsignificant" should be interpreted as "_____" or "_____ _____ _____."

"inconclusive"
"not yet proved"

23. The skepticism of scientists is reflected in their use of the _____ _____ .

null hypothesis

24. A type I error leads to a _____ _____ conclusion. In a court of law, this translates to _____ an _____ defendant.

false positive
convicting
innocent

25. Legally, a type II error associated with making a _____

false negative

convict
guilty

_____ conclusion would result in a failure to _____ the _____ defendant.

Bayesian Method

26. A mathematical basis for expressing one's beliefs in the language of probability *prior* to data collection is called the _____ _____.

probabilities
prior
data
posterior

27. The Bayesian method requires the establishment of three kinds of _____ . These are: (1) _____ , (2) _____ , and (3) _____ probabilities.

previous

28. Unlike inferential statistics, Bayesian methods incorporate within the analysis information from _____ samples.

probability

29. Bayesian statisticians would argue against discounting a finding simply because it falls below a preordained _____ value.

prior
posterior

30. A major strength of the Bayesian method is that it permits the comparison of _____ with _____ distributions of data over time.

paradigm

31. A _____ shift involves a new way of "looking at the world."

data
hypothesis
theory

32. According to Sidman, that which is most important in any experiment is a question that leads in the end to good _____ owing allegiance to no particular _____ or _____ .

groups
individual

33. Inferential statistics are predicated on comparing the performance of _____ of subjects, not _____ subjects.

systematic replication

34. One way to generalize the results of small-N research is through _____ _____ .

5. Planning and Designing Research

Identifying a Topic

Conducting a Literature Review

Stating the Research Problem

Choosing a Research Design

Nonexperimental Designs

—*Descriptive Studies*

—*Predictive Studies*

—*Probability Studies*

True Experimental Designs

—*Pretest-Posttest Control Group Design*

—*Posttest-Only Control Group Design*

—*Solomon Four-Group Design*

—*Multigroup Designs*

Quasi-Experimental Designs

—*Nonequivalent Comparison Group*

—*Interrupted Time-Series Designs*

—*Small-N Quasi-Experiments*

Pre-experimental Designs

—*One-Shot Case Study*

—*One-Group Pretest-Posttest*

—*Static-Group Comparison*

Selecting a Sample of Subjects

Random Assignment versus Random Selection

Types of Populations

Random Sampling Methods

—*Simple Random Sampling*

—*Systematic Sampling*

—*Stratified Sampling*

—*Cluster Sampling*

Nonrandom Sampling Methods

—*Consecutive Sampling*

—*Convenience Sampling*

—*Purposive Sampling*

—*Matched Samples*

Controlling Variables

Maximizing Experimental Systematic Variance

Minimizing Random and Systematic Errors

Specifying Measurements

Measurements Utility

Measurement Precision

Measurement Accuracy

Measurement Scales

Recording Measurements

Response Frequency

Response Latency

Response Duration

Response Amplitude-Intensity

Thus far, we have attempted to make clear some of the conceptual and philosophical cornerstones of scientific thinking that underlie the action processes of research. In this chapter, we wish to extend our discussion to include a concise review of the actual steps taken in planning and designing a research study prior to its implementation. We have listed

Table 5.1.

Basic Steps in Planning and Designing a Research Study

1. **Identify the topic:**   Choose the topic you wish to investigate based on the need or desire to solve an interesting and important problem.
2. **Conduct a literature review:**   Read efficiently and selectively, focusing on the facts most necessary for developing a rationale for your study.
3. **State the research problem:**   State the problem in operational terms as either a research question or a hypothesis.
4. **Choose a research design:**   Choose a research design appropriate for answering the question or testing the hypothesis.
5. **Select a sample of subjects:**   Select subjects as appropriate for your investigation and study and assign them to groups or treatment conditions.
6. **Control the variables:**   Control the independent and dependent variables, maximizing experimental systematic variance while minimizing random and systematic errors.
7. **Specify the measurements:**   Specify the measurements in terms of their utility, accuracy, precision, and scaling power.
8. **Record the measurements:**   Record the measurements according to the type of scoring procedures selected (e.g., frequency, latency, duration, or amplitude-intensity.

eight such steps in Table 5.1. Several of these operations have been discussed in previous chapters and will be briefly summarized. Other items will require more extensive commentary.

The number of tasks included is somewhat arbitrary and may vary depending on the unique requirements of a particular investigation. Furthermore, although the steps are listed in a linear sequence, the reality of any fixed arrangement of this kind can be debated as we have emphasized throughout this book. Using what he believed to be an apt analogy, one colleague remarked that "the gait of science can be quite staggering, often not unlike that seen in drunkenness!" Although some might object to such a comparison, even on metaphorical grounds, most experienced investigators would no doubt agree that the actual operations of planning and designing research are often performed in an overlapping if not circuitous fashion. With this understanding, the following outline should be viewed as a general guide rather than a detailed map of the steps involved in formulating a research plan.

IDENTIFYING A TOPIC

The first step in the research planning process is choosing a general topic that one wishes to investigate. Choosing the subject matter for an investigation entails describing the broad parameters of a research area or potential field of inquiry. The decision on a subject for research typically reflects motivations and preferences having a myriad of origins based on one's cumulative personal or subjective opinions, clinical observations and experiences, and interactions with fellow students and professors, as well as on the complex interplay of reading, writing, and thinking processes.

At the initial stage of research planning, students usually can express some overall interest in a particular research topic but often little more. This is frequently the case for those who are attempting to decide on a particular subject matter for a master's thesis or doctoral dissertation. When asked about the subject of their interest, most students can verbalize **what** global interest they might want to pursue: "I'm interested in the area of stuttering" (or child-language disorders, aphasia, cochlear implantation, etc.). Occasionally, the interest is more fully articulated or focused in terms of **where** they would like to direct their attention, e.g., "I'm interested in the role of anxiety in stuttering," or "the influence of socioeconomic factors in child-language disorders," or "gains in hearing level following cochlear implantation," etc. However, at such an early stage of the planning process, it is indeed rare when one can fully explain **why** a particular subject area has been selected for research. The reason or rationale for selecting a particular topic can usually be established only after a thorough review of the research literature.

CONDUCTING A LITERATURE REVIEW

Having chosen a subject matter for research, the next step in the planning process is conducting a thorough literature review relevant to the area of interest. The ways and means of organizing an efficient search as opposed to meandering aimlessly through tangential literature were discussed in the previous chapter. The goal is to read broadly enough to uncover present trends and controversies pertinent to the research topic but also selectively with the aim of discovering gaps in existing knowledge and problems needing further study.

Hypothetically, suppose that one is interested in the role that early speech-language impairments might play in later-occurring learning/reading disabilities. In the process of reviewing the literature, one learns that the research has consistently shown that children with speech-language impairments are at risk for reading disabilities. One wonders about the precise relationship between certain verbal disabilities and later-occurring reading failure. A continued review of the literature reveals that this question is highly complex. In fact, some evidence suggests that different types of speech-language impairments are related to (i.e., predict) different kinds of reading outcomes. More specifically, the results of previous research seem to suggest that standardized measures of language ability are better predictors of reading comprehension than measures of phonologic awareness. On the other hand, such research also seems to indicate that measures of phonologic awareness are better predictors of written word recognition than are standardized measures of language ability. As one distills these facts, a possible therapy implication begins to emerge in the form of a tentative research question: Does phonologic awareness training (e.g., sound blending, segmentation, rhyming exercises, etc.) differentially affect the skills associated with reading achievement—i.e., reading recognition versus reading comprehension? Determining the relative influence of such training on the different components of reading competence is a question that has developed out of the framework of the selected literature review. Still other types of problems might have emerged from the interplay of reading and pondering other research studies. Indeed, sometimes a topic might change entirely as you discover new untapped areas for investigation.

It is important to bear in mind that the purpose of a literature review done in preparation for a research study may be quite different from one connected with a term paper or similar academic project. Whereas the latter activities may be directed toward achieving a critical review and evaluation of a subject area, they seldom involve the kind of problem distillation process necessary for funneling a body of diverse facts into a well-delineated testable question or research hypothesis. Like a court attorney, increasingly one must exclude irrelevant evidence by focusing on only the facts most necessary for establishing the case for the study.

STATING THE RESEARCH PROBLEM

Merely reviewing literature in a particular subject area and determining the need for additional inquiry (problem making) falls short of the criteria necessary for performing systematic research (problem solving). In addition, the problem must be defined by specifying the experimental variables of which it is constituted. As we have already emphasized, this requires establishing operational definitions of the independent and dependent variables and the conditions of their control (see Chapter 2).

Prior to formulating a hypothesis, stating the overall purpose(s) of an investigation is a useful strategy for clarifying general goals. This initial step is exemplified in the prospectus for a dissertation written by an Emerson College doctoral student (Barresi, 1996). In conjunction with her review of relevant research literature pertaining to the naming abilities of older and younger adults, she stated:

> The purposes of the present study are twofold:
> (1) to investigate the effects of age on learning and recalling common and uncommon proper names, and
> (2) to investigate the effects of age on reported strategies for learning and recalling proper names and proper nouns.

After formulating a purpose statement, an investigator may elect to frame the problem in a question format before proceeding to develop specific research hypotheses. As stated before, three major categories of questions are possible: (1) descriptive questions that simply ask what the attributes of a particular variable look like based on specific types of observations and measurements; (2) relationship questions that seek to determine when or under what circumstances a change in one variable may predict the direction of change in another; and (3) difference questions that attempt to uncover causal factors by comparing the effect of an independent variable on a dependent variable under different experimental conditions. Most research studies are concerned with the latter two types of questions. In Barresi's study, she proceeds to ask the following questions:

- What effect does age have on recall of common and uncommon names and occupations?
- What is the effect of a second learning trial on recall of common and uncommon items for each age group?
- What effect does age have on reported use of strategies for learning common and uncommon names and occupations?
- What is the association between reported use of strategies and recall of names and occupations in younger and older adults?

The first three questions noted above are difference questions to the degree that they inquire about the effect of an independent variable (age) or treatment (second learning trial) on several dependent variables. The fourth question is a relationship question because it asks about the association between certain dependent variables (use of certain strategies and recall abilities).

As noted previously, questions like those used by Barressi are often preliminary to stating formal research hypotheses. In fact, some investigators may prefer the former type of format over the latter as a style of expressing problems. Such a preference might be justified on logical grounds when considerable ambiguity surrounds a problem or in cases of exploratory studies of phenomena about which few facts are known. In the case of Barressi's dissertation proposal, several previous research studies related to her problem were cited, serving as a foundation for certain predictions that she made in the form of the following research hypotheses:

- Both younger and older subjects will recall common names (e.g., "Owens") and occupations (e.g., "surgeon") better than uncommon names (e.g., "Reisman") and occupations (e.g., "tuner") . . . Further, older adults will recall fewer items than younger adults.
- Both age groups should recall more names and occupations on the second learning trial than on the first.

- Both age groups will report using similar strategies, but the older adults will use them less frequently, resulting in lower scores than those of the younger adults.
- There will be a significant positive correlation between frequency of reported strategy use and recall of names and occupations for both younger and older adults.

Note that the independent and dependent variables have been made apparent in the research hypotheses along with the type of measure to be used (i.e., frequency) in assessing the predicted findings. Barressi could have carried the definition of her research one step further by expressing her hypotheses in the null form as statements of **statistical equality.** Nevertheless, the fact that hypotheses are not explicitly stated in such a manner does not mean that researchers will fail to conduct appropriate statistical tests in order to reject the implicit assumption of "no difference" if warranted. No matter how a research hypothesis is stated, unless Bayesian or descriptive statistics are used, it must imply a null hypothesis that is subject to a probability estimate.

Unfortunately, journal editors commonly accept articles for publication when their authors have neglected entirely the importance of defining the problem as either a question or a formalized research hypothesis. Some might contend that such an omission does not constitute neglect but an unspoken understanding that "seasoned researchers" will automatically understand the parameters of a problem despite the lack of its formal explication. In our opinion, although writing good research questions and research hypotheses can be a laborious and time-consuming task, there is no better means available for defining and clarifying the variables to be studied in an experiment. As an investigative tool, the well-formulated question or hypothesis is to a researcher what the scalpel is in the hands of a surgeon. It creates the conditions for cutting through the vagaries of words and ill-conceived ideas to focus sharply on a scientific problem. It likewise establishes the operative boundaries of an experiment and defines the limits for interpreting successes and failures. Finally, it discourages small bands of specialized investigators from becoming what Francis Bacon (1561–1626) called the "Idols of the Tribe," who, for the most part, talk only to one another.

CHOOSING A RESEARCH DESIGN

Researchers commonly speak of research designs to denote the kind of plans or schemes that are used in meeting the aims of various types of investigations. As the working plans for the study of phenomena, some designs are tightly organized and highly detailed; others are loosely sketched.

Sorting out the confusing array of multitudinous terms and taxonomies used to describe and categorize various research designs is a formidable task even for seasoned investigators. Among the ways in which designs are commonly classified relate to the **purpose** or aim of a study; its **setting** or place of occurrence, whether in a laboratory, clinic, or natural setting; the dimension of **time,** determined by examining phenomena prospectively (longitudinally) as they unfold or retrospectively after they occur; the degree to which **quantitative versus qualitative** observations and judgment are emphasized; the **number** of subjects or groups involved; and the degree to which variables are **experimentally** controlled.

We have attempted to logically organize the elements that constitute basic nonexperimental and experimental design strategies according to the schema shown in Table 5.2. In addition to the name of a particular design, we have used the notation system of Campbell and Stanley (1966), wherein the symbols X = treatment by the independent variable, 0 = observation of the dependent variable, and R = randomization.

Table 5.2.
Classification of Research Designs

Nonexperimental			Experimental		
Studies that seek to describe and/or relate events through passive observation.			*Studies that seek to identify causal relations through manipulation of independent variables.*		
Descriptive Studies	Predictive Studies	Probability Studies	True Experiments	Quasi Experiments	Pre-Experiments
Examples	*Examples*	*Examples*	*Examples*	*Examples*	*Examples*

• Surveys
• Case studies
• Prevalence/ Incidence
• Field studies
	• Correlation
	• Regression
		• Sensitivity
		• Specificity
		• Bayesian probability
			• Randomized pretest-posttest control group
			  - ROXO
			  - RO O
			• Randomized posttest control group
			  - RXO
			  - R O
			• Solomon four-group
			  - ROXO
			  - RO O
			  - R X O
			  - R O
			• Multi-group (ANOVAR designs)
			• Factorial (Treatment by level designs)
				• Nonequivalent comparison group
				  - OXO
				  - O O
				• Interrupted time-Series
				  - $O_1O_2O_3XO_4O_5O_6$
				• Small-N
				  - A B
				  - A B A
				  - A B A B
				  - multiple baseline
					• One-shot case study
					  - XO
					• One-group pretest/ posttest
					  - OXO
					• Static-group comparison
					  - X O
					  - O

As a preamble to the discussion that follows, we wish to make clear that, as a general rule, no one study method is necessarily better than another but should be selected on the basis of the type of question asked and the level of understanding that the researcher hopes to achieve.

Nonexperimental Designs

Descriptive Studies

According to our view, studies can be best classified based on the degree to which they explain the causal relations among variables. In achieving this goal, the weakest of the lot are **descriptive studies,** or those intended to observe, illustrate, record, classify, or by other means attempt to clarify the distinctive features of research variables. The methods of description include surveys, case histories, clinical reports, prevalence/incidence studies, and field studies. Such studies often result in a better understanding of phenomena as they exist *in the here and now,* thereby establishing the conditions for later scientific work when questions as to the relationship among variables might arise.

Predictive Studies

Predictive studies are those aimed toward fulfilling the second main goal of scientific research—determining relationships among variables. Many clinically based problems start out at the level of description, involving efforts to classify the characteristics of a disorder, and then proceed to explore how variations in one characteristic may relate to another. Such might be the case in a disorder like cleft lip and palate, wherein clefts of the lip alone appear to occur more frequently in association with nasal deformities than do clefts of the palate alone. On the other hand, clefts of the palate alone may be a better predictor of Eustachian tube dysfunction than isolated clefts of the lip.

A quantitative index of the strength of a relationship between two or more variables can be established by computing correlation coefficients in accord with various statistical tests. As noted earlier, such correlational relationships may indicate the direction of variance (change) among two or more measures. A positive correlation suggests that as the value of one measure either increases or decreases, the other measure(s) do(es) likewise. On the other hand, a negative correlation results as the consequence of the values expressed by two or more measures moving in opposite directions.

As a measure of association, correlations are intended to assess (1) the *magnitude* of the relationships among variables (the degree to which they covary) and (2) the *direction* of the relationship (whether they move positively together or depart negatively from one another). In accord with our previous example, suppose one is interested in knowing whether or not a certain type of orofacial cleft in children is a "good predictor" of Eustachian tube dysfunction. The criteria offered by Guilford (1950, 3rd ed.) for evaluating a correlation coefficient can serve as a general guide:

< .20, slight; almost negligible relationship
.20–.40, low correlation; definite but small relationship
.40–.70, moderate correlation; substantial relationship
.70–.90, high correlation; marked relationship
> .90, very high correlation; very dependable relationship

For practical purposes, whether or not a correlation coefficient is judged to be a good predictive index of a relationship among variables depends to some extent on the purposes of the experiment. Even a low correlation may be statistically significant but lack the associative strength the investigator had hoped to find. Also, it is important to avoid the common mistake of viewing correlation coefficients as percentages of relationship. A .80 correlation does not mean that one can expect to find a relationship between two variables 80 percent of the time. Furthermore, because a correlation coefficient does not represent an actual scale of measurement, it is inappropriate to say that a coefficient of .80 is exactly twice the magnitude of a .40 coefficient.

A correlation is best viewed as a *general index* of association, having limited mathematical power. A more refined basis for prediction involves the use of a statistic called **regression analysis.** In cases in which it is already known or suspected that an association exists between variable X and variable Y, one might wish to carry the analysis one step further by asking, "What particular values of X are predictive of particular values of Y?" In such cases, X is termed the **predictor variable** and Y is called the **criterion variable.**

Sometimes, the researcher might wish to predict the criterion variable in a stepwise fashion by progressively adding additional predictor variables to the analysis. Thus, in an effort to predict Eustachian tube dysfunction, one might begin by asking about the extent to which clefts of the palate alone are predictive of the abnormality. Assume that clefts of the palate alone are found to be a strong predictor of Eustachian tube dysfunction. Next, one adds to the computation clefts of the lip as well as the palate. In such a case, the addition of the new predictor variable (cleft lip) will increase the accuracy of prediction *only* if it is *not* correlated with the previous predictor variable (cleft palate). In evaluating the predictive power of two or more variables, a procedure called **multiple regression analysis**

Table 5.3.

Two-by-two Contingency Table that Cross-Tabulates Eustachian Tube Functioning in Various Orofacial Clefts (Hypothetic Data)

	Cleft Lip	Cleft Palate	Row Subtotal
Eustachian tube dysfunction	a	b	a+b
Non-eustachian tube dysfunction	c	d	c+d
Column subtotal	a+c	b+d	Grand total a+b+c+d=n

where: a = frequency of cleft lip and eustachian tube dysfunction

   b = frequency of cleft palate and eustachian tube dysfunction

   c = frequency of cleft lip and non-eustachian tube dysfunction

   d = frequency of cleft palate and non-eustachian tube dysfunction

   n = total number of subjects

can be used. The statistical rationale and methods for its calculation are discussed more thoroughly in Chapter 6.

Another means of examining predictive relationships among two or more variables is through **cross tabulation** procedures in which the frequency distributions of data sets are arranged into categories. The distribution of scores on the dependent variable, as they stand in relation to the independent variable, are often organized and portrayed within a **contingency table.** A simple 2×2 (two-by-two) form of this table is shown in Table 5.3. The data of our hypothetical study, involving the relation between certain orofacial clefts and Eustachian tube functioning, could be arranged within columns and rows, with each cell in the table representing different categories of the independent variable (type of cleft) in combination with the dependent variable (Eustachian tube functioning). Statistically, the **"goodness of fit,"** or extent to which our observed observations follows a theoretical distribution of some kind, can be evaluated subsequently by a procedure called the **chi-square test** (see Chapter 8).

Probability Studies

Given the nature of their professional work, clinicians in the field of communication disorders often ask questions about the *probability* for certain types of outcomes. For example, we might ask,

- "How probable is it that a particular sign or symptom is predictive of a certain disorder or disease process?"
- "How probable is it that a particular client will improve in response to a certain therapy program?"
- "How probable is it that clinical gains can be generalized across various situations, setting or spans of time?"

Although we frequently ask these and many other "probability" questions in the course of our professional and personal lives, the definition of probability is a complex matter. Mathematically, the term is relatively easy to define as a simple ratio. The numerator is the expected frequency of an event and the denominator gives the total number of possible outcomes. A classic example is the "law of averages" expressed mathematically as the likelihood of a tossed coin turning up heads or tails. For any one toss, the probability for a head turning up is 1/2, as is the probability for a tail. The 1 in the numerator is the expected frequency for the head or tail and the 2 in the denominator represents the total number of possible occurrences.

Statistically, there are at least two understandings of the term probability. The first of these is based on what is commonly called the **"frequentist definition,"** in which probability is understood to be the expected frequency for an event *in the long run*—i.e., in repeated trials under similar conditions. Such probabilities are generally assessed through the process of null of hypothesis testing and the use of inferential statistics.

An older but less commonly known view of probability is based on **Bayes' Theorem** (1763). As noted in Chapter 4, Bayesian statistics provide a basis for describing and testing the accuracy of one's personal or subjective views in the mathematical language of probability. Clinically, the kinds of probabilities that can be expressed relate to such *prognostic statements* as, "The chance for this client having a particular disorder . . . improving in response to therapy . . . generalizing clinical gains . . . are, lets say, 30% or 50% or 80%," etc. Such statements reflect **a priori probabilities** versus **empirical probabilities**—the latter being the observed or actual frequency of an event in a given number of trials. Further information pertaining to Bayesian methods is found in Chapter 7, where the principles and clinical applications of this approach are discussed in relation to specific clinical issues.

Another approach to probability relates to determining conditional probabilities, or the probabilities for events provided that certain other events hold true. This particular issue is relevant to determining the *accuracy* of a particular diagnostic test. Two aspects of test accuracy relate to its **sensitivity** and **specificity.** These concepts pertain to the ability of a test to identify the presence or absence of a particular disorder or disease. The probability of a client with a disorder or disease testing positive relates to the sensitivity of the test. On the other hand, test specificity relates to the probability of a nondisordered/diseased client testing negative. For obvious reasons, research concerned with the development of diagnostic test instruments is concerned with maximizing both of these measurement parameters. Issues pertaining to test sensitivity and specificity are discussed later in this chapter and also in Chapter 7.

As with descriptive approaches to research, predictive and probability studies involve **nonexperimental scientific methods** that are best viewed as preliminary, yet generally necessary, steps in the search for causal explanations, which is the *third and most important goal of science*. Although nonexperimental methods are important in many research plans, they do not allow for an examination of hypothesized causal relations among variables. The latter goal can only be achieved by determining the influence of an independent variable on a dependent variable as *purposefully manipulated or designed to occur under conditions arranged and controlled by an experimenter.*

True Experimental Designs

Some types of research aimed at isolating causative relations among variables are better than other types at achieving this end. Along this continuum, the strongest of the research designs is called a **true experiment** (Campbell and Stanley, 1966). In such a design, there are three requirements. These include:

1. Random assignment of subjects to at least two groups or treatment conditions.
2. The use of one of the groups or conditions as a control mechanism to examine the relative influence of an independent variable as compared to its absence.
3. Deliberate and active manipulation of an independent variable by the experimenter.

Pretest-Posttest Control Group Design: $\quad R\ O_1\ X\ R\ O_2$
$$R\ O_3 \qquad R\ O_4$$

The most commonly used of the true experimental designs is the pretest-posttest control group design. Two groups of subjects are randomly assigned to either an experimental condition, in which they will receive treatment (X), or to a control condition, in which no treatment will be given. This design permits an assessment of the degree of change that occurs from the pretest to the posttest in response to a treatment factor as compared to the absence of treatment. In this case, because the experiment involves the comparison of only two groups, it is likely that a statistical analysis called a ***t*-test** would be carried out to determine if the independent variable had a significant effect. If statistical testing reveals that the amount of change is significantly different between the two groups, such change is causally inferred to have resulted from a treatment effect.

Posttest-Only Control Group Design: $\quad R\ X\ O_1$
$$R \qquad O_2$$

An even more basic version of a true experiment is the posttest-only control group design. The rationale for this design is based on the assumption underlying random assignment procedures intended to minimize extraneous pre-existing differences between groups. If such procedures are truly effective in accomplishing this goal, then pretesting subjects could seem redundant and unnecessary. Furthermore, posttest-only designs are advantageous when pretesting is impossible to accomplish or when the effect of such testing might unduly sensitize subjects to the experimental treatment or bias posttest scores as the result of repeated measurement. Despite the legitimacy of the posttest-only design for many experimental situations, it is not widely used, perhaps because of the prevailing belief in the value of a pretest as a "fail-safe mechanism" to guard against the possible failure of randomization to establish group equivalency.

Solomon Four-Group Design: $\quad R\ O_1\ X\ O_2$
$$R\ O_3 \quad O_4$$
$$R \qquad X\ O_5$$
$$R \qquad O_6$$

A popular experimental design that incorporates aspects of both the previously discussed pretest-posttest and posttest-only control group designs is the **Solomon four-group design.** The strength of this design lies in its ability to control for certain **interaction effects** between a pretest and an independent variable that combine to affect a dependent variable in a way that neither might have done when operating alone.

    To use a concrete example of such an unwanted interaction, imagine that you wish to investigate the attitudes of classroom teachers toward providing direct assistance to children with speech or language disorders by reinforcing the goals and procedures of a therapy program designed by a speech-language pathologist. Suppose further that you develop a questionnaire to uncover positive and negative attitudes toward such involvement; it is completed by a targeted sample of first grade teachers in a school system. Subsequently, these same teachers will be assigned to either an experimental or a control group. Teachers assigned to the experimental group will participate in a workshop to learn about various speech and language disorders and how communication deficits can impede educational achievement. Teachers assigned to the control group will not participate in the workshop. Thereafter, both groups are posttested and the results indicate that teachers who completed the workshop now show a significant reduction in negative attitudes and a reciprocal increase in positive attitudes. No such changes are found in the control group.

Although you may be inclined to conclude from the results that the workshop had a favorable effect in altering attitudes, such a conclusion may not be valid because of a possible interaction between the pretest and the experimental treatment. More specifically, in the course of completing the workshop, the experimental group may eventually surmise that the purpose of the experiment is to alter their attitudes in a particular manner, leading them to respond accordingly on the posttest. Thus, their posttest performance actually reflects the insights gained from the *combined influence* of pretesting and exposure to treatment.

The Solomon four-group design allows the experimenter to assess the influence of pretesting on a particular experimental result. This is accomplished by comparing the posttest results of two experimental groups and making the same comparisons for two control groups. The experimental and control groups are arranged in pairs with one pair pretested and the other pair not pretested. If the posttest results of the two experimental groups are comparable, you can be relatively confident that the interaction effects of pretesting and treatment were negligible.

Multigroup Designs: (ANOVAR and FACTORIAL)

In addition to the type of control procedures used, experimental designs can also be described according to the number of groups involved and the nature of the statistical analysis. For example, in addition to the control of randomization, we also can speak of **multigroup designs** in which *three or more groups* are used to examine different treatment effects resulting from alternative independent variables or from different levels of the same independent variable. Such a design would be appropriate for comparing the relative efficacy of three or more different therapy approaches. On the other hand, the question posed might concern whether or not the effectiveness of a single treatment approach varied as a function of the number of therapy sessions per week (e.g., one, two, three, etc.). Designs that require the comparison of three or more groups are sometimes called **ANOVAR designs** because they involve the use of statistical techniques called an **analysis of variance (ANOVA).**

The most complex of all the experimental designs are called **factorial designs** because they allow for administering more than one independent variable at a time to a subject. More specifically, within the framework of this design, different **treatment factors** and **level effects** can be studied simultaneously. Given the example provided above, we might choose to study the interaction of three treatment factors (therapy approaches A, B, or C) with three treatment levels (once, twice, or three times a week) on a clinical outcome. These interactions can be diagrammed as shown in Table 5.4. As can be seen, factorial de-

Table 5.4.
General Structure of Three-by-Three Factorial Design

Number of Sessions (J)		Treatments (I)		
		A	B	C
	1	Y_{A1}	Y_{B1}	Y_{C1}
	2	Y_{A2}	Y_{B2}	Y_{C2}
	3	Y_{A3}	Y_{B3}	Y_{C3}

where: Y_{IJ} = An outcome with the treatment I and J sessions
I = A, B, or C; J = 1, 2, or 3.
For example, Y_{B2} represents the outcome with the treatment "B" and "2" sessions

signs involve at least two dimensions of analysis involving the number of treatments employed (independent variables) and the number of levels for each application of a treatment. Our example can be described as a 3×3 factorial design.

Theoretically, there is no limit to the number and levels of independent variables that can be employed in an experiment. However, the complexity of statistical analysis will grow logarithmically with increments in the number of interactions to be investigated. Because of the complexity of the statistical calculations required, computer assistance can greatly ease the burden of what might otherwise prove to be an onerous and time-consuming task.

Quasi-Experimental Designs

Quasi-experiments are those that satisfy all of the requirements of a true experiment *with the exception of random assignment.* Although these designs are less powerful than true experiments, quasi-experiments are rated second best, particularly in cases in which (1) only preformed groups or specific individual cases are available for study, and/or (2) ethical issues may preclude withholding treatment from certain individuals. For example, this might be the most appropriate design in a clinical situation in which you wish to evaluate the effect of a specific treatment for a group of cases already admitted to therapy as compared to the absence of such treatment for other cases on a waiting list. Often, the pre-assemblage of such comparison groups is the natural consequence of scheduling factors beyond the control or interests of the experimenter. In other words, lacking randomization, such a design allows for "when and to whom" certain measurements are made but not "when and to whom" treatment is given (Campbell and Stanley, 1966).

Nonequivalent Comparison Group Design: O_1 **X** O_2
$$O_3 \quad O_4$$

A design typical of the type discussed above is known as the nonequivalent comparison group design. It entails the use of at least two nonrandom comparison groups, the members of both of which are pretested with respect to some dependent variable. The experimental group then is treated according to the independent variable while the comparable group goes untreated. Subsequently, a posttest is again administered to both groups, and their performance scores are compared. If statistical testing indicates that the performance of the experimental group is significantly better than that of the comparison group, some level of confidence can be placed in the efficacy of the treatment in question.

Interrupted Time-Series Design: $O_1 \, O_2 \, O_3 \, O_4$ **X** $O_5 \, O_6 \, O_7 \, O_8$

Other types of quasi-experimental studies include **interrupted time-series designs** in which **repeated measures** of a dependent variable are made prior and subsequent to the administration of an independent variable. More specifically, this design involves periodic measurements over a time span in order to establish either an **average** performance value (in the case of groups) or a **baseline** (in the case of individual subjects) prior to introducing an experimental treatment. Subsequently, a series of ongoing measurements are taken to determine whether or not a change in the dependent variable has occurred. The basic concept of what is called a **multiple time-series design** for group experiments is graphically portrayed in Figure 5.1.

Small-N Quasi-Experiments

Quasi-experimental studies involving what have been variously called small-N designs, N-of-1 designs, intensive designs, single-case designs, etc. are especially adaptable to many clinical research problems. Group studies, by comparison, can have major limitations as

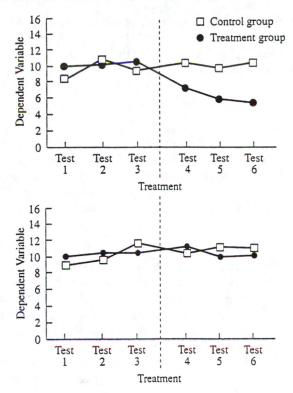

Figure 5.1. Two possible outcomes of a multiple time-series design. *Top,* Results suggest that treatment had an effect on the dependent variable; *Bottom,* Results supply no evidence that treatment affected the dependent variable. From *Research Methods and Statistics for Psychology* by W.A. Schweigert. Copyright © 1994 Brooks/Cole Publishing Company, Pacific Grove, CA 93950, a division of International Thompson Publishing Inc. By permission of the publisher.

their findings apply to therapeutic situations. In the process of attempting to assure generality of group data to the targeted population, investigators typically employ sampling procedures designed to include *all* relevant population characteristics in the sample. In so doing, the relevance of such data to specific subjects may be substantially diminished (Herson and Barlow, 1976). Statistically, this is comparable to observing that many individual scores in a distribution may depart substantially from an average score used to represent such a distribution as a whole.

Small-N designs should not be confused with more primitive case study methodologies. The latter type of investigations are typically characterized by uncontrolled sources of variation, inadequate descriptions of independent and dependent variables, and are usually impossible to replicate. Unlike time-series research, case studies often involve "one shot" measurement approaches, usually in the form of a posttest followed by a treatment intervention. On the other hand, time-series research generally extends over a period of time in which the behavioral target is measured almost continuously. As we noted in Chapter 1, the scientific basis of time-series research of individual subjects owes much to B. F. Skinner, who was among the first to emphasize the importance of the experimental analysis of human behavior using repeated measurements under controlled conditions.

A-B design. The most basic of the time-series designs involving individuals is the A-B design. In this paradigm, observations are made over a period of time to establish a "baseline" of retest data. Subsequently, a treatment is introduced and changes in the dependent variable are noted. Suppose one wishes to study the effect of a verbal cueing procedure on the naming ability of patients with Broca's aphasia. Using an A-B design, one could establish a baseline during pretreatment phase A; treatment then could be introduced during phase B in an effort to increase the number of correct responses. This design differs from a case study by virtue of establishing a baseline prior to intervention and by repeated measurement of the dependent variable throughout both the baseline and treatment phases of the experiment.

A-B-A design. An improvement over the basic design is to add a second A in a third phase of the experiment in which the dependent variable is measured again after treatment has been withdrawn. The advantage of this A-B-A design over the simpler A-B approach is that it affords greater experimental control. By withdrawing the treatment during the third phase and observing the effect on the dependent variable, the researcher can conclude with greater confidence that the independent variable was indeed responsible for the observed change in behavior.

A-B-A-B design. Still a further elaboration of the A-B design is the A-B-A-B design, which is the most frequently employed design in behavioral or "operant" research. (Glass et al., 1975). By adding a second B phase, the last two phases of the design are a replica of the first two phases. Thus, A-B-A-B studies are sometimes called **replication designs.** A common form of this design involves **withdrawal of treatment** during the third phase so that phase one represents *baseline*, phase two represents *treatment* and phase three represents *withdrawal* as in the A-B-A design. However, the A-B-A-B design adds a fourth phase in order to determine what happens to the dependent variable when the treatment is *reinstated* (Figure 5.2). In effect, the A-B-A-B sequence involves the study of the treatment effect as it both *precedes* and *follows* a baseline condition. Clinically, the fourth phase of such a design is highly desirable because it avoids the negative consequences of the A-B-A experiment that leaves the client/patient at the end of the study as they were in the beginning—i.e., in a state comparable to their original baseline level of responding. Further variations of the A-B-A-B design may involve additional subtypes as follows:

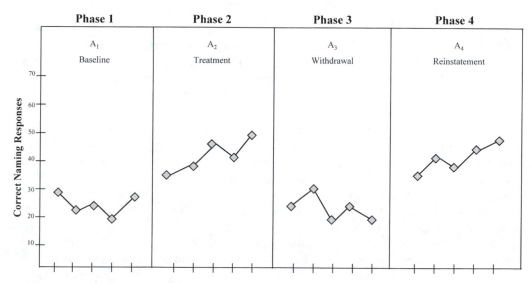

Figure 5.2. Representative A-B-A-B design. The addition of a fourth phase enhances the internal validity of the treatment effect, demonstrated in phase 2, by restoring the desirable behavior following the withdrawal of treatment (phase 3).

• **Alternating Treatment Design:** The effects of two alternating treatments are studied, first A, then B. Instead of using a baseline as traditionally defined, two treatments (A and B) are presented randomly. A clinical advantage of this design is that some type of treatment is always being used in contrast to a withdrawal design that returns to baseline following treatment. Thus, treatment effectiveness can be assessed by comparing differences between alternative treatments for a comparable series of data points. An example of an alternating treatment design in which the efficacy of two language treatment methods were compared can be found in an investigation by Weismer and associates (Weismer, Murray-Branch, and Miller, 1993). Two teaching methods, modeling versus modeling *plus* evoked production techniques, were taught in a semi-random order during group and individual instruction. Although not a required component of an alternating treatment design, the authors choose to use a baseline phase before individual (but not group) instruction. This was done " . . . to further document the lack of target vocabulary in a child's repertoire before teaching." (p. 1040). As shown in Figure 5.3, more correct productions generally occurred in response to modeling alone than for the combined treatment approach. This was true under individual as well as group instruction, although overlap in the curves for the two treatments is evident for both types of instruction.

• **Reversal Design:** This design is similar to withdrawal with an important exception. During the third phase, instead of withdrawing treatment, a second form of intervention can be applied and the effect of the two treatments then compared. For example, two incompatible behaviors such as fluency and disfluency in a stuttering individual might be selected for treatment (Figure 5.4). After establishing a baseline in phase one, the first con-

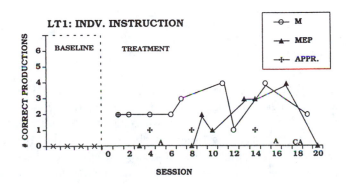

Figure 5.3. Frequency data for subject LT1 on the production probes following individual instruction (top panel) and group instruction (bottom panel). M = modeling treatment; MEP = modeling plus evoked production treatment; APPR = approximation; A = subject absence; CA = clinician absence.

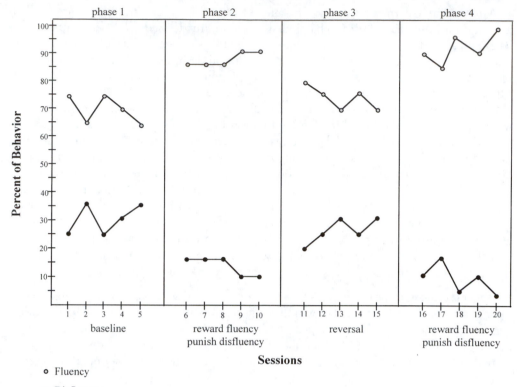

Figure 5.4. Reversal design for treating stuttering and the hypothetic results. The contingencies of phase 2 (reward of fluency/punishment of disfluency) were reversed in phase 3 (punishment of disfluency/reward of fluency). In phase 4, the phase 2 contingencies were reinstated.

tingency could be applied—e.g., reward of fluency/punishment of disfluency. Subsequently, in phase three, these contingencies might be reversed (reward of disfluency/punishment of fluency). Phase four of the reversal design typically entails reinstatement of the same treatment contingency as administered in phase two in order to terminate the experiment by once again producing the *desired* treatment effect. In the case of our hypothetical experiment, this would involve rewarding fluency and punishing disfluency. Although a strength of the reversal design is its power in illustrating the efficacy of a clinical intervention, a weakness is the possibility of being unable to reverse some negative consequence associated with the effort to demonstrate experimental control over the targeted behavior (Gelfand and Hartmann, 1984). Thus, for practical and ethical reasons, caution should be exercised in the use of this particular design.

Multiple-Baseline Design. In cases in which it is undesirable to leave the subject in the original baseline state or to augment some behavior incompatible to the intended treatment outcome merely to demonstrate the ability to reverse such a negative effect, a multiple-baseline design might be used instead. Commonly used variations of this design are applicable to the study of efforts to modify different behaviors across two or more situations or the same behavior across two or more situations or settings.

A simplified graphic representation of the basic paradigm for a multiple-baseline design is shown in Figure 5.5. As illustrated, a stable baseline is established on two or more behaviors in the series. After a predetermined number of sessions, the treatment is next applied to the second behavior in the series while the first behavior continues to receive treat-

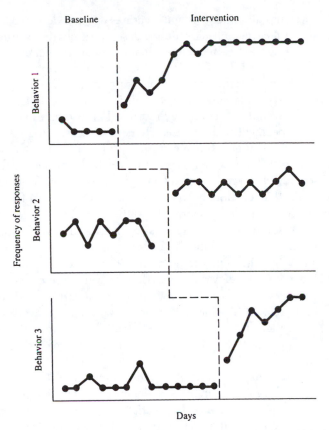

Figure 5.5. Hypothetic data for a multiple-baseline design across behaviors in which the intervention was introduced to three behaviors at different points in time. From *Single Case Research Designs.* Copyright © 1982 by A. Kazdin. Used by permission of Oxford University Press, Inc.

ment. In this manner, sequential applications of treatment continues across all behaviors to be assessed. Similarly, treatment efficacy can also be evaluated across two or more situations, settings, or time periods by the sequential application of the intervention to different baselines. As Kazdin (1982) pointed out, multiple-baseline designs are essentially "mini A-B experiments" involving successive comparisons between treatment and no-treatment conditions. More specifically, he noted, "Each time the intervention is introduced, a test is made between the level of performance during the intervention and the projected level of the previous baseline." (p. 128) In this way, each baseline serves as a control condition against which the influence of subsequent interventions can be evaluated.

Typically, these designs involve " . . . keeping data on two or more behaviors that are to be modified sequentially with the same treatment procedure" (Gelfand and Hartmann, 1984) (p. 69). The main steps in the use of any multiple-baseline design are as follows:

1. Establish reliable and stable baselines on all behaviors selected for modification.
2. Randomly select a behavior (or subject or setting) for treatment while simultaneously observing an untreated behavior (or subject or setting).
3. Randomly select another untreated baseline and introduce the experimental treatment.
4. Continue until all baselines have been treated.
5. Demonstrate treatment effectiveness by showing systematic modifications in performance across more than one baseline.

Multiple-baseline designs can also incorporate features of other designs such as the **Changing Criterion Design.** Like the multiple-baseline design, the changing criterion design uses each phase of an experimental treatment to evaluate subsequent phases of treatment. However, in the latter design, a step-wise criterion rate of responding is determined for each phase of treatment, which subsequently serves as a baseline for the next phase in the series.

An example application of a single-subject multiple-baseline design that incorporated a changing criterion is found in a study by Pratt and her associates (Pratt, Heintzelman, and Deming, 1993). Specifically, these researchers investigated the efficacy of the IBM SpeechViewer's Vowel Accuracy Module for treating vowel productions in hearing-impaired children. The children were treated individually by providing feedback to them concerning the accuracy of 10 productions of a targeted vowel. Subsequently, the children were required to make 10 additional productions without benefit of feedback from the computer program. Eight levels of contextual difficulty were employed, ranging from vowel productions in isolation to productions in phrases, in which the children could strive for three progressively more difficult levels of production accuracy. The easiest criterion was defined as a "goodness metric" of no more than 3.0, and the most difficult was set at 1.4. An 80% accuracy level was required on two consecutive sessions without feedback before the children were allowed to progress from one criterion to the next.

An example of individual treatment data for the vowel /u/ is shown in Figure 5.6. As can be seen, a treatment effect was demonstrated for all three criteria through level 6 (picture labeling with a CVC word). However, all criteria were not met at higher levels of contextual difficulty that involved the use of the vowel in phrases.

As noted previously, a major advantage of multiple-baseline designs is that they do not necessitate withdrawal of treatment in order to demonstrate treatment efficacy as do A-B-A-B designs. Thus, they are well suited to a variety of clinical applications, particularly when the clinical researcher is interested in monitoring several target measures concurrently. A potential disadvantage associated with their use arises when different baselines are not independent so that the effects arising from treating the first behavioral target or situation/setting spread across to influence performance in other experimental conditions. Other problems might arise from the inability to achieve stable baselines prior to intervention and the large amount of time that may be needed to collect data.

Although both group and single-subject quasi-experimental designs fall short of meeting the randomization requirement of true experiments, they nonetheless have many useful applications to clinical or applied settings in which random assignment of individuals to treatment groups or conditions is impractical or impossible to achieve. As Campbell so aptly stated,

> The general ethic is . . . to use the very best method possible aiming at "true experiments" . . . But where randomization is not possible . . . we must do the best we can with what is available to us. (Campbell, 1969, p. 411).

Pre-experimental Designs

Pre-experimental designs involve studies that fail to meet at least two of the criteria of a true experiment. As forerunners of stronger experimental designs, the present day value of such studies is limited because of their almost total lack of control of numerous extraneous variables that can invalidate an experiment.

One-Shot Case Study: X O

Among the pre-experimental designs, the weakest of all is the **one-shot case study,** which has practically no scientific value for drawing causal inferences. This approach, also known

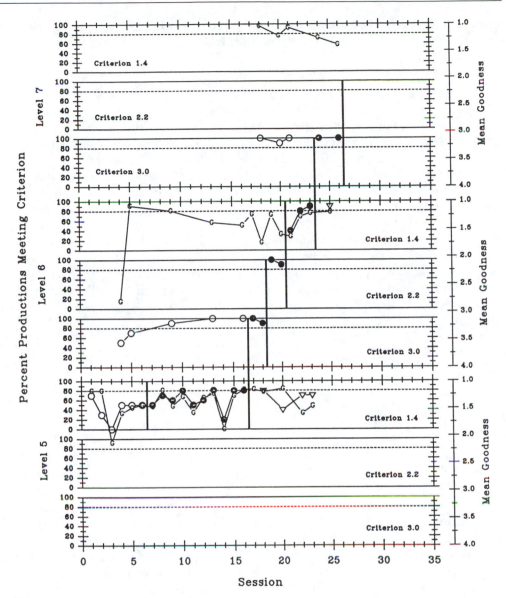

Figure 5.6. Individual treatment data for Subject 1 for vowel /u/. The open circles represent pretreatment data points, the filled circles treatment data points, and the inverted open triangles represent posttreatment data points; all are referred to the left-hand axis. The letter G represents the average goodness of the productions and is referred to the right-hand axis. The 80% level of performance is marked by a dashed line. Four of the five judges indicated an overall treatment effect.

as the **one-group posttest design,** involves studying the presumed effect of an independent variable in a single group of subjects by administering a posttest after some intervention(s). Although used extensively in various clinical studies, there are serious pitfalls to this approach. Suppose you are treating a number of cases whose clinical progress is below your level of expectation. You decide to increase the number of clinical contacts from one to two therapy sessions per week. After a certain period, you measure the achievement of these cases and observe improvements as consistent with your therapy goals. Can you conclude that increasing the amount of therapy (level of the independent variable) was an effective strategy? Unfortunately, there is no valid basis for drawing this conclusion.

One-Group Pretest-Posttest: $O_1 \; X \; O_2$

One major hindrance to determining causal relations in a one-shot case study is the lack of a pretest, so that conclusions must take the form of **retrospective suppositions** about what the results might otherwise have been in the absence of the independent variable. Most clinicians are knowledgeable about the importance of pretesting; therefore, we wisely would have included this step in our hypothetical study. Had this occurred, the design would be called a **one-group pretest-posttest design.** Is this design, by virtue of including a pretest, markedly improved over the one-shot case study? Again, we must say no. There are still many extraneous variables that can seriously confound the interpretation of findings. Indeed, by the inclusion of a pretest, this design introduces another potential problem not present in the posttest-only design, namely, that of pretest sensitization with the possibility of accompanying interaction effects that are impossible to evaluate because of the absence of an appropriate comparison group. Posttest scores may simply reflect the influence of practice or learning how to be a better "test taker" the second time around. In order to avoid this complication, one might decide to omit the pretest and use a control group.

Static-Group Comparison: $\; X \; O_1$
$$O_2$$

Opting for the control group approach, perhaps we would select a design called **static-group comparison** wherein two preformed groups would be selected—one group receiving additional therapy sessions and the other not. However, this goes back to the problem of lacking two important criteria for inferring causal relations. What is now missing is *both* random assignment and the use of a pretest as a control mechanism. Should we decide to add both factors to our study design, we have once again established the requirement for performing a true experiment!

Because appropriate statistical comparisons cannot be performed on the results of preexperimental studies, such investigations are essentially limited to descriptive questions of the type discussed previously. Perhaps they might be more appropriately described as **pseudo-experiments** that sometimes convey the misleading impression of belonging to more rigorous and powerful kinds of experimental methodologies that are better equipped for observing lawful relationships and drawing plausible explanations with greater confidence.

SELECTING A SAMPLE OF SUBJECTS

The main purpose of the majority of clinical investigations conducted in the field of communication disorders is to generalize the findings obtained from the study of one group of subjects **(sample)** to a larger group of similar individuals **(population)** that the sample was chosen to represent. For example, in a study to examine the role of speech perception training in the correction of phonologic errors, Rvachew (1994) randomly assigned preschoolers with phonologic impairment (misarticulated /ʃ/) to one of three groups involving various clinical treatments. In summarizing the results of her investigation, she concluded that " . . . this study demonstrates that interpersonal speech perception training can facilitate sound production learning for some children who are phonologically impaired." Rvachew's belief in the generalizability of her findings to a population of similar children was reflected in her concluding statement,

Although further research is required, some suggestions for clinical application of this approach can be made on the basis of the currently available information . . . Speech perception training should *probably* [ital. added] be provided concurrently with speech production training. (p. 355)

Rvachew's conclusion is indicative of having inductively inferred certain results to a population of children based on a sample of children who were believed to be representative of the population as a whole. The use of the word "probably" in Rvachew's concluding statement implies that consideration was given to the statistical probability of being wrong—i.e., one cannot be sure that *all* children with such a pattern of phonologic errors will respond to the treatment(s) found effective even though a significant number are predicted to respond favorably.

Random Assignment versus Random Selection

Rvachew's experiment is representative of a random assignment design in which an effort is made to form comparable groups prior to treatment. **Random assignment** is to be distinguished from **random selection** procedures. The goal of random assignment is to establish equivalent groups by balancing subject characteristics on the basis of the available subject pool. On the other hand, random selection involves drawing observations from a population defined as all members of any well-defined class of people, events, or objects in such a way that each observation has an equal chance of being represented (Kerlinger, 1986).

Types of Populations

In many investigations, there actually are two types of populations that an experimenter might wish to represent. First, there is an **infinite** number of observations that could conceivably be made in reference to certain populations of persons, objects, or events under specified conditions. Hypothetically, such a population is without limit, consisting of all possible observations of interest. For example, in the experiment discussed previously, an infinite population of preschoolers with /ʃ/ misarticulations would consist of all similar children that could conceivably be subjected to the same treatment conditions. By definition, such a population must be conceptualized in **ideal** rather than **actual** terms because the probability that all possible members of a population could ever be studied is negligible. Furthermore, even if possible to accomplish, few investigators would undertake such an enormous task.

A second type of population can be defined in **finite** terms based on the number of individuals, objects, or events that are known to actually exist at a given time. For example, such a population might consist of all preschool children with a particular type of phonologic disorder living in a certain town or school district from which a smaller sample of children might be taken.

Random Sampling Methods

Random sampling methods are designed to eliminate or reduce systematic bias in the selection of subjects that otherwise might limit the generality of research findings. Sampling methods of this kind are sometimes called **probability sampling** because they allow for estimating how closely a sample statistic represents the population parameter from which it was drawn (see Figure 5.7 for the basic steps in drawing a random sample). Nonrepresentative samples can threaten the validity of an experiment. There are several alternative methods for drawing a random sample so that it is representative of a given population. Four of these methods are discussed here.

Goal: Estimate the general characteristics of an infinite population (or general population) based on the sample from a finite population (or some defined population).

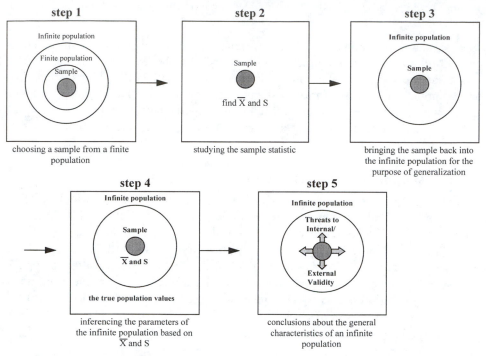

Figure 5.7. Steps in estimating a population parameter from a sample statistic. Symbols $\overline{X}$ and S represent the mean and standard deviation, respectively.

Simple Random Sampling

Perhaps the least complicated means of obtaining an appropriate sample is called simple random sampling or, less commonly, unrestricted random sampling. There are two basic assumptions underlying this approach. First, each member of a population must have a chance of being selected for a sample equal to that of every other member. Second, one's chance for inclusion must not be diminished as the consequence of other individuals having been selected. One well-known way for obtaining such a sample is the "hat technique" in which the names of all members of a population are written on individual slips (or more conveniently coded by numbers) and then drawn one by one from the hat or some other container after being thoroughly mixed. Each name or number would be returned after every draw in order to maintain equal probabilities for being chosen throughout the selection process until a sample of the desired size has been obtained.

An even more straightforward and convenient method is to use a table of random numbers available in many statistical texts. The numbers composing such lists are computer-generated using special equations so that the odds for each one's placement in the list is independent of the odds for the preceding and following number. An example subset of random numbers taken from a random number table is shown in Table 5.5.

Suppose you are interested in randomly selecting children for audiometric screening in an elementary school system. The first step would be to clearly define the specific population of interest. Do you wish to sample all grades or a particular grade level? What proportion of the population do you wish to sample? For illustration, assume that you have decided

Table 5.5.
Subset of Random Numbers

Row Number										
00080	59580	06478	75569	78800	88835	54486	23768	06156	04111	08408
00081	38508	07341	23793	48763	90822	97022	17719	04207	95954	49953
00082	30692	70668	94688	16127	56196	80091	82067	63400	05462	69200
00083	65443	95659	18238	27437	49632	24041	08337	65676	96299	90836
00084	27267	50264	13192	72294	07477	44606	17985	48911	97341	30358
00085	91307	06991	19072	24210	36699	53728	28825	35793	28976	66252
00086	68434	94688	84473	13622	62126	98408	12843	82590	09815	93146
00087	48908	15877	54745	24591	35700	04754	83824	52692	54130	55160
00088	06913	45197	42672	78601	11883	09528	63011	98901	14974	40344
00089	10455	16019	14210	33712	91342	37821	88325	80851	43667	70883

to limit your population to grades 1–3, for which you have a list containing 90 names. You wish to evaluate one third, or 30, of these children. The second step would entail assigning consecutive numbers to each member of the population. The third and final step would entail the actual use of the table in order to obtain a random sample of 30 children.

The actual use of a random number table is a simple process by which one closes his or her eyes and brings the point of a pencil down at a place on the page chosen arbitrarily. Numbers in the table are arranged in columns and rows; one may proceed either horizontally or vertically as long as the direction does not change. Imagine that you decide to proceed down columns. Assume further that your pencil points to the third set of numbers shown opposite row number 00084. The numbers listed in the table contain five digits but only the first two digits of the number sets will be needed to meet our selection requirement of 30 subjects. We begin by listing our initially selected number (50). We then proceed to move down the column, listing the first two numbers found in a row while ignoring duplicate numbers. When we hit the bottom of the column, we move to the top of the next one and proceed down it. In so doing, the initial 10 subjects of the 30 needed to complete our sample are selected accordingly:

Subject #	Subject #
50	75
6	23
15	18
45	13
16	19
	etc.

Remember that the number of digits used depends on the number of subjects to be selected from a particular **sampling frame,** defined as a full listing of all subjects in a targeted population that one wishes to sample. In the case of our example, the sampling frame consisted of 90 students from which the actual sample of 30 students was drawn. Had we wished to randomly select one hundred or more subjects from the sampling frame, we would have elected to use three-digit rather two-digit numbers while proceeding in the manner as described.

Systematic Sampling

Another type of sampling method is called systematic sampling, which is a parsimonious way of drawing a sample from a large population when a membership list is available. For example, in a study designed to survey the attitudes of ASHA members toward some professional issue, every tenth name appearing in the membership directory could be selected. In using this technique, investigators need to be wary of the potential danger of using a sampling interval that varies in some preordained fashion. If the ASHA directory was arranged so that every tenth name listed was a male, the survey might yield a very distorted view the issue under study. One means of reducing the possibility of some bias introducing an unwanted influence in sampling is to use a randomization procedure for deciding where in the list to begin the selection process. For example, if there are 30 names on the first page of the directory, use the "hat method" or a random number table as described previously to select the name of the first person to be surveyed. Thereafter, systematically select every tenth or another constant number of your choosing until the end of the directory listing.

Stratified Sampling

Another form of sampling is called stratified sampling. This technique involves dividing a population into subgroups called strata in order to assure that certain segments of the population are adequately represented in a sample. Suppose in the previously mentioned survey of ASHA membership attitudes, we wanted to assure adequate representation according to the factor of gender. For purposes of illustration, let us further assume that we learn that the professional membership is approximately 80% female and 20% male. Given this knowledge, we decide that we want our sample to represent the same gender proportion. One way to accomplish such a sampling distribution is to divide the population into two groups and then randomly select four females for every male using a random numbers table. The same stratified random sampling procedure could be used to assure adequate representation of age, race, employment setting, and specialty area, among other factors.

Cluster Sampling

In order to expedite the efficiency of data collection, cluster sampling may be also used in some combination with any of the sampling techniques mentioned above. Cluster sampling typically involves a multistage procedure in which smaller samples are selected from larger units or clusters. Referring once more to our attitudinal study of the ASHA membership, we might decide to conduct an area sampling survey in clusters of people based on geographic location. For example, using simple random selection procedures discussed earlier, we might initially select a predetermined number of states. Based on the states randomly selected (clusters), we would then randomly select from the appropriate geographic listings in the ASHA directory the desired number of names necessary for purposes of the survey. As noted previously, this could be done in combination with other sampling techniques. Although the use of clusters can reduce the time, effort, and expense involved in sampling, the risk for bias or sampling error can be relatively high, particularly when a small number of clusters are used.

Nonrandom Sampling Procedures

The sampling techniques discussed thus far have involved random sampling procedures designed to distribute extraneous influences in a chance fashion that might otherwise produce differences between groups or treatments unrelated to the independent variable. Several other types of sampling techniques may be used in research studies, but their scientific application is more limited.

Consecutive Sampling

This technique involves selecting all individuals who agree to participate, provided they meet pre-established criteria, until the number of subjects desired have been recruited. For example, an author of this text once conducted a study of the verbal memory of adult dyslexics who were recruited by means of several techniques including appeals through newspaper and radio advertising. In order to qualify as subjects, several criteria had to be satisfied pertaining to age, IQ level, educational achievement, history of remediation, mental and physical status, and scores on standardized tests of reading ability, among other factors. Consecutive sampling can be highly useful when the available subject pool is limited or when using selection criteria so stringent as to reduce the number of subjects to a point that threatens the generality of findings. Although consecutive sampling methods are typically stronger than other nonprobability techniques in controlling sampling bias, such confounding influence cannot be ruled out. **Response rate,** the proportion of subjects willing to participate of those selected, may also influence the validity of inferences. For instance, subjects who agree to participate may have different motivations or life circumstances than those who do not. Such bias can result in a nonrepresentative sample.

Convenience Sampling

Convenience sampling, sometimes called "on-the-street" or "opportunistic sampling," is another technique commonly used by the media to poll attitudes or opinions about current events. Often, the general public may be invited to write or telephone to express their opinion about a particular issue. Obviously, such survey data is potentially fraught with bias because of the restricted pool of respondents who may just happen to be available at a given time.

Purposive Sampling

A third type of nonrandom sampling is called **purposive or judgment sampling.** A small group of "key" individuals are used to focus or represent the attitudes, interests, or attributes of a larger group. In such a case, the researcher might deliberately select certain respondents based on a knowledge of their characteristics. For example, one might make judgments about the suitability of recognized authorities in a particular field to summarize current clinical or research trends. This type of sampling is also used in the study of relatively infrequent phenomena such as rare genetic diseases or disorders existing in individuals judged to be representative of the problem. As with other types of nonrandom sampling procedures, the generality of purposive samples may suffer if they fail to adequately represent the population as intended.

Matched Samples

Another type of sampling procedure used to establish equivalent groups in an experiment is called **matching**. Matching is a control procedure designed to restrict the degree to which subjects in different groups are allowed to differ by pairing them according to particular characteristics. Matching is frequently used in cases in which randomization is not possible or in experiments in which the number of available subjects are so few that random selection and assignment cannot be trusted to achieve equivalent groups representative of the population.

Quasi-experimental designs commonly match subjects on key characteristics that are likely to exert some unintended systematic influence on the dependent variable over and above that intended by the independent variable under investigation. For example, in clinical studies designed to improve various aspects of language ability, subjects assigned to different groups are often matched on the basis of verbal intelligence factors in an effort to balance such potential mitigating influences. Such variables as age, gender, socioeconomic status, physical and emotional status, and type and severity of disorder are among others frequently used in matching subjects to reduce potential between-group bias. To do so may be especially important when a researcher knows in advance that such pre-existing extraneous factors may impact the dependent variable.

Although matching techniques are often used in place of randomization, one procedure does not necessarily exclude the use of the other. Indeed, the strength of a design can be augmented by a combination of these methods. Liebert and Liebert (1995) described matched random assignment procedures, sometimes called **blocking,** as involving three steps:

1. Rank-order the subjects according to the variable for which control is desired.
2. Segregate the subjects into matched pairs (blocks) so that each pair member has approximately the same score on the variable to be matched.
3. Randomly assign pair members to the conditions of the experiment.

When matching procedures are used, they should be carried out on an *a priori* basis—i.e., before the actual treatments are administered. In cases in which the independent variable cannot be manipulated because the phenomenon of interest has already occurred, efforts to match individuals **ex post facto** (after the fact) can lead to serious errors in interpreting research findings. Conceivably, this could result in a case study of some communication disorder in which the investigator is looking to establish the relation between a certain predictor variable and currently manifested symptoms. Suppose we wish to examine the factor of age in relation to recovery of language in aphasia resulting from head trauma. After carefully matching subjects on the basis of the loci and severity of brain damage as determined from preexisting records, we conclude on the basis of current test results that the degree of language recovery is greater for children and adolescents than for middle-aged and older adults. Such findings are explained on the basis of differences in brain plasticity—the ability of new brain regions to acquire functional abilities previously subsumed by others. However, such a conclusion is unwarranted because of the possible confounding influence of a third variable that is impossible to isolate on the basis of hindsight. Between-group differences in motivation, intelligence, type and extent of therapy, availability of family support systems, and pattern of recovery over time are but a few of the extraneous factors that might have influenced the outcome. Trying to second guess (ex post facto) which of these or other factors might have played a role in recovery, and thereby match subjects accordingly in order to control potential confounding influences, is usually a waste of effort.

CONTROLLING VARIABLES

The ultimate power of an experiment can be assessed according to the degree that it is able to effectively maximize the variance associated with systematic manipulation of an independent variable while minimizing error variance through the use of various control procedures.

Maximizing Experimental Systematic Variance

The systematic influence of the independent variable can best be maximized by assuring that the treatment effect is sufficient to produce the intended result. In considering an independent variable for use in an experiment, some factors to evaluate are

- The amount or strength of the stimulus variable to be administered
- The number of trials or sessions involved
- The duration of treatment
- The degree to which treatment influences can be operationally specified and linked to changes in the dependent variable

Once manipulation of the independent variable has been shown to be sufficient to produce changes in the dependent variable, modifications in its size or manner of control can be explored in future experiments. However, its influence on the dependent variable must first be demonstrated. Experimental variations or refinements in an independent variable, to determine its range of effectiveness in producing desirable changes in behavior, are typically explored in more advanced stages of research.

Minimizing Random and Systematic Errors

In earlier chapters, we discussed the concept of error variance as it pertains to random fluctuations in scores. Such variance is associated with **random errors** owing to unknown factors. Systematic variance, on the other hand, includes sources of variance resulting from **systematic errors** that consistently *cause* the scores in a distribution to lean in one direction or another. Both types of errors culminate in the wrong result but, whereas random errors are due to chance alone, systematic errors are the result of certain bias that may or may not be known to the experimenter. Although no research study is immune to the influence of certain types of errors, the ultimate goal is to maximize the internal and external validity of its findings to the greatest extent possible (see Chapter 3).

Random Errors: Control of random errors can be partially achieved through the **method of constancy**. Factors that can undermine constancy in an experiment include:

- inconsistency in measurements
- inconsistency in subject responses during the repeated performance of the same task
- inconsistency in the conditions of testing

To illustrate efforts to control errors arising from inconsistency in measurement, imagine that you wish to investigate the duration of stuttering moments during oral reading. Prior to such a study, observers could be trained in the use of a stop watch to improve their **intraobserver reliability** (consistency within self) and **interobserver reliability** (consistency with others) in starting and stopping the watch in accordance with the task demands. Without such training, observers might start and stop the watch at different times even though subject responses remain the same. Also, clear agreement must be established among observers as to the units of behavior to be measured and the exact way measurements are to be made. In measuring instances of stuttering, it is important to know whether *whole word* or *part word* disfluencies are to be counted; perhaps some combination of these features will be evaluated in conjunction with such *accessory behaviors* as facial tics, dysrhythmic phonation, interjections, etc. Will measurements be made under a standard set of recording conditions involving direct observation, or will a tape recorder or audio video tape be used? Of course, the calibration and precision of all measuring devices (e.g., stop watch, electronic timer, etc.) should be determined before the experiment.

Efforts must also be made to reduce individual subject variability resulting from uncontrolled influences. At the outset of an experiment, some amount of variation in subject responses can always be expected owing to a myriad of factors such as innate learning ability, attention, emotional state, motivation, fatigue, etc. Nevertheless, consistency in performance can often be improved by training trials designed to familiarize and give subjects prior practice with a similar task to that required in the actual experiment. For example, if we wish to investigate stuttering severity in relation to some variable like *voice initiation time*, all subjects could be given training prior to studying potential group differences to improve "readiness to respond." Such preliminary training may also be used in conjunction with a pretest or to establish a baseline of responding that can be compared to subsequent behavior changes observed in response to treatment.

Another source of random error can result from the failure to hold constant the conditions of testing in an experiment. Uncontrolled variations can arise from numerous sources such as distracting noise, breakdowns in equipment, marked changes in temperature, and physical rearrangements in the testing environment, or the researcher may fail to treat all subjects participating in a particular condition in the same manner. The latter problem is less likely to occur if the researcher gains practice in administering the experimental procedures prior to an experiment. For this reason, a **pilot investigation** can be useful in planning and rehearsing exactly how the independent variables are to be administered, how measures of the dependent variables are to be recorded, and how subjects can best be instructed on the tasks they are asked to perform. A written protocol or outline that specifies all experimental procedures and the sequence for carrying out each step can greatly expedite precision of control over the variables of a study. The main value of pilot investigations is that they aid in solving many problems that might otherwise be unanticipated in the course of an actual experiment.

Systematic Errors: As noted previously, uncontrolled systematic errors can bias the findings of an experiment so that it is impossible to separate the intentional effects of the independent variable from inadvertent influences. One means of controlling the potential biasing influence of one experimental treatment or condition preceding another is through the **method of counterbalancing.** Suppose you wish to investigate the influence of some drug like haloperidol (treatment X) against a placebo (treatment Y) on the severity of stuttering behavior wherein each participant receives both treatments. A problem of **within-subject designs** of this kind involves **order effects**—i.e., interactions arising from one treatment variable preceding another. If treatment X precedes Y, there is the possibility of a drug residue being carried over to influence performance during the placebo condition. On the other hand, should treatment Y precede treatment X, certain pretesting factors such as practice may combine with the effects of the drug to augment its apparent influence on performance. To counterbalance such interactions, the researcher can reverse the order of treatments from one subject to the next. Thus, the first subject would be given treatment X followed by treatment Y; the second subject would then receive treatment Y followed by treatment X; and thereafter treatments would alternate in this manner for each new subject.

An extended application of counterbalancing used to guard against systematic errors is known as a **cross-over design,** sometimes called a **Latin Square.** In this design, two groups are typically used to evaluate the influence of a particular treatment versus another with each group serving as its own control. For example, to test the effect of a tranquilizer like haloperidol on stuttering, the following design could be used:

$$\text{Group 1:} \quad O_1 \quad X \quad O_2 \quad Y \quad O_3$$
$$\qquad\qquad\quad \text{drug} \qquad \text{placebo}$$

$$\text{Group 2:} \quad O_1 \quad Y \quad O_2 \quad X \quad O_3$$
$$\qquad\qquad\qquad \text{placebo} \qquad \text{drug}$$

As can be seen, subjects who originally received the drug crossed over to the placebo condition. Conversely, subjects who first received the placebo crossed over to the drug condition.

Provided that *both* groups illustrate significant gains after drug treatment as compared to placebo, we can be relatively confident that the independent variable had the intended effect.

Another control procedure for dealing with systematic sources of error is the **method of elimination**. Selection biases that lead to unwanted differences in the composition of control and experimental groups can be largely eliminated through careful matching of subjects on salient dimensions that might potentially confound the results prior to an experiment. Obviously, if the goal is to examine a particular element of language processing in children with a *specific* type of learning disability, one would want to exclude those subjects with *gross* cognitive impairment.

As we have noted, confounding factors pertaining to differences in subject characteristics can best be eliminated or diminished through random assignment or matching techniques aimed at producing **homogeneous samples.** Nevertheless, despite the researcher's wish to achieve group equivalence, there are some experiments in which naturally occurring categories of variables such as intelligence, race, and gender are beyond one's ability to control. In other cases, groups may have been formed with little attention to how these or other factors might influence the dependent variable under investigation, hoping, perhaps, that randomization or matching would eliminate any untold bias. The unwanted influence of problems such as these can sometimes be eliminated or greatly diminished through **statistical control.** One such method is the **Analysis of Covariance (ANCOVA)** designed to remove the influence of secondary variables of the type noted above on the dependent variable. This is accomplished by treating secondary variables that are predicted to have such an influence as **covariates** to be measured and then, through the use of combined correlational and analysis of variance procedures, removing their influence as uncontrolled sources of variation. In essence, the analysis of covariance is a mathematical correction procedure that is highly useful for eliminating unwanted influences in an experiment.

A second technique has statistical control implications, more so for random than for systematic errors; this is simply to increase sample size, thereby augmenting the likelihood of finding a significant result, if present. Selecting an appropriate sample size for detecting a significant association or difference between two or more measured variables is a complex matter that is discussed more fully in Chapter 8. For the time being, keep in mind that as sample size increases, the likelihood correspondingly decreases for certain chance factors or selection biases that threaten the validity of inductive inferences.

Finally, an important control procedure designed to eliminate the potential influence of *experimenter bias* should be mentioned. Imagine that a particular researcher has a vested interest in *proving* the effectiveness of some clinical program over another. To improve the potential for drawing objective conclusions, perhaps three graduate students are appointed to judge treatment outcomes. If the judges are aware of which subjects receive the favored treatment versus those who receive the alternative approach, they may be prone to see more improvement in the former cases than in the latter. These biasing influences can be controlled by using independent judges who are **blind** with respect to the anticipated outcome and to what treatment a particular subject was assigned. An even greater degree of control can be achieved in a **double-blind investigation.** For example, in the previously mentioned hypothetical study of the effect of haloperidol on stuttering, *both* the judges and the subjects would be kept blind as to the type of treatments (drug or placebo) being used as well as to the results that might be anticipated.

SPECIFYING MEASUREMENTS

A major concern in any experimental study is the manner of measurement of the dependent variable. Such measurements are a means for numerically representing the characteristics of objects or events of interest to the researcher. The measurement procedures selected are largely determined by the type of information one wishes to record.

In selecting a particular measurement for an experiment, four important factors to consider pertain to its (1) utility; (2) precision; (3) accuracy; and (4) scaling power.

Measurement Utility

The first and perhaps most important question to ask in assessing the overall usefulness of a measurement is whether or not it is *appropriate* given the aims of the study. If the desire of a researcher is to investigate the role of memory in language comprehension, it is important to specify further which kind of memory and language comprehension processes one actually wants to examine. Is the type of memory operation of interest related to short-term phonologic memory or to long-term semantic memory? What aspect of language will be evaluated in reference to memory proficiency—oral or written comprehension? And what specific tasks and performance measurements are most appropriate given the particular investigative goals? For these questions to be answered, the aims of the study must be stated as clearly as possible and in operational terms that define the parameters of the independent and dependent variables. Only then can suitable measurements be selected.

The utility of measurements can also be evaluated in reference to the **sensitivity** and **specificity** of test results. A **sensitive test** is one that rarely fails to identify a disorder or disease. In mathematical terms, such a test can be defined as the proportion of people with a disorder or disease who likewise test positive for that disorder or disease.

In a study by Jerger and his colleagues (1993), the utility of acoustic reflex measurements in predicting hearing threshold levels was examined in 1043 ears. The overall sensitivity of reflex testing was found, in the words of the authors, to be "amazingly good." Of the 453 ears that showed some level of audiometric hearing loss, 372 ears were correctly predicted to have abnormal audiograms. This result, corresponding to the sensitivity of the acoustic reflex screening test, was calculated as $\frac{372}{453} = 82.12\%$. As in the case of this example, a sensitive test is one that "casts a wide net," rarely missing people who have a disorder or disease. Test sensitivity must also be evaluated in relation to test specificity. A **specific test** is one that seldom erroneously identifies a person as having a disorder or disease when they do not. Mathematically, this translates into the ratio of people who test negative on a screening test to people without the disorder or disease. Referring again to the study just mentioned, of the 590 ears that showed normal audiometric test results, 349 ears were correctly predicted to have normal hearing. This result, corresponding to the specificity of the acoustic reflex screening test, was calculated as $\frac{349}{590} = 59.15\%$.

Generally speaking, a "good test" is one that is both sensitive and specific. Nevertheless, the practical reality is that leveraging a test in one direction correspondingly diminishes its utility in the other. With increased sensitivity, more false-positive identifications are likely as opposed to a highly specific tests in which false-negative identifications prevail.

Closely related to the concepts of test sensitivity and specificity are **ceiling effects** and **floor effects.** Ceiling effects result when scores on a test pile up at the high end of a distribution because the test is too easy or the dependent variable is too sensitive to the treatment employed. Conversely, a floor effect occurs when the majority of scores fall near the lower limit of a distribution, indicating that the test may be too difficult or perhaps the dependent variable is insensitive to the experimental treatment. Both ceiling and floor effects are undesirable sources of variation that can obscure the influence of the independent variable on the dependent variable.

Measurement Precision

The precision of measurement relates to the ability of a test instrument, whether mechanical or human, to render consistently similar or identical values on repeated applications or observations. The lack of precision is reflected in variability of measurement. Statistically, precision can be expressed as the correlation coefficients reflecting the reliability of measurement.

In addition to the need for determining **intraobserver** and **interobserver reliability,** as discussed previously in this chapter, other aspects of measurement precision to consider include **test-retest reliability** and **internal consistency reliability.** Each of these indices is typically assessed in evaluating and selecting a test instrument for use whether for diagnostic or research purposes. The psychometric assessment of three of these reliability measures is exemplified by the Childhood Autism Rating Scale (CARS) developed by Eric Schopler and his colleagues (1988). The main purpose of this scale is to reliably distinguish children with the autistic syndrome from children with other developmental disorders. Interobserver reliability was assessed by correlating individual item scores obtained from two trained independent observers. The overall interobserver reliability was calculated to be .71 based on an average correlation coefficient for 15 individual CARS items.

In order to assess test-retest reliability, scores on the first administration of the test were compared with those obtained from a second administration approximately one year later. The resulting correlation of .88 indicated that the CARS yielded temporally stable measurement.

The internal consistency of reliability of the CARS was also assessed to determine the degree to which the 15 scale items were related to one another as opposed to representing different facets of behavior. The resulting correlation of .94 provided justification for combining scale item scores into a single score.

From the previous discussion of measurement errors in this chapter, it will be recalled that a loss of precision is generally the result of random errors. Many such errors can be controlled through several means. Precise measurements can greatly reduce the variability of individual scores in a data set, thereby increasing the power of statistical tests to yield significant research findings as warranted.

Measurement Accuracy

As a concept, accuracy of measurement applies to issues involving both validity and reliability. For a measurement to be valid, it must accurately reflect the nature of the underlying variable that it is intended to represent. To be reliable, it must do so consistently with repetition over a span of time.

Whereas precision of measurement is threatened by random errors, accuracy is largely influenced by systematic errors in the form of certain biases. As we have noted, **experimenter bias** stemming from either unintended or willful actions in recording data can seriously distort the outcome of an investigation. Such distortion can also result from **subject bias,** in the form of the previously discussed Hawthorne Effect, and **instrument bias,** resulting from poorly calibrated equipment. In evaluating the accuracy of measurements for possible use, each of these biasing influences must be evaluated along with the means of their control (e.g., blinding, unobtrusive measures, instrument calibration, etc.).

The degree to which a variable adequately represents the phenomenon of interest to the researcher and how accurately it is measured pertains to its validity. Three aspects of validity are important in assessing the accuracy of measurement procedures. The first of these, **predictive validity,** concerns the success of a measurement in accurately estimating a particular outcome. Such validity is based on the extent to which test results are correlated with performance measures. Although such validity was not assessed in the case of the Childhood Rating Scale cited above, it might have been by evaluating how successful it *actually* was in predicting educational achievement, language development, emotional adjustment, or other significant factors. Predictive validity is often difficult or unfeasible to establish because prospective studies of subjects may be needed that require data analysis over a lengthy time span.

When predictive validity is not established, the next best alternative is to establish **criterion-related validity (convergence or concurrent validity),** a closely related concept. Such validity is established by collecting test measurements along with other criterion data almost simultaneously to determine their degree of agreement. Referring once again to the CARS, criterion-related validity was established by comparing total scores to clinical ratings of the degree of abnormality made during the same diagnostic sessions. The resulting correlation was .84, indicating high validity with respect to the criterion clinical ratings. High agreement (.84) was also found between the CARS and "expert clinical judgments" rendered by a child psychologist and psychiatrist.

Perhaps the most desired yet difficult-to-establish form of measurement validity is termed **content validity.** Such validity must be based largely on subjective opinion as to whether or not a test actually measures what it has been designed to test. Using the CARS once again to illustrate this concept, the scale ought to reflect the underlying attributes of autistic syndromes in a true and comprehensive manner. Commenting on this matter, Prizant (1992) noted that a strength of the CARS is that its content was derived from behavioral characteristics of autistic children over the last four decades. He further noted that a content weakness is found in its failure to sufficiently emphasize measurement of reciprocal social relations, communication, and imaginative activity. Such criteria are weighted heavily in current diagnoses of autistic syndromes. Prizant's review of the CARS appear in the *Buros Mental Measurement Yearbook,* a standard and highly useful reference for gaining reliability and validity information relating to published tests and measurements in current use.

Measurement Scales

Measurement involves the assignment of numerical values to observations made directly by an investigator or indirectly by a test instrument or recording device. Underlying the theory of measurement are certain assumptions pertaining to the suitability and power of different numerical scales for representing the data of an investigation. These assumptions form the basis for a set of rules that specify the admissible operations for the mathematical manipulation and statistical analysis of data that can be (1) named or categorized only; (2) ordered or ranked; (3) arranged along a numerical line, possessing equal intervals and an arbitrary zero point; or (4) treated as a ratio, possessing all the previous features in addition to a nonarbitrary zero point. Each of these classes of data along with their respective measurement scales are discussed further in the next chapter.

RECORDING MEASUREMENTS

Researchers in the field of communication disorders are primarily interested in the speech, language, and hearing abilities of human subjects and the means of their measurement. A major avenue of recording data with respect to these and related phenomena entails the observational use of the sensory apparatus of the observer—i.e., his or her own eyes and ears. Such observations often require **binary judgments** about the *presence or absence* of certain characteristics that are important in categorizing various types of disorders and related attributes of the subjects' physical or psychological makeup (e.g., age, sex, gender, cognitive functioning, etc.).

In many studies, simple **checklists** are sufficient for satisfying the purpose of coding the targeted behavior, perhaps supplemented by the use of tape recorders, audio-video recordings, or hand-held computers. In more complex investigations in which a number of behavioral or physiologic responses may be of interest, electrical or mechanical devices can often facilitate the precision and accuracy of recorded observations.

An example of a useful method for recording overt verbal or nonverbal behaviors as they occur was developed by Robert Bales (1950) who designed a 12-category system for classifying different types of goal-oriented and socioemotional interactions among individuals in small group settings (Table 5.6). To expedite the goals of such studies, Bales developed a recording device consisting of a driving mechanism and a movable tape that rolls across the top surface of the casing at a constant speed. Space is provided for an observer to tabulate interactions according to the 12 categories, within which a unit of behavior is judged to fall. Bales Interaction Process Analysis has been applied in the study of several aspects of human communication, including some problems in the field of communication disorders. For example, Weinberg (1968) found the approach to be a useful tool in observing and analyzing the fluency of stutterers in relation to certain patterns of social interaction occurring in small groups. Other useful applications of such categorical recording procedures in observational research might be found in studies of patterns of parent-child interaction in relation to various aspects of language development.

Computerized event recorders are now available that are capable of recording frequencies or durations of several categories of behavior. Observations pertaining to the qualities of various social interactions, of the type described by Bales, can now be recorded at regular intervals in response to a series of simple keyboard commands. For a description of a general purpose software package that can be adapted to a wide range of observational data, see Noldus (1991). For various physiological measurements, such as heart rate, electromyography (EMG), or electroencephalography (EEG), biotelemetry techniques now make possible the remote recording of responses from sensors and electrodes with the resulting signals fed to computers or analogue-to-digital converters.

Four common measures of behavioral/physiological responses include the following: (1) frequency; (2) latency; (3) duration; and (4) amplitude/intensity.

Response Frequency

The most common unit of measurement in the behavioral sciences is **response frequency,** referring to the total number of response units observed to occur. Perhaps the popularity of this measure is due to its relative simplicity of use and broad range of research and clinical applications. Frequency measures are especially useful in describing the characteristics of dichotomous observations that have only two categories (nominal data) or that can only be ranked according to which observation occurred more often than another (ordinal data). In the field of communication disorders, we are typically interested in measuring the number of correct versus incorrect responses with respect to various types of speech, language, or hearing behavior. We might also wish to use the frequency of certain errors to rank a disorder according to severity level (e.g., mild, moderate, or severe).

Table 5.6.
Bales' Category System for Assessing and Recording Goal-Oriented and Socioemotional Interactions

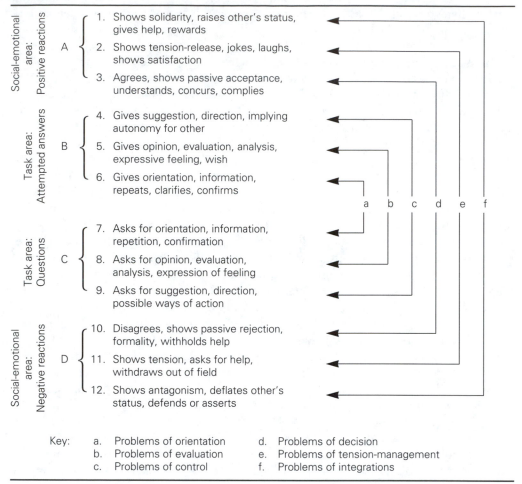

1. Shows solidarity, raises other's status, gives help, rewards
2. Shows tension-release, jokes, laughs, shows satisfaction
3. Agrees, shows passive acceptance, understands, concurs, complies
4. Gives suggestion, direction, implying autonomy for other
5. Gives opinion, evaluation, analysis, expressive feeling, wish
6. Gives orientation, information, repeats, clarifies, confirms
7. Asks for orientation, information, repetition, confirmation
8. Asks for opinion, evaluation, analysis, expression of feeling
9. Asks for suggestion, direction, possible ways of action
10. Disagrees, shows passive rejection, formality, withholds help
11. Shows tension, asks for help, withdraws out of field
12. Shows antagonism, deflates other's status, defends or asserts

A — Social-emotional area: Positive reactions
B — Task area: Attempted answers
C — Task area: Questions
D — Social-emotional area: Negative reactions

Key: a. Problems of orientation   d. Problems of decision
      b. Problems of evaluation   e. Problems of tension-management
      c. Problems of control   f. Problems of integrations

To have meaning, the frequency of an observed event must be specified in terms of some time frame. Thus, we often describe the **rate** of responding as the total number of occurrences per unit of time (minutes, hours, days, etc.). In discussing the history of time-series research, McGuigan (1993) cited B. F. Skinner, who said that, with respect to progress in the behavioral sciences, his development of a rate of responding measures was the most important of his own contributions. Small-N research paradigms of the type previously discussed in this chapter often display the results of an experiment in the form of a **cumulative graph.** Such a graph shows the total frequency of responses whereby changes in the dependent variable are attributed to systematic changes in the independent variable.

Frequency measures also have utility in studies of auditory physiology such as the investigations of the characteristic frequency of discharge (Cfs) of cochlear neurons in response to acoustic stimuli. Figure 5.8 is a neurogram representing the Cfs of 50 individual neurons in response to brief clicks. Recordings of neurons having Cfs in the lower-frequency range (cochlear apex) are located toward the front of the neurogram, whereas those with higher frequency Cfs (cochlear base) are located toward the rear.

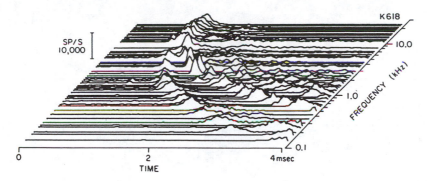

Figure 5.8. Neurogram display of spike activity for 50 individual neurons in a single animal. The stimulus was a brief click presented at a peak SPL of 100 dB. From Kiang NYS. Stimulus representation in the discharge pattern of auditory neurons. In: Tower DB, ed. The nervous system. Vol. 3. Human communication and its disorders. New York: Raven Press, 1975.

Response Latency

Measurements of **response latency** also are used in recording physiological or behavioral observations in accord with some predetermined unit of time. Such measures are recorded in accord with how long it takes for a specified response to occur following some specified event. In the neurogram shown in Figure 5.8, Cfs with the shortest latencies in response to clicks are located toward the rear of the neurogram, whereas those with the longest latencies are found toward the front.

Latency measures likewise have many applications in acoustic studies of speech. For example, in studies of the acoustic cues that may be used in making perceptual distinctions among speech sounds, measures of **voice onset time** (VOT) have been employed often in conjunction with sound spectrography. VOT measures are based on the time period between the start of vocal fold vibration and the occurrence of a noise burst or some other articulatory event (Fry, 1979). Sound spectrograms can be highly useful in the analysis of the temporal features of speech production and perception. Figure 5.9 illustrates the VOT intervals, denoted by a vertical bar and arrow, for four speakers producing the word *dad*. The first spectrogram (a) is for a normal speaker, and the remaining three spectrograms (b-d) are for speakers with apraxia of speech. As can be seen, the interval preceding voicing was relatively long for the neurologically impaired speakers as compared to the normal speaker, with speaker (d) showing the longest VOT. Spectrographic records such as these can help to make possible an objective examination of speech disorders (Kent & Reed, 1992). In addition to VOT, several other reaction time measures of response latency have been employed in studies of laryngeal dynamics associated with the study of speech fluency disorders (Adams, Freeman, and Conture, 1984).

Behavioral response latency measures also are applied in clinical studies designed to assess naming or word retrieval abilities in populations with various types of cognitive and language disorders. A representative and well-known test instrument often used for this purpose by speech-language pathologists is the Boston Naming Test (Kaplan, Goodglass, and Weintraub, 1983).

Response Duration

Measures of **response duration** also have utility in both behavioral and physiological studies. A common measure of stuttering severity involves recording the duration of stuttering moments as assessed, for example, on the *Riley Stuttering Severity Instrument for Children and Adults* (1986). A simple stop watch may be used for this purpose, or more

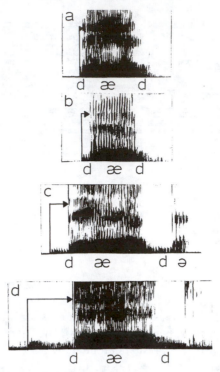

Figure 5.9. Spectrograms of the word *dad* produced by (a) a person with normal speech, and (b–d) persons with apraxia of speech. The interval marked by the arrow is the voice onset time (VOT) for the initial (d). From Kent R, Read C. The acoustic analysis of speech. San Diego: Singular Publishing Group, 1992.

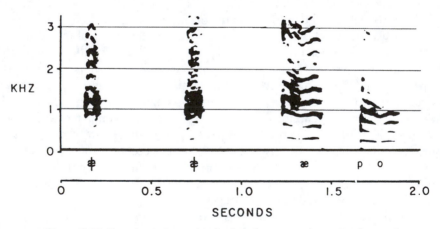

Figure 5.10. Sound spectrography display of separate elements of stuttering.

sophisticated instrumentation such as sound spectrography could be employed in the analysis of the separate elements of stuttering as shown in Figure 5.10.

Total response duration can also be expressed as a proportion (percentage) of time spent in emitting a particular behavior during a defined period. For example, we might wish to calculate the proportion of speaking time marked by stuttering behavior during a 60-minute session. If the total response duration, based on measuring all stuttering moments, was found to be 10 minutes, then the proportion of time spent stuttering would be calculated as 10/60 = .16 or 16 percent. Because some stuttering moments are likely to be

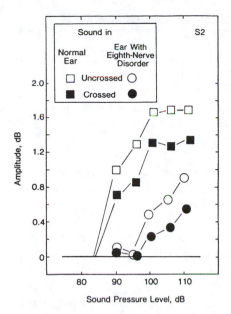

Figure 5.11. Amplitude-intensity function for acoustic reflex amplitude in a patient with an acoustic tumor. From Jerger J, Hayes D. Latency of the acoustic reflex in eighth-nerve tumor. In: Alford BR, Jerger S, eds. Clinical audiology: the Jerger perspective. San Diego: Singular Publishing Group, 1993:357.

longer than others, we might likewise wish to calculate their **mean duration.** This would involve a simple matter of dividing the total response duration time for stuttering by the number of stuttering moments noted to occur.

Response Amplitude-Intensity

The final measure that we wish to mention is based on physical or behavioral recordings of the **amplitude or intensity** of a response. Using a sound level meter with the decibel (dB) as a standard unit of sound measurement, we might investigate the average intensity level of conversational speech (about 60 dB) as compared to shouting (about 75 dB) or very quiet speech (approximately 35–40 dB) as measured 3 feet from the sound source (Fry, 1979). We might compare these values to inanimate sound sources such as a jet plane (130 dB at a distance of 120 feet) or the ticking of a watch next to the ear (20 dB).

Alternatively, we might decide to measure the amplitude-intensity function of the ear itself in response to sound. A recording of the acoustic reflex is an example of the response of the auditory system to a sound wave that increases with the intensity of the stimulus. Figure 5.11 shows the acoustic reflex for a normal ear and for an ear with eighth nerve disorder. Note that the maximum amplitude reflex of the abnormal ear is substantially reduced as compared to the normal ear.

A more general meaning of amplitude-intensity pertains to the amount or level of a quality as it is perceived or judged to exist by an observer. We might speak of the intensity of an anxiety reaction in a speaker and apply various rating scales such as low anxiety, moderate anxiety, or high anxiety based on our observation of a proscribed set of behaviors.

In considering the response measures discussed above, remember that no one of these is better than another but is selected as appropriate for recording the specific characteristics of the particular dependent variable under study. Furthermore, no matter how precise they might be, empirical measurements cannot replace the discerning judgments of the human observer who ultimately is responsible for analyzing and interpreting the recorded data in a reliable and valid manner.

SELF-LEARNING REVIEW

1. When asked to indicate their research interests, most graduate students know _____ global area they want to investigate. Sometimes they can also say _____ they might look for an answer. However, prior to reviewing the literature, it is rare that the question as to _____ a topic has been selected can be fully stated.

what
where
why

2. Prior to formulating a hypothesis, stating the overall _____ of an investigation is a useful strategy for clarifying general research _____ .

purpose
goals

3. After formulating a purpose statement, the investigator can elect to frame the problem as either a _____ or a _____ .

question
hypothesis

4. _____ questions attempt to uncover _____ factors by comparing the effect of an _____ variable on a _____ variable under different experimental conditions.

Difference
causal
independent
dependent

5. The fact that null hypotheses are not explicitly stated does not mean that researchers will fail to administer appropriate _____ tests.

statistical

6. Surveys, case histories, clinical reports, and prevalence/incidence studies are all examples of _____ study methods. Such studies can lead to a better understanding of phenomena as they exist in the "_____" and "_____."

descriptive

here   now

7. _____ studies are aimed at determining the relationships among variables. The strength of such relationships can be expressed as _____ _____ .

Predictive

correlation
coefficients

8. Both descriptive and predictive studies are _____ scientific methods. Such methods do not allow for determining _____ relations among variables.

nonexperimental
causal

9. Studies aimed at isolating causal relations involve the use of _____ designs. The strongest of these designs is called a _____ experiment.

experimental
true

10. The most commonly used experimental design is a _____-_____ control group design.

pretest-posttest

11. The analysis of the statistical significance of research findings often involves the use of a _____-test.

t

correlation
coefficient

12. In practical terms, whether or not a _____ _____

is judged to be a good predictive index of an association among variables depends on the _____ of the experiment.

purpose

13. When we ask, "What values of X are predictive of values of Y?", X is the _____ _____ and Y is the criterion variable.

predictor variable

14. A statistic termed _____ _____ is used to evaluate the predictive power of _____ or more variables.

multiple regression
two

15. A _____ table provides a means of examining a two-dimensional _____ distribution.

contingency
frequency

16. The _____ definition of probability is based on the expected _____ for an event in the long run.

frequentist
frequency

17. _____ theorem provides a basis for describing and testing subjective views in the mathematical language of _____ .

Bayes'
probability

18. Two aspects of test accuracy relate to its _____ and _____ .

sensitivity
specificity

19. The strongest of all research designs is a _____ experiment. Such designs require _____ _____ of subjects to at least two groups or treatment conditions.

true
random assignment

20. A design that attempts to control for interaction effects between a pretest and an independent variable is the _____ _____-_____ design.

Solomon four-group

21. ANOVAR designs involve the use of a statistical technique called the _____ of _____ , abbreviated _____ .

analysis
variance
ANOVA

22. The most complex of all experimental designs are termed _____ designs because they allow for administering more than two _____ _____ at a time.

factorial
independent variables

23. Factorial designs allow for different _____ factors and _____ effects to be studied simultaneously.

treatment
level

24. _____-_____ satisfy all the requirements of a true experiment with the exception of random assignment.

Quasi-experiments

25. The non_____ comparison group design entails the use of at least two non_____ groups, members of both of which are _____ before administering treatment.

equivalent
random
pretested

26. Designs in which repeated measures of a _____ _____ are made prior and subsequent to administering an

dependent variable

interrupted time-series

independent variable are called _____ _____ - _____ designs.

groups
individuals

27. Time-series designs are applicable to the study of both _____ and _____ .

Small-N
case study

28. _____ - _____ or N-of-1 designs should not be confused with more primitive _____ _____ methodologies.

A-B
A-B-A

29. The most basic time-series design involving individuals is called the _____ paradigm. An elaboration of this design in which the dependent variable is measured again after withdrawing treatment is the _____ design.

withdrawal
replication or
reinstatement

30. The A-B-A-B design can involve both _____ and _____ of treatment. This makes the design clinically more appealing than the A-B-A design.

alternating treatment
different
randomly

31. A design used in evaluating alternative treatment approaches is the _____ _____ design. In such a design, _____ treatments are alternated _____ with a single person.

reversal
practical
ethical

32. A design in which alternative incompatible behaviors can be treated is called _____ . For _____ and _____ reasons, this design should be used with caution.

Multiple-baseline

33. _____ - _____ designs are used to evaluate the effect of an independent variable across several behaviors, subjects, or situations.

changing criterion

34. When the ratio of responding for each phase of treatment serves as a baseline for the next phase in the series, the study is called a _____ _____ design.

true experiment
one-shot

35. Pre-experimental designs fail to meet at least two of the criteria of a _____ _____ . The weakest of these is the _____ - _____ case study.

static-group

36. A pre-experimental design that omits both random assignment and the use of a pretest is called _____ - _____ comparison.

random assignment
random selection

37. Whereas the goal of _____ _____ is to establish equivalent groups, _____ _____ attempts to draw a representative sample from a population.

infinite

38. An _____ population contains an unlimited number of

observations as opposed to a _____ number of individuals, objects, or events known to exist at a given time.

finite

39. Two assumptions of simple random sampling are: (1) each member of the population must have an _____ _____ of being selected and (2) one's chance for inclusion must not be reduced because of others having been _____ .

equal chance

selected

40. The number of digits chosen for use in a table of random numbers depends on the size of the _____ frame. Such a frame contains a full listing of all subjects in a _____ population.

sampling
targeted

41. A procedure in which smaller samples are selected from larger units is called _____ sampling.

cluster

42. _____ _____ involves selecting all participants who agree to participate in a study provided that they meet established criteria.

Convenience
sampling

43. A control procedure designed to restrict the degree to which subjects in different groups are allowed to differ is called _____ .

matching

44. _____ is a procedure that involves _____ pairs and _____ assignments.

Blocking
matched
random

45. In an _____ _____ _____ study, efforts are made to match subjects after the fact.

ex post facto

46. Controlling variables helps to maximize experimental _____ _____ while minimizing _____ and _____ errors.

systematic variance
random
systematic

47. A study that is useful in planning and rehearsing how the independent variables are to be administered is termed a _____ investigation.

pilot

48. Systematic errors involving order effects can be controlled through _____ or the use of a _____ design.

counterbalancing
crossover

49. Confounding differences in subject characteristics can be eliminated by the use of _____ samples.

homogenous

50. A statistical control procedure designed to remove the influence of secondary variables extraneous to the interests of an investigator is termed the _____ of _____ .

analysis covariance

double blind

51. A _____ _____ investigation is one in which neither the experimenter nor the subject is aware of what particular treatment is being administered.

false positive
false negative

52. Sensitive tests are associated with _____ _____ identifications, whereas specific tests yield more _____ _____ identifications.

Ceiling effects
floor effects

53. _____ _____ are caused by scores piling up at the high end of a distribution whereas _____ _____ occur when scores fall near the lower limit of a distribution.

reliability
validity
reliability

54. Test precision reflects the _____ of measurement. Test accuracy relates to issues involving both _____ and _____ .

Predictive validity

55. _____ _____ concerns the success of a measurement in accurately estimating a particular outcome.

Criterion validity

56. _____ _____ is established by collecting test measurements along with other criterion data to determine their degree of agreement.

Content validity

57. _____ _____ is largely based on subjective opinion as to whether a test actually measures what it was designed to test.

check lists

58. In many studies, simple _____ _____ are used for recording and coding the target responses.

latency

59. Recording how long it takes for a particular response to occur pertains to its _____ .

rate

60. The total number of responses occurring within a given unit of time is a measure of _____ .

duration

61. The percentage of time spent emitting a particular response is a measure of its _____ .

amplitude-intensity

62. A general meaning of _____-_____ pertains to the level of a quality as it is perceived or judged to exist by an observer.

6. Describing and Analyzing Data

Two major categories of statistics are commonly identified as **descriptive** and **inferential** techniques. Descriptive statistics essentially involve what the term implies. They are used for classifying, organizing, and summarizing a particular set of observations in a manner convenient for numerically evaluating the attributes of *available* data. On the other hand, inferential statistics are designed to allow an investigator to generalize findings from a subset of subjects (**sample**) to a similar group (**population**) from which the subset was drawn. Making inferences about the probability of possible outcomes in the *future* is the main goal of inferential statistics. This chapter provides an overview of basic concepts and methods that underlie descriptive statistical techniques; this forms a preliminary basis for the discussions of probability theory and statistical inference in Chapters 7 and 8.

TYPES OF DATA

Before undertaking the analysis of a data set, it is important for a researcher to know the properties of the *measurement scale* used to represent the variables under study and the manner of their distribution. As we noted in the previous chapter, not all data collected share the same qualities. Enumerating the spoken opinions of jurors about "guilt" or "innocence" in a court of law is not the same as measuring the acoustic spectra of their various speech sounds. Data of the first type are best represented by *frequency counts*, whereas only the second type of data possess properties amenable to formal mathematical operations.

Nominal and Ordinal Data

Frequency data are representative of the kind of distributions in which observations have been (1) placed in certain categories or (2) arranged in a meaningful order.

As clinicians we may be interested in describing various individuals or groups within our work settings according to certain qualitative categories such as children/adults, male/female, normal/impaired, and improvement/no improvement. Observations that can only be named and counted are called **nominal data.** Such data are sometimes described as **dichotomous** in nature because they involve "either/or" judgments about the presence or absence of a particular quality. Although such data may allow for some degree of numerical representation in terms of the frequency of the observations that fall within a given category, they have little or no quantitative meaning. For example, we can arbitrarily assign the number 1 to males and the number 2 to females as a means of designating the quality of gender. The reversal of the order of the two numbers would not make any difference in the type of gender involved.

Nominal data are commonly represented in various diagrams, charts, and graphs that illustrate the frequency or relative frequency (percentage) of observations that fall within certain categories or groups. For example, Figure 6.1 illustrates the use of a **pie diagram** to summarize the results of a survey of audiologists in the state of California who were asked about their desire to upgrade their level of professional training to the Doctor of Audiology (AuD) degree. Data were coded simply in terms of the percentage of yes or no responses. The results of the study can be readily interpreted to mean that the most frequently expressed desire among the audiologists was to upgrade their level of professional competence through additional education.

To summarize the major characteristics of a nominal scale, it can be said that:

- It classifies without arranging data in a logical order.
- Data categories are mutually exclusive in that a numerical value can belong to one and only one category.

In addition to placing observations into particular categories, we often are interested in arranging them in relation to one another. Unlike the nominal scale, ordinal measurement involves the ranking or logical ordering of categories. For example, should one wish to explore factors contributing toward student decisions in selecting a particular graduate program, the study might be done by devising an appropriate questionnaire. Figure 6.2 illustrates the actual results of such a study completed by Lass and his associates (1995) in

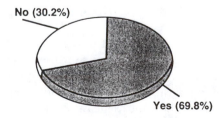

Figure 6.1. Desire to upgrade to AuD (N=494).

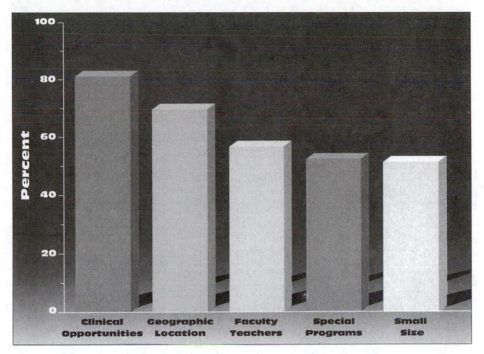

Figure 6.2. Illustration of a bar graph.

which students in communication disorders at several universities were asked to rank the importance of five factors in selecting a training program. A **bar graph** was used to depict the findings so that the percentage of students who considered a factor to be important was displayed on the vertical axis **(ordinate),** whereas the factors themselves were displayed along the horizontal axis **(abscissa).** Typically, in using a bar graph, the variable of interest **(X)** is scaled on the horizontal axis, whereas the tabulated results for the **(Y)** variable are depicted on the vertical axis. In terms of the results shown in Figure 6.2, the factor of clinical opportunities was ranked most important followed by geographic location, faculty/teachers, special programs, and small size, respectively.

Trend charts can also be used to illustrate frequencies or percentages of change in a data set arranged in a temporal or developmental order. In a study by Shriberg and his associates (1994) of speech sound normalization, " . . . the processes and behaviors by which speech become normally articulated over time," was examined in two groups of phonologically impaired children: those who "normalized" and those who failed to "normalize" sound productions over a one-year period. Figure 6.3 illustrates the results of this study for three categories of consonant comparisons from the *original* profiles of these children and ranked according to their developmental order of emergence (early, middle, or late). Visual inspection is suggestive of "intertwined trends" in the data for each category of sounds tested. The validity of this observation was supported by the failure of the researchers to uncover statistically significant differences between the normalized and nonnormalized groups of a specific profile of speech sound development that might otherwise have discriminated among them.

To summarize the features of an ordinal scale:

- Data are arranged in a distinctive order.
- Data categories are mutually exclusive.

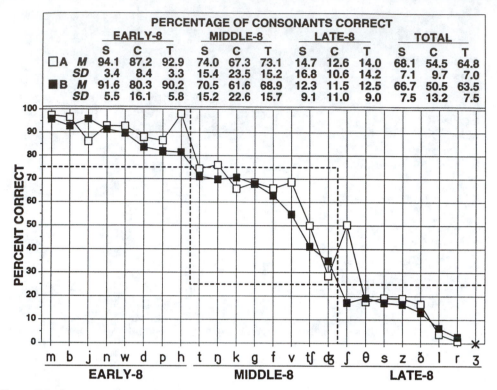

Figure 6.3. Consonants comparison for children who normalized (Group A) and for those who did not normalize (Group B).

- Data categories are logically ranked on the basis of the amount of the characteristic possessed.

Interval and Ratio Data

An **interval scale** of measurement possesses two added features that are missing from the nominal and ordinal scale. Interval measurements are characterized by both equal intervals between data points and an arbitrary zero point. Whereas nominal and ordinal scales involve the measurement of **discrete variables,** those that can only be represented by integers (e.g., whole numbers 1, 2, 3, . . .), interval and ratio scales can represent **continuous variables** *theoretically capable* of taking on any value, including fractional units of measurement (e.g., 1.2, 1.22, 1.23, . . .). In actual practice, continuous data are often rounded to the nearest appropriate value.

As noted in the previous chapter, interval scales contain an equal amount of distance between any two comparable points of measurement along the scale. Relating this fact to many tests involving psychological measurement, we could say, for example, that the difference between 90 and 100 points of intelligence is equal to the difference between 100 and 110 points of intelligence. Although some interval scales may contain an arbitrary zero point, such a designation is actually without meaning. Thus, in the same way that it would make no sense to conclude that the zero point on the Fahrenheit or Celsius scale means "no temperature," the idea of finding a living human without any measurable intelligence, personality, motivation, or language is equally implausible.

Nevertheless, it is often the case that both clinicians and researchers count the frequency of correct and incorrect responses without understanding whether or not the units of behavioral measurement are truly equal. For example, in the measurement of stuttering, one may not know the exact quantitative relation between one moment of stuttering and another, as these might be perceived and recorded by an observer. Yet, in many investigations, such disfluencies are often counted, averaged, and treated statistically as though they were the same. Similar dilemmas arise in the perceptual rating of other types of communication disorders in which the assumption of equal intervals in the scale of measurement is tenuous. Too often, the summated ratings of a **Likert-type scale** (e.g., 1= very mild, 2= mild, 3= moderate, 4= severe, 5= very severe) are treated statistically as though the intervals between these numerical values are equal when there may be no established basis for this conclusion. The principle to remember is that, as much as possible, assumptions about the applicability of any measurement scale should be consistent with the characteristics of the variables being measured. Unless equality between intervals can be determined, there is no basis for determining mathematical relations in a data set. Furthermore, regardless of the type of mathematical operations that might be permissible, good judgment must always be exercised in the interpretation of a data set. To conclude on the basis of a general test score that a person with a measured IQ of 100 is twice as intelligent as another individual having an IQ of 50 would do little to enlighten our understanding of specific differences in their cognitive abilities.

In summary, the major features of an interval scale are:

- It has distinctive and logically ordered data categories.
- Data categories are mutually exclusive.
- Comparable differences between any two points on the scale are equal regardless of their position along the line of data points.
- An arbitrary zero point in the scale denotes neither the presence of a starting point for measurement nor the absence of the quality being measured.

A ratio scale not only allows numbers to be classified, ordered, and linearly specified at equal intervals, but also contains an absolute zero starting point. Measurements of length or weight are examples of physical attributes that can be interpreted using the ratio scale. Starting at zero, we can say that four inches is exactly twice two inches; the same could be said for four pounds as compared to two pounds. Thus, ratio scales permit not only the addition and subtraction of measurement units but also their division and multiplication both as whole numbers or fractions. Although infrequently used in the study of most psychological phenomenon (Stevens, 1960), certain psychophysical procedures, as in the **method of constant stimuli,** do incorporate ratio scales of measurement. This particular method requires that several comparison stimuli be paired at random with a fixed standard. The observer is required to judge whether each comparison is greater or less than the fixed standard. Relevant examples of this procedure might include studies of loudness or pitch in which listeners have scaled these perceptions according to fractional units of measurement called the *sone* and *mel*, respectively.

ORGANIZING AND PORTRAYING DATA

A convenient way to begin summarizing an unorganized set of data is with a frequency table. Suppose we wish to determine the vocabulary comprehension of first grade students in a particular elementary class using the Peabody Picture Vocabulary Test-Revised (PPVT-R) (Dunn and Dunn, 1981). The following is a sample of scores that might be found:

Peabody Picture Vocabulary Scores
(30 First Grade Students)

100 87 84 100 98 89 67 115 80 76
72 70 91 110 94 79 86 91 93 105
83 89 92 84 100 81 105 86 95 80

As these scores are presently arranged, they provide the reader with little useful information. In order to make better sense of this **ungrouped data,** the first step is to arrange the scores into a frequency table. Such a table provides a convenient format for summarizing and presenting data within a series of predetermined **class intervals** along with a **tally** of the number of observations that fall within each class interval.

An illustration of a frequency table and tally of the data shown above is provided in Table 6.1. Also illustrated are the class intervals into which the data are grouped. In deciding the size and number of class intervals to be used in an investigation, chief among the factors to consider is the *degree of detail* that is desired. Greater detail in describing data is provided by smaller class intervals, whereas larger interval sizes are useful should the investigator wish to achieve greater condensation of data. Thus, the selection of a particular class interval depends on the goals of the investigation and the purposes that the data will serve.

Generally, 10 to 20 class intervals are used to portray data in research studies. A convenient method for determining the size of a class interval is based on the following:

$$\text{Interval Size} = \frac{\text{highest score} - \text{lowest score}}{\text{number of class intervals}}$$

Using this method, the **range** of scores (highest and lowest) is simply divided by the number of class intervals selected for use. Given the raw ungrouped data that we listed previously, we note that the high score achieved on the PPVT-R was 115 and the low score was 69.

To find the interval size for about 10 class intervals, we would calculate the following:

$$\frac{115 - 69}{10} = 4.6$$

Rounding the decimal to the nearest place, the class interval size is 5.

Table 6.1.
Frequency Distribution of Hypothetical Test Scores Obtained on the Peabody Picture Vocabulary Test-Revised (PPVT-R)

Class Interval	Exact Limits	Midpoint	Tally	Frequency	Cumulative Frequency	Relative Frequency (in %)
115–119	114.5–119.5	117		0	0	0.00
110–114	109.5–114.5	112	||	2	2	6.67
105–109	104.5–109.5	107	|||	3	5	10.00
100–104	99.5–104.5	102	||||	4	9	13.33
95–99	94.5–99.5	97	|||||	5	14	16.67
90–94	89.5–94.5	92	||||||	6	20	20.00
85–89	84.5–89.5	87	||||	4	24	13.33
80–84	79.5–84.5	82	||	2	26	6.67
75–79	74.5–79.5	77	||	2	28	6.67
70–74	69.5–74.5	72	|	1	29	3.33
65–69	64.5–69.5	67	|	1	30	3.33
60–64	59.5–64.5	62		0	30	0.00
				n = 30		**100.00**

In some cases, an investigator may wish to transform the data of a grouped frequency distribution into a **relative frequency distribution.** Such a distribution shows the percentage of scores that fall within each class interval. This can be determined by dividing the frequency of scores falling within each interval by the size of the sample (n) and multiplying the result by 100. For example, in the case of the frequency data found in Table 6.1, the results indicate that 6.67% of the cases achieved language scores falling within the 110–114 interval.

Graphic Displays of Frequency Distributions

Previously, we noted that numerically discrete data, as found on nominal or ordinal scales, are often presented graphically by means of a bar chart with spaces between the horizontal bars to depict separate categories or different ranks. Continuous data, on the other hand, are often displayed as **histograms** that are much like bar charts in their visual appearance, except the data are partitioned along the abscissa (horizontal or X axis) so as to fall within several equal class intervals. As in the case of the bar graph, the frequencies of occurrence are shown on the ordinate (vertical or Y axis).

Figure 6.4 is a histogram of the grouped data shown in Table 6.1. Scores are depicted in terms of the percentages of cases falling within a particular interval. The same data are also graphically portrayed in the form of a **frequency polygon.** The latter figure is a line graph that can be used in portraying all types of scaled measurements with the exception of nominal data. Such a graph is formed by connecting the midpoint of each class interval with straight lines.

Although graphs can be useful in providing a visual and readily interpretable summary of data, they can also convey a misleading impression if not thoughtfully constructed. Figure 6.5 contains two line graphs that represent an identical data set. Both reflect a decrement in the relative frequency of stuttering that might occur during the repeated oral reading of the same passage (adaptation effect) by a hypothetical group of stutterers. However, as can be seen, by extending the length of the ordinate and shortening the length of

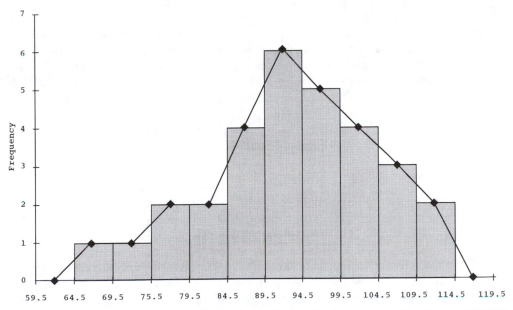

Figure 6.4. Histogram of hypothetical test scores on the Peabody Picture Vocabulary Test-Revised (PPVT-R).

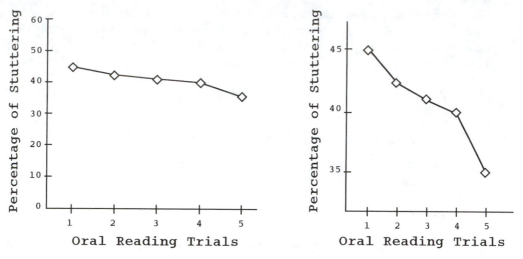

Figure 6.5. Two line graphs depicting the same hypothetical data: the percentage of stuttering during five oral reading trials.

the abscissa in the second graph, the impression of a greater decline in the frequency of stuttering is thereby conveyed. Although there are no specific standards for constructing a graph according to a uniform size or scale, the graph should convey an impression that accurately reflects the data it is intended to represent. The following additional guidelines are offered in preparing and evaluating the utility of tables, charts, and graphs:

- First, all such means of displaying and summarizing data should be made as simple as possible and easy to understand by conveying only the essential facts.
- The title of a table should be stated at the top of a horizontal line that extends the length of the table, preceded by a number reflecting its consecutive order in the article (Table 1, 2, 3, etc.) or book chapter, e.g., Table 1.1, 1.2, 1.3, etc.). Numerical information is placed below this line in clearly labeled rows and columns.
- The same need for clarity obviously applies in constructing graphs in which titles are typically placed at the bottom instead of at the top of the figure. This is a logical placement because, unlike tables that are read from the top down, graphs are usually read from the bottom to the top. As with tables, figures should be consecutively numbered, and all of the variables depicted must be identified using distinctive symbols, legends, and keys.
- All such methods of data presentation should be self-explanatory while serving the primary purpose of supplementing rather than substituting for cogent narrative descriptions of the research findings.

Shapes of Frequency Distributions

Histograms and polygons are used, in part, to gain some idea of the shape of a frequency distribution. As shown in Figure 6.6, the **normal distribution curve** is bell shaped with data points symmetrically distributed along a horizontal line to the left and right of center. Several departures from this normal shape also are shown. Asymmetrical distributions are said to be **skewed.** A **negatively skewed distribution** is one in which the tail points to the left (negative) side of the curve, signifying that the proportion of high scores in the distribution is greater than for low scores. Conversely, a **positively skewed distribution** is found in cases in which the tail points to the right (positive) side because the frequency of

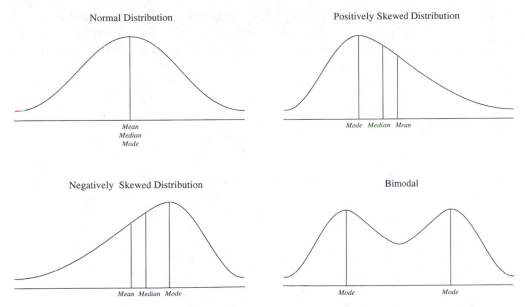

Figure 6.6. Various shapes of frequency distribution curves depicting relationships among different measures of central tendency.

low scores greatly outnumbers that of high scores in the distribution. A **bimodal distribution** curve characterized by the presence of two modes is suggestive of two distinct populations. In cases in which a distribution is not **homogeneous,** serious misinterpretations of data are possible. For example, if we set out to test the knowledge of graduate students at a particular college or university about certain communication disorders, and this population was made up partly of students with an undergraduate background in that field and partly of students having no academic preparation, a bimodal curve might result.

As we shall see in Chapter 8, populations that lack **homogeneity** in a distribution can limit or contraindicate the application of some types of inferential statistical procedures to the analysis of data sets.

CENTRAL TENDENCY OF DATA

In representing frequency distributions numerically, researchers are commonly interested in the extent to which scores cluster around the center of a distribution.

Measures of the Center

Measures of central tendency that represent the average size of a frequency distribution include the **mean** (the arithmetic average value), the **median** (the mid-score value), and the **mode** (the most frequently occurring value).

Suppose a researcher is interested in comparing the performance of five groups of subjects (A,B,C,D,E) on a test of Auditory Sequential Memory (ASM). Assume that the following scores were obtained (higher scores indicate better memory performance).

Group	A	7,	5,	4,	4			
Group	B	6,	8,	10,	4,	9,	5,	8,	6
Group	C	3,	7,	9,	5,	6			
Group	D	9,	10,	8					
Group	E	1,	0,	4,	4				

To answer questions such as "Does group A have better memory than group B?" or "Which group shows the lowest score?," data values representing the performance of each group would be needed. This one numerical measure, called a measure of **central tendency,** can be used to represent where a particular group of scores in a distribution "stands out." As mentioned previously, there are three different measures of central tendency (mean, median, mode) that can be used to represent what is sometimes called the *"center of gravity"* in a data set. The most important thing to determine is which measure can *best be used* for this purpose.

The Mean

The mean is known as the **arithmetic average** of a set of data values. The formula for calculating the mean is the ratio of the total sum of data values to the total number of subjects, denoted by **N (population size)** or **n (sample size).** Symbolically, the general formula for the mean is:

$$\mu = \Sigma X / N \qquad \text{(population mean)}$$

$$\bar{X} = \Sigma X / n \qquad \text{(sample mean)}$$

where Σ (sigma)represents "the sum of"
$\quad$ **X** represents "score"
$\quad$ μ (mu) specifies the mean from the population of scores
$\quad$ $\bar{X}$ (X bar) specifies the mean from the sample of scores.

For purposes of calculation, there is no difference between μ and $\bar{X}$. Thus, the mean for the group D is given by $(9+10+8) / 3 = 27 / 3 = 9$.

The mean can also be calculated from *grouped* data by dividing the product of the midpoint of the class interval and its corresponding frequency by the sample size (n). Let us now illustrate this particular calculation using the midpoint values for PPVT-R scores shown in Table 6.1. The steps in calculating the mean of our grouped data are as follows:

Step 1. Construct a table to include the midpoint (X), frequency (f), and the product of X and f (X · f). (See Table 6.2.)

Table 6.2.
The Product of Hypothetical Midpoint Values and Their Corresponding Frequencies on the Peabody Picture Vocabulary Test-Revised (PPVT-R)

X	f	X·f
117	0	0
112	2	224
107	3	321
102	4	408
97	5	485
92	6	552
87	4	348
82	2	164
77	2	154
72	1	72
67	1	67
62	0	0
Σ	30	2795

Step 2. Enter the appropriate values into the standard formula for calculating the mean of grouped data. The formula is given by:

$$\overline{X} = \frac{\Sigma \overline{X} \cdot f}{n}$$

Hence, after entering the appropriate values into the above formula, $\overline{X} = $ **93.17.**

As a general rule, the mean is preferred over other measures of central tendency because of its greater accuracy and reliability in representing a data set and its suitability for a wider range of arithmetic computations. However, two qualifications to this statement are important to consider in the evaluation of any data set. First, the *normal* shape of the distribution about its center ought to be *symmetrical* so that the mean closely approximates the values obtained for other measures of central tendency as discussed below. As noted previously, if the distribution is relatively *skewed* in either a positive or negative direction, the mean may not be a good reflection of central tendency because of the biasing effects of extreme scores. Second, it is important to consider the scale of measurement as appropriate for a particular data set. The mean is best applied in cases in which the data can be assumed to have at least interval characteristics that are subject to quantitative manipulation.

The Median

The **median** is the mid-value in a distribution of scores. The easiest way to identify the median is to rearrange all data values in order of magnitude (from smallest to largest). One must be sure to list all data values even though some values may repeat more than once. Ordering group C's scores gives:

3,   5,   6,   7,   9

Next, one must determine whether or not N is odd. When N is odd, there exists a single value in the middle of the distribution. Symbolically, the location of the median is given by $((N+1)/2)$ number from the left. Therefore, $(5+1)/2 = 6/2 = 3^{rd}$ number from the left or the median of 6 for this distribution. When N is even, the location of the median is expressed as half-way between $(N/2)$ number and $((N/2)+1)$ number from the left. For example, should we wish to calculate the median of group A's distribution, all data values must first be arranged from smallest to largest, thereby yielding:

4,   4,   5,   7

Next, we determine two numbers that correspond to $(N/2) = (4/2) = 2^{nd}$ and $(N/2) + 1) = 3^{rd}$ from the left. They are 4 and 5, respectively. We then average 4 and 5, or $(4 + 5)/2 = 4.5$. The median is 4.5, although 4.5 did not appear in the original data set.

As in the case of the mean, it is also possible to calculate the median from grouped scores shown in Table 6.1. The steps for this calculation are as follows:

Step 1. Find (1) the lower exact limit of the interval containing $n \cdot (.50)$, denoted by II; (2) the cumulative frequency of the interval below the one containing $n \cdot (.50)$, denoted by cf_b; (3) the frequency of the interval containing $n \cdot (.50)$, denoted by f_i; and (4) the width of the class interval, denoted by w.

Step 2. Enter the appropriate values into the standard formula for calculating the median of grouped data. The formula is given by:

$$\text{Median} = \text{ll} + \left[\frac{n \cdot (.50) - cf_b}{f_i} \right] \cdot w$$

Thus, after entering the appropriate values into the above formula, the median is equal to 90.17.

Because the median is less sensitive than the mean to the biasing influence of extreme scores in a data set, it is best used when a distribution is known to be asymmetrical or when its shape is otherwise unknown. The median is particularly suitable for scales of measurement having ordinal characteristics and when the validity of assumptions about equality in the size of the intervals between data points is questionable.

The Mode

The **mode** is constituted by the data value in a set of scores that occurs most frequently. By definition, the mode is represented by a number that must occur more than once. The mode could represent more than one data value if (1) there is a tie, and (2) each value occurs at least twice. Referring to the ASM scores previously listed for group A, the data value 4 occurred most frequently (twice). Therefore, 4 is the modal score for this distribution. On the other hand, there is a tie for the most frequently occurring value in the distribution of scores of group B. Two values, 6 and 8, occurred equally often and, in this case, both values are identified as modes. Thus, although it is common for most distributions to contain exactly one mode, it is possible for more than one mode to exist. A distribution having one mode is called **unimodal.** A distribution having two modes is called **bimodal.** For groups C and D, no mode can be said to exist because no value occurred more than once in either case.

As an index of central tendency, the mode often provides a crude and limited representation of the characteristics of a distribution as compared to the mean and median. This is true because, in some cases, the mode may be the lowest or highest value in a distribution. For example, the following three distributions have the same mode:

Group F	6,	6,	7,	8,	9,	10
Group G	0,	1,	2,	3,	6,	6
Group H	6,	6,	25,	26,	27,	28

As can be seen, the differences in the magnitude of the scores in each group are quite large and not well represented by the mode. Furthermore, because the mode is extremely sensitive to fluctuations in the distribution, different samples from the same population can have widely divergent modes. For example, in the case of group H, if one of the 6's is changed to 28, the mode likewise becomes 28, swinging from the extreme low end to the high end of the distribution.

As the weakest measure of central tendency, the use of the mode is restricted to nominal scales of measurement and is seldom reported except in association with other indices of central tendency.

VARIABILITY OF DATA

In the nineteenth century, the German mathematician Carl Gauss formulated the **"law of errors,"** which holds that the majority of repeated measurements made on the same subject *normally* cluster about the center of a distribution to form a bell-shaped curve with progressively fewer values dispersed symmetrically toward the tail ends on the left and right of center. A distribution that conforms to this shape is suggestive of good measurement reliability. If measurements are made on a number of individuals, they can be said to constitute a **homogeneous group** provided there is little variability among scores. More specifically, the scores should follow a predictable bell-shaped pattern of distribution with the majority of values clustering in the center.

Measures of Variability

Three important measures of variability that describe the shape of the distribution include (1) the **range** (the difference between the highest value and the lowest value); (2) the **variance** (the mean of the squared deviation from the mean); and (3) the **standard deviation** (the square root of the variance). The range is the difference (span) between the lowest and highest value in a distribution. However, like the mode, the range is extremely sensitive to fluctuations in a data set because, with the exception of the two extreme scores (the lowest and highest values), all other scores in the distribution are completely neglected. Therefore, another measure of dispersion is needed that can take into account the magnitude of *every* value of a distribution, not just the two extremes.

Mathematically, this measure of variance must calculate the **deviation** (the difference between each data value and the mean) and the **mean of these deviations.** For a population, the mean of these deviation scores is expressed as $\Sigma(X - \mu) / N$. For group D, $\Sigma(X - \mu) / N$ is given by:

$$\frac{(9 - 9) + (10 - 9) + (8 - 9)}{3} = 0$$

$$\left(\text{because } \mu = \frac{9 + 10 + 8}{3} = 9\right).$$

In fact, the sum of the deviations from the mean is always equal to zero. This is because the values above the mean must have positive deviations and the values below the mean must have negative deviations, resulting in a kind of mathematical cancellation effect. This problem surely affects the status of the mean as the "center of gravity" for the distribution. As a result, a solution is required to deal with this zero-sum deviation to confirm the fact that *"The more spread out the distribution, the larger the mean deviation from the mean."*

A solution is found in squaring each deviation from the mean and summing these squared deviation scores. The result is called the **mean squared deviation from the mean,** symbolically expressed as $\Sigma(X - \mu)^2 / N$, or simply called **variance(σ^2).** Therefore, with the data values of group D,

$$\sigma^2 = \Sigma(X - \mu)^2 / N = \frac{(9 - 9)^2 + (10 - 9)^2 + (8 - 9)^2}{3} = \frac{2}{3} = .67$$

where σ^2 represents *population variance* and is pronounced as "sigma square."

The formula for sample variance, denoted by s^2, is given by:

$$s^2 = \frac{\Sigma(X - \overline{X})^2}{n - 1}$$

The variance is quite useful for ratio measures but has one disadvantage. Large deviations in values farthest from the mean may outscore small deviation in values nearest to the mean. Squaring a large deviation would result in a disproportionately greater value than squaring a small deviation. This disadvantage in the use of variance as a measure of dispersion can be repaired (or compensated for) simply by taking the square root. The resulting value is called the **standard deviation,** denoted by σ (for a population) or **s** (for a sample). The standard deviation is sometimes denoted by the symbols **SD** in describing the spread among a set of measurements about the mean. The standard deviation for the population and sample is calculated by one of the following formula:

$$\sigma = \sqrt{\Sigma\,(X - \mu)^2/N} = \sqrt{\sigma^2} \quad \text{(population SD)}$$

$$s = \sqrt{\frac{\Sigma(X - \overline{X})^2}{n - 1}} \qquad \text{(sample SD)}$$

The standard deviation is useful in indicating the position of data values that are this "mean distance" away from the mean μ or $\overline{X}$. However, the most practical use of the standard deviation can be observed in relation to a **normal distribution curve,** which has a characteristic bell shape (see Figure 6.7). In such a distribution, approximately 68.26% of the data values lie within one standard deviation from the mean, denoted by $(\mu - \sigma, \mu + \sigma) = .6826$; 95.44% of the data values lie $\pm\,2\sigma$ from the mean μ, denoted by $(\mu - 2\sigma, \mu + 2\sigma) = .9544$; and 99.74% of the data values lie $(\mu - 3\sigma, \mu + 3\sigma)$.

In general, regardless of the shape of the distribution, the standard deviation is the key measure of dispersion of scores.

Chebyshev's Theorem

According to Chebyshev's theorem, for any set of data, at least $100 \cdot (1 - (1\,/\,K)^2)\%$ of the data values are lying within K standard deviation of the mean, where $K > 1$.

Although many frequency distributions have different patterns of variation, it is true of all sets of data values that at least $100 \cdot (1 - (1/2)^2)\% = 75\%$ are lying within 2 standard deviations and at least $100 \cdot (1 - (1/3)^2)\% = 88.9\%$ are lying within 3 standard deviations from the mean. The importance of Chebyshev's theorem is that it helps guide us to where the major portion of the data values are located and how much variation there is in a set of data. A small standard deviation indicates that the data values are clustered near the mean. A large standard deviation indicates that the data values are widely dispersed about the mean.

Coefficient of Variation

To determine whether a set of data values has much variation (spread) or whether a number of measurements are precise, the ratio of the mean to the standard deviation is calculated. This value, called the **coefficient of variation,** is determined by the following:

The coefficient of variation = $100 \cdot (s/\overline{X})\%$.

For example, the coefficient of variation of the set $\overline{X} = 10$ and $s = 0.3$ is $100 \cdot (0.3/10) = 3\%$. This data set has very little variation. On the other hand, for the set $\overline{X} = 10$ and $s = 3$, the coefficient of variation is determined to be $100 \cdot 3/10 = 30\%$, suggesting that this latter data set is relatively varied.

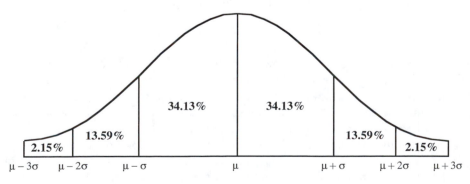

Figure 6.7. Areas under the standard normal curve.

Calculating Standard Scores and Percentile Ranks

The standard score, denoted by **Z,** refers to the number of standard deviation units away from the mean that its raw-score (X) equivalent lies. Standard scores are very useful in comparing raw scores in different distributions of the same shape. Raw scores (X) can be converted into standard scores (Z) and expressed as the number of standard deviations units away from the mean through the following formula:

$$Z = (X - \mu) / \sigma$$

A positive Z-score indicates that the raw score is above the mean, and a negative Z-score indicates that the raw score is below the mean. For example, given the standardization data of the PPVT-R, it is known that the national mean score (μ) for this test is 100 and the standard deviation (σ) is 15. (See Figure 6.8.)

Suppose a randomly selected subject has a PPVT-R score *above* the mean of 100, with a score of 124. What is his/her Z-score? Such a score can be calculated as follows:

$$Z = (124 - 100) / 15 = 1.6$$

The result indicates that the subject's score is 1.6 standard deviations above the mean. For ease of interpretation, it is common practice in the standardization of tests to convert standard scores into **percentile ranks.** A percentile rank is simply a number on a particular measurement scale at or below which a given percentage of the remaining distribution of scores can be found. Percentiles range from 1 to 100, with 50 being the median score in the distribution. For example, the 45th percentile in a distribution of scores would be interpreted as the score at or below which 45% of all scores in the distribution falls. Percentile ranks are highly useful in interpreting the results of many clinical tests and measuring instruments because they are readily interpretable indices of an individual's performance.

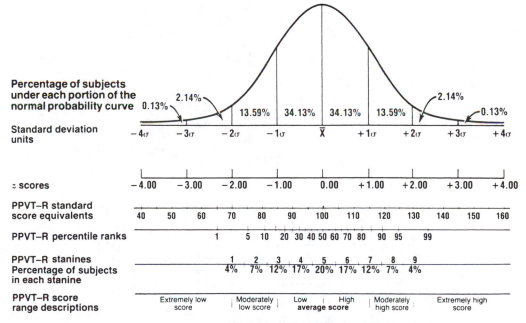

Figure 6.8. Interchangeability of different types of deviation norms when the distribution of raw scores is normal, or has been normalized, as in the case of the PPVT-R. Peabody Picture Vocabulary Test-Revised. © 1981 by Lloyd M. Dunn and Leota M. Dunn. American Guidance Service, Inc., 4201 Woodland Road, Circle Pines, MN 55014-1796. Reproduced with permission of the authors. All rights reserved.

How do we determine the percentile rank for a raw score on the PPVT-R of 124, when the corresponding Z = 1.6? To answer this question, three important properties of a normal distribution must be understood. These are as follows:

1. The entire area under the curve is 100%.
2. The normal distribution curve is symmetrical around the center: Z = 0.
3. The percentage of data values between the mean and any given Z-score in a normal distribution can be derived through a Z-table like that found in Appendix C.1. Such a table consist of two major components, namely a Z score and the percentage of a distribution that falls between Z = 0 and some specific positive value for Z. This area is called a **table area,** as will be described more fully in relation to our example.

As we can see in Figure 6.9a, a Z-score of 1.6 appears on the positive side of a normal curve. The shaded area of the graph is the percentage of data values derived from the table for Z. This was determined by consulting Appendix C.1. A portion of a Z table applicable to our example is shown in Figure 6.9b. More specifically, the percentage of the distribution that falls between Z = 0 and Z = 1.6 was derived by locating:

1. The number in the left hand column of the Z table that contains the same units and tenth's digits as 1.60 (1.6).
2. The number that has the same hundredth's digit, which, in the case of our example, is .00.
3. The intersection of the row containing 1.6 and the column .00. This number is .4452 or 44.52%.

In order to determine the percentile rank for the Z score in question, we then add 50% of the area to the left of Z = 0, yielding 44.52% + 50% = 94.52%. The result of our example can be interpreted to mean that approximately 94.52% of all PPVT-R scores fell at or below a score of 124.

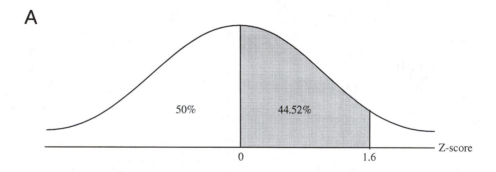

A, Interpreting a Z-score under the normal curve

B

Z	0.00	0.01	0.02	.	.	.
0.00						
0.10						
0.20						
.						
.						
.						
1.60	0.4452					

Figure 6.9. A, Interpreting a Z-score under the normal curve; **B,** Finding the corresponding area from a portion of a Z-table.

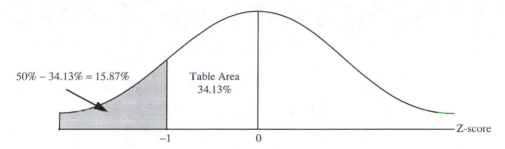

Figure 6.10. The area under the normal curve that falls at or below Z=−1.

To use another example, suppose we wish to determine the percentile rank for a PPVT-R score falling *below* the mean of 100, say a score of 85. First, we must convert the raw score X of 85 into the corresponding Z-score by the formula:

$$Z = (85 - 100) / 15 = -1$$

Second, we must draw a diagram of $Z = -1$ in order to better conceptualize the data in graphic terms (Figure 6.10).

Third, we find the **table area.** As noted previously, this area is defined as the percentage of a distribution that falls between Z=0 and a given Z score. In the case of our example, the table area is the percentage of the distribution that falls between the mean ($Z = 0$) and ($Z = -1$). We subtract it from 50% with the following result:

$$50\% - 34.13\% = 15.87\%$$

From this example, we can conclude that 15.87% of all PPVT-R scores fell at or below the score of 85.

Calculating Proportions from Two Standard Scores

Suppose we wish to calculate the percentage of all PPVT-R scores falling between two raw scores in a distribution. In illustrating how to accomplish this task, we will use two examples.

Case 1

In the first case, imagine that we have two raw scores, with one score, a score of 85, falling below the mean of 100 and the other, a score of 130, falling above the mean. Initially, in order to solve this problem, we must calculate the corresponding Z scores of 85 and 100, namely −1 and 2, respectively. When two Z-scores are on *different* sides of the mean, such as the area between $Z = -1.0$ and $Z = 2.0$, we add the two table areas (34.13% for $Z = 0$ and $Z = -1.0$; 47.72% for $Z = 0$ and $Z = 2.0$) (Figure 6.11). The area between $Z = -1$ and $Z = 2$ can be calculated as follows:

$$34.13\% + 47.72\% = 81.85\%$$

Hence, we can see that 81.85% of all PPVT-R scores fall within the interval of 85 and 130.

Case 2

Suppose that we have two raw scores. Let us say that one of these scores is 115 and the second score is 130. In this case, both of these scores are *above* the mean of 100. First, we must calculate the corresponding Z scores of 115 and 130. This results in Z scores of 1 and 2, re-

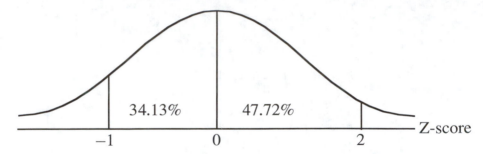

Figure 6.11. The area of the normal curve that falls between Z=−1 and Z=2.

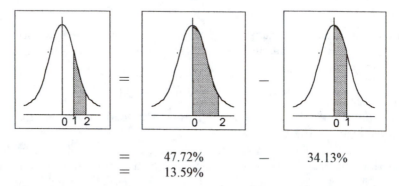

Figure 6.12. The area under the normal curve that falls between Z=1 and Z=2.

spectively. When two Z-scores are on the same side of the mean, we subtract the smaller table area from the larger table area. For example, in order to determine the percentages of Z = 1.0 and Z = 2.0, we must first consult the Z-table in Appendix C.1 to find the table area of Z = 1.0 (34.13%) and the table area of Z = 2.0 (47.72%). Next, we subtract 34.13% from 47.72% to find the percentage. The results of this calculation are graphically displayed in Figure 6.12.

It can be seen that 13.59% of all PPVT-R scores fall within the interval of 115 and 130. Note that the same technique is used in determining the percentage of data values between two negative Z-scores.

Calculating Raw Scores from Proportions

In constructing a test, a clinical researcher might wish to know the specific score that separates or "cuts off" a category of individuals from another category of individuals. For example, we might wish to use a certain percentage as a cut-off score to categorize certain speech-language-hearing disorders as mild, moderate, or severe. Suppose you are given a certain percentage of PPVT-R scores and asked to solve the raw score that distinguishes one such category from another. Given our knowledge that the bottom 10% of the test scores obtained on the PPVT-R falls within the *moderately low score range* (see Figure 6.8) when the mean (μ) and standard deviation (σ) of the test were 100 and 15, respectively, then what is the cut-off raw score for this range? In order to answer this question, we must first draw a diagram, like that illustrated in Figure 6.13.

Next, we need to determine the table area. From the above figure, it can be seen that the table area is 40%. In order to find the corresponding Z value that contains this particular table area, we will need to look up the closest table area to 40% in a Z Table like that

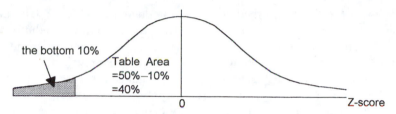

Figure 6.13. The area under the normal curve that represents the bottom 10% of the distribution.

found in Appendix C.1. By consulting Appendix C.1, one can determine that the closest value to 40% (.4000) is .3997 or 39.97%. This value corresponds to a Z score of 1.28. Because the desired raw score appears on the negative side, Z = 1.28 must be interpreted as Z = −1.28. Next, substitute all numbers into the appropriate places of a Z-score formula and solve for X:

$$-1.28 = (X - 100) / 15$$
$$X = (-1.28) \cdot 15 + 100$$
$$= 80.8$$

Therefore, given these data, the hypothetical cut-off score for the *moderately low score range* of the PPVT-R is 80.8. It is noteworthy that this particular value closely approximates the actual cut-off score for the identical range on the PPVT-R test.

DESCRIBING RELATIONSHIPS AND PREDICTING OUTCOMES: CORRELATION AND REGRESSION

Thus far, several descriptive statistical methods have been reviewed that are useful in summarizing observations on a single variable or **univariate** characteristic of a sample. However, it is often the case that an investigator wishes to describe or predict the relationship between two variables (**bivariate relationship**) or more (**multivariate relationship**). This can be accomplished by means of correlation and regression techniques.

Although the overall goals of correlation and regression methods bear close resemblance, these techniques must be distinguished as they apply to different types of sampling procedures and to the definition of variables in an experiment. Generally, we can say that if the main goal of an experiment is to simply examine the association between two or more variables without regard to distinguishing between the independent and dependent variable, then correlational methods are used. If the specific goal is to predict one variable from another, then regression analysis methods are the better choice.

To illustrate some of the distinguishing features of correlation and regression more clearly, suppose we obtain two sets of observations on a group of children, in which values of X represent scores on a language comprehension measure, such as hearing vocabulary, and Y reflects their performance on some standardized test of intelligence. Suppose further that we have no preconceived idea about the causal relations among these variables such that X is believed to influence the direction of Y or vice versa. In other words, for any individual in our sample, values of X and Y are merely assumed to represent joint or "coexisting" events that are in no way controlled or manipulated by the experimenter. In such a case, values of X and Y are *not* selected in advance of an experiment but are allowed to vary freely as inherently found in a sample of n individuals drawn from some population.

In contrast to correlational problems of the type just described, the use of regression techniques requires that the independent variable be selected and defined *prior* to an experiment. If the question asked concerns the degree to which Y (the dependent or criterion variable) can be predicted from X (the independent or predictor variable), then **simple linear regression** analysis can be used. Thus, in the case of our example, we might inquire about the extent to which certain measured levels of vocabulary comprehension are predictive of IQ. Had additional language measures been used as predictor variables, **multiple regression** methods might also be incorporated given the aims of a more comprehensive analysis. The concepts and statistical applications underlying correlation and regression problems are discussed in greater detail in the following sections.

Correlation

Correlational problems pertain to observations made under conditions in which an observed change in one variable appears to be associated with a concomitant change in another. Such variables form a joint distribution of data sets that are said to be **mutually dependent** or **related.** The following properties of correlational statistics are important to understand as a basis for their application.

1. **Linearity of correlations:** When two variables are plotted alongside one another in such a way that they follow a straight line, they are said to be linearly related. The correlation coefficient, denoted by **r**, describes a **linear relationship** between two variables. This means that a straight line can be drawn through the number of given points when a scatterplot of the joint variables is constructed. As shown in Figure 6.14, three main types

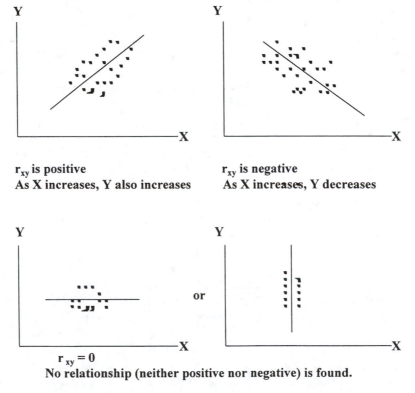

r_{xy} is positive
As X increases, Y also increases

r_{xy} is negative
As X increases, Y decreases

$r_{xy} = 0$
No relationship (neither positive nor negative) is found.

Figure 6.14. Three main types of correlational relationships.

of r can be observed, indicative of (1) a positive relationship; (2) a negative relationship; or (3) no relationship.

2. **Magnitude of correlations:** A quantitative index of the degree of dependence (relatedness) between variables is the **correlation coefficient.** The range of a correlation coefficient falls between -1 ($r = -1$, absolute negative) and $+1$ ($r = 1$, absolute positive). Very often, r can be translated into the shape of a linear equation. For example, $r = .50$ means that Y increases by .50 unit while X increases 1 unit. And $r = -.33$ means that Y decreases .33 unit while X increases 1 unit. If the absolute value of r, denoted by $|r|$, is greater than .80, then it is said to be a *strong correlation.* If $|r|$ is less than .40, then it is said to be a *weak correlation.* If $|r|$ falls between .40 and .80, it is said to be a *moderate correlation.* Lastly, as mentioned before, there is *no correlation* if $|r| = 0$. The closer the correlation is to 0, the weaker the relationship. The closer the correlation is to -1 or $+1$, the stronger the relationship between the variables.

3. **Correlations versus causation:** As we have emphasized in previous chapters, correlation coefficients can only be interpreted as indices of *association* between variables—not as evidence that one such variable is *causative* of the other. An amusing example might help the reader to keep this important fact in mind. Students in a research class taught by one of the authors of this text were once asked to list, on *separate* slips of paper, two variables that they would like to study using correlational methods. After making their choices, the slips were collated and placed in a hat; two slips then were randomly selected by each student, resulting in an interesting assortment of paired variables. One student had by chance selected two seemingly unrelated variables for study involving the number of passengers arriving on planes during a particular time of day at Boston's Logan International Airport and the number of births occurring around the same time in the City's hospitals. Subsequently, the results of the student's correlational study turned up a Pearson r of approximately .60, suggestive of a moderate association between the two variables. Perhaps the results reflected the efforts of anxious dads scampering home as quickly as possible to meet their newborns. More likely, because both variables involved time-related events, the results were merely indicative of a spurious association between them. In thinking about the meaning of correlations, remember the adage, "If you wait long enough, almost any thing can happen."

Calculation of the Pearson Product-Moment Correlation Coefficient

Let us now illustrate an application of correlational methods in the analysis of a hypothetical data set involving the association between hearing vocabulary scores and IQ scores. For this purpose, imagine that we have randomly selected a group of nine subjects, for whom scores on the Peabody Picture Vocabulary Test-Revised (PPVT-R) and the Stanford-Binet Intelligence Scale (SBIS) were obtained. Given both of these data sets consisting of X and Y, respectively, we assume that the test scores for each instrument forms a continuous distribution. It will be recalled that the values of such a distribution possess fractional numerical properties as measured on an interval or ratio scale. For data of this kind, the **Pearson Product-Moment Correlation** is a suitable technique for calculating the correlation of interest. The formula and steps involved in the computation of our example are given below:

Step 1. Draw a scatterplot like that shown in Figure 6.15 to verify that X and Y are linearly related.

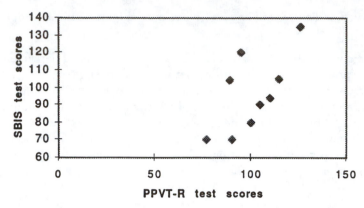

Figure 6.15. Scatterplot showing the relationship between hypothetical test scores obtained on the Standard Binet Intelligence Scale (SBIS) and the Peabody Picture Vocabulary Test-Revised (PPVT-R).

Step 2. Construct a table, as illustrated in Table 6.3, to include:

X = PPVT-R test scores   ΣX = Sum of X values
Y = SBIS test scores   ΣY = Sum of Y values
X² = Square of X values   ΣX² = Sum of square of X
Y² = Square of Y values   ΣY² = Sum of square of Y
XY = Product of X and Y values   ΣXY = Sum of XY

Step 3. Enter the appropriate values into the standard formula for calculating the correlation coefficient. The formula for the Pearson Product-Moment Correlation Coefficient, denoted by **r**, is given by:

$$r = \frac{N(\Sigma XY) - (\Sigma X)(\Sigma Y)}{\sqrt{N(\Sigma X^2) - (\Sigma X)^2]\cdot [N(\Sigma Y^2) - (\Sigma Y^2]}}$$

Hence, after entering the appropriate values into the above formula, r= .69 (verify this number if desired).

As we noted previously, a correlation in this range is indicative of a moderate relationship between two variables. Based on the analysis of our hypothetical data, the resulting coefficient is very close to results of actual studies that have collectively yielded a median correlation of .62 between the PPVT and SBIS (Dunn et al., 1981).

Table 6.3.
Calculation of the Pearson Product-Moment Correlation Coefficient Based on Hypothetical Data for PPVT-R Test Scores (X) abd SBIS Test Scores (Y).

X	Y	X²	Y²	XY
115	105	13225	11025	12075
105	90	11025	8100	9450
110	94	12100	8836	10340
95	120	9025	14400	11400
89	104	7921	10816	9256
126	135	15876	18225	17010
77	70	5929	4900	5390
100	80	10000	6400	8000
90	70	8100	4900	6300
ΣX = 907	ΣY = 868	ΣX² = 93021	ΣY² = 87602	ΣXY = 89221

N = 9

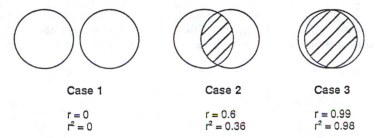

Case 1   Case 2   Case 3

$r = 0$ $r = 0.6$ $r = 0.99$
$r^2 = 0$ $r^2 = 0.36$ $r^2 = 0.98$

Figure 6.16. Illustration of the degree of the common variance shared by three cases.

Correlation as an Index of Common Variance

As we noted earlier, a correlation coefficient is simply an index of the relationship between variables. It does not express the amount of variance that X and Y share. However, when r is squared (r^2), it can be interpreted as the proportion of variability in Y that can be predicted based on a knowledge of X, or vice versa. The actual percentage of variance in Y accounted for by X can be found by the following formula:

% of variance in Y accounted for by knowing X = $r^2 \cdot 100$

Therefore, based on our previous example, with a correlation of .69, the proportion of variance in Y (SBIS) predictable from X (PPVT-R) is 47.61% because $(.69)^2 \cdot 100 = 47.61$. The common variance shared by X and Y variables is illustrated graphically in Figure 6.16.

Other Correlation Techniques

The basic assumption underlying the use of the Pearson r is that both variables reflect a continuous distribution that is normally distributed. More specifically, the shape of the distribution for both variables should conform to the bell curve, lacking skewness. If this assumption is violated, a nonparametric correlation technique should be used as an alternative to the Pearson r.

    When the level of measurement for both data sets is ordinal, the **Spearman Rank (Rho)** correlation coefficient, denoted by ρ, may be employed. Let us illustrate the application of this particular technique, as it might be used in determining the relationship between two components of stuttering severity, as defined on the Stuttering Severity Instrument (SSI) (Riley, 1986). Specifically, we will determine the correlation between two parameters of the SSI, namely (1) the physical concomitants of stuttering, e.g., distracting sounds and facial grimaces, and (2) the frequency of stuttering occurrences. The following steps are outlined to illustrate the actual calculation of the Spearman correlation coefficient based on some fictitious SSI results.

Step 1.   **Construct a table, as shown in Table 6.4, to include:**

     X = physical concomitant test scores, as defined
     Y = frequency of stuttering, as defined
    $\mathbf{X_r}$ = rank of X
    $\mathbf{Y_r}$ = rank of Y
     d = $X_r - Y_r$
   $\mathbf{d^2}$ = square of d
  $\mathbf{\Sigma d^2}$ = total sum of d^2
     N = number of pairs of ranks

Table 6.4.

Calculation of the Spearman Rank Correlation Coefficient Based on Hypothetical Data for Physical Concomitants of Stuttering as Measured (X) and Frequency of Stuttering Occurrences (Y).

X	X_r	Y	Y_r	d	d^2
3	5	14	8	−3	9
2	3	10	5	−2	4
1	1.5	8	3	−1.5	2.25
5	10	12	6	4	16
3	5	4	1	4	16
1	1.5	9	4	−2.5	6.25
4	8	6	2	6	36
4	8	18	10	−2	4
3	5	16	9	−4	16
4	8	13	7	1	1

N = 10

Σd^2 = 115

Step 2. Enter the appropriate values into the standard formula for calculating the correlation coefficient. The formula for the Spearman Rank Correlation Coefficient is given by:

$$\rho = 1 - \frac{6 \cdot (\Sigma d^2)}{N \cdot (N^2 - 1)}$$

Thus, after substituting the appropriate values into the formula above, ρ is equal to 0.33. This coefficient indicates that there is a weak positive correlation between X (physical concomitants) and Y (frequency of stuttering). This correlation is identical in magnitude to that actually found in the standardization of the SSI.

A number of alternative correlation techniques are available as appropriate for a particular scale of measurement. Some of the commonly used correlational techniques are listed in Table 6.5.

Regression

As noted previously, when the main goal of an investigation is to quantify the relationship between variables, correlation coefficients are the most useful tool for this purpose. How-

Table 6.5.

Types of Correlation and Their Statistical Applications

Type of Correlation	Statistical Application
• Pearson product-moment (r):	Two continuous or normally distributed variables on an interval or ratio scale.
• Spearman rank or rho (ρ):	Two discrete variables on an ordinal (rank order) scale. Nonparametric equivalent of the Pearson r.
• Contingency coefficient:	Two dichotomous variables on a nominal (categoric) scale.
• Point biserial r:	Two variables when one is on an interval scale and the second is on an ordinal scale.
• Multiple correlation:	One single variable and some combination of two or more other variables. Applications for parametric and nonparametric statistics.
• Partial correlation:	Two variables are studied while holding constant the influence of a third or several other variables.

ever, provided that the correlation observed between two data sets is reasonably high, next we might want to estimate individual scores on one of two correlated variables from scores obtained on the other. Such an estimate is made possible by the use of a **regression equation** to calculate what is called "*the best fit*" of the data points of the X and Y variables as they are scattered about a **regression line.**

The general equation for a regression line consists of the following three major components: (1) the slope; (2) the Y-intercept; and (3) a predicted score of Y. The sloping line shown in Figure 6.17 approximates the general configuration of a regression line. Each of the components of such a line are described below.

Slope

The slope of a line is sometimes called "average rate of change" or "the average ratio of Y to X," which means the amount of change in Y that corresponds to a change of one unit in X. For example, given the regression line shown in Figure 6.17, the statement "the slope equals 3" indicates that, on the average, a gain of 3 units in Y corresponds to a gain of 1 unit in X. The mathematical formula for determining the value of the slope (b) is given as

$$b = \frac{N(\Sigma XY) - (\Sigma X)(\Sigma Y)}{N(\Sigma X^2) - (\Sigma X)^2}$$

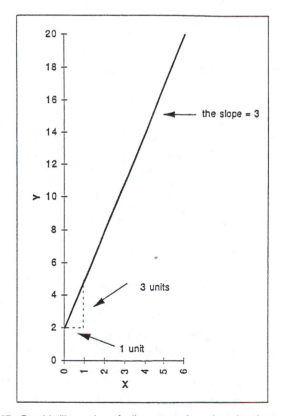

Figure 6.17. Graphic illustration of a linear equation when the slope equals 3.

Y-Intercept

The intercept of a line is defined as the value of Y when X equals 0. In other words, the Y intercept is the value of Y where the line intercepts (crosses) the Y axis. Thus, as shown in Figure 6.17, the average gain of 2 units along the Y axis, when X is equal to 0, corresponds to the term "Y intercept is equal to 2." The mathematical formula for determining the value of the Y intercept is given by:

$$a = \overline{Y} - b\overline{X}$$

Predicted score of Y: The regression line is used to estimate the value of Y for a given value of X. The mathematical equation of a regression line expresses a *functional relationship* between two variables X and Y. In predicting the value of Y from the value of X, we can say that "Y is a function of X." This equation is given by:

$$\hat{Y} = bX + a$$

where $\hat{Y}$ = predicted value of Y
  b = slope of the regression line
  a = Y-intercept of the regression line

Clinical Application of Regression

Let us now illustrate the use of linear regression techniques in predicting an individual's SBIS score from a test score obtained on the PPVT-R. For this purpose, assume that the PPVT-R score was found to be 103. Given this knowledge, how can we use this score to estimate the SBIS score obtained by the same individual? The following steps represent the calculation of the slope and Y-intercept using the data given in Table 6.3 and the appropriate formula for each parameter as noted above.

Step l.   Enter the appropriate values into the standard formula for calculating the slope and the Y-intercept.

$$b = 1.08 \text{ and } a = -12.4$$

Therefore, the general equation of the regression line that allows us to predict Y from X can be written as

$$\hat{Y} = 1.08X - 12.4$$

A graphic representation of the results from the above equation is shown in Figure 6.18.

Step 2.   Replace X in the equation above by the PPVT-R score of 103. This yields the predicted SBIS score (approximately 99). Given these hypothetical results, we can conclude that hearing vocabulary, as assessed by the PPVT-R, was a good predictor of intelligence, as measured by the SBIS.

In conclusion, there are many types of regression techniques in addition to simple linear regression that have application to a variety of clinical and research problems. In this chapter, we have illustrated the application of simple linear regression to estimate a criterion variable from a single predictor variable. However, there are several clinical and research problems that necessitate the use of more comprehensive regression techniques. As noted earlier, one of these methods, called multiple regression, permits the simultaneous estimation of a criterion variable from several predictor variables. Thus, instead of using only the scores obtained on the PPVT-R to predict IQ, we might have incorporated such other semantic language measures as found on the Clinical Evaluation of Language Fun-

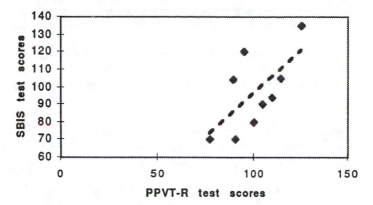

Figure 6.18. Scatterplot illustrating the line of best fit between hypothetical test scores obtained on the Stanford Binet Intelligence Scale (SBIS) and the Peabody Picture Vocabulary Test-Revised (PPVT-R).

damentals (CELF-R) and the Woodcock-Johnson Psycho-Educational Battery (WJ-R), among many others.

There are a number of *multivariate* techniques that can be used to predict a binary dependent variable from a set of independent variables. Among these, multiple regression techniques have numerous applications in answering a variety of clinical and research questions, such as: What factors in a client's history best predict a certain speech-language-hearing disorder? What clinical and laboratory data best identify patients with such disorders? What therapy procedures are most likely to predict favorable clinical outcomes? etc. On the other hand, such techniques have major limitations when the dependent variable has dichotomous values—e.g., an event either occurs or does not occur. In this situation, the assumptions required for performing multiple regression analysis, such as normality in the distribution of data, will be violated.

Another difficulty is that the predicted values cannot be calculated as *probabilities* falling in the interval between 0 and 1 (see Chapter 7). In this situation, another multivariate technique called **logistic regression** might be used instead. The mathematical derivation and illustration of the latter technique is beyond the scope of this chapter. Generally, it can be said that logistic regression is useful in estimating the probability that an event will occur when the independent variables in an experiment include both quantitative and nonquantitative measures and the criterion or outcome variable is dichotomous.

SELF-LEARNING REVIEW

descriptive
inferential
Descriptive

1. Two major categories of statistics are commonly identified as _____ and _____ techniques. _____ statistics are used for classifying, organizing, and summarizing a particular data set.

Frequency
categories
order

2. _____ data are representative of the kinds of distributions in which observations have been placed in certain _____ or arranged in a meaningful _____ .

nominal
dichotomous
presence
absence

3. Observations that can only be named and counted are called _____ data. Such data are sometimes described as _____ "either/or" judgments about the _____ or _____ of a particular quality.

classifies
order
mutually exclusive

ordinal
ranking
ordering

4. A nominal scale _____ without arranging data in a logical _____ . Its data categories are said to be _____ _____ in that a numerical value can belong to only one category.

5. Unlike the nominal scale, _____ measurement involves the _____ or logical _____ of data categories.

bar graph
ordinate
abscissa

6. A _____ _____ can be used to graphically depict the percentage of subjects who consider a certain factor to be important. Such a percentage is typically displayed on the vertical axis, or _____ , whereas the factors themselves are displayed along the horizontal axis, or _____ .

order
mutually exclusive
amount

7. Three characteristics of an ordinal scale are (1) data categories are arranged in a distinctive _____ ; (2) data categories are _____ _____ ; and (3) data categories are logically ranked on the basis of the _____ of the characteristic possessed.

equal
zero

8. An interval scale contains two added features missing from a nominal scale. These are (1) _____ intervals and (2) an arbitrary _____ point.

ratio
absolute

9. A _____ scale not only allows numbers to be classified, ordered, and linearly specified at equal intervals, but also contains an _____ zero point.

dichotomous
discrete
continuous

10. Although nominal and ordinal scales involve the measurement of _____ or _____ variables, both interval and ratio scales can represent _____ variables.

frequency

11. In order to organize ungrouped data in a logical manner, the first step is to arrange the scores within a _____ table.

Such a table provides a convenient format for summarizing the data within a series of predetermined _____ _____ .
The number of observations that fall within each class interval is called a frequency _____ .

class intervals
tally

12. In deciding the size and number of _____ _____ to be used in an investigation, chief among the factors to consider is the degree of _____ desired.

class intervals
detail

13. A convenient method for determining the size of a class interval is to _____ the _____ of scores by the number of class intervals.

divide
range

14. A _____ frequency distribution shows the percentage of scores that fall within each class interval. This can be determined simply by dividing the _____ of scores falling within each interval by the size of the _____ and multiplying the result by _____ .

relative
frequency
sample
100

15. Continuous data are often presented graphically as a _____ that is much like a _____ chart except the data are partitioned along the abscissa as to fall within _____ intervals.

histogram
bar
equal

16. A line graph that is useful in portraying all types of scaled measurements except nominal data is a _____ _____ . Such a graph is formed by connecting the _____ of the class intervals with a straight line.

frequency polygon
midpoints

17. The normal distribution curve is _____ -shaped with data symmetrically distributed to the _____ and _____ of _____ .

bell
left
right
center

18. A _____ skewed distribution is one in which the tail points to the _____ side of the curve. This signifies that the proportion of _____ scores in the distribution is greater than for _____ scores.

negatively
left
high
low

19. A _____ skewed distribution is found in cases where the tail points to _____ side of the curve because the frequency of _____ scores greatly outnumber _____ scores in the distribution.

positively
right
low
high

20. Two characteristics of frequency distributions that commonly are of interest to researchers relate to (1) the tendency for the scores to cluster around the _____ and (2) their degree of _____ or spread. The first characteristic is often summarized by measures of _____ _____ and second by measures of _____ .

center
dispersion
central tendency
variability

mean
median
mode

21. Measures of central tendency include the _____ (arithmetic average), the _____ (midscore value), and the _____ (most frequently occurring value).

symmetrical
central tendency
interval
quantitative

22. In using mean scores, two important qualifications are important to consider. First, the shape of the distribution should be _____ so as to approximate the values for other measures of _____ _____ . Second, the data should have _____ measurement characteristics that are subject to _____ manipulation.

middle
(N+1)/2

23. The median is the _____ value in a distribution of scores. Symbolically, the location of the median is given by _____ .

limit
cumulative
class interval

24. In order to calculate the median from grouped scores, we must find (1) the exact _____ of the interval containing n · (.50); (2) the _____ frequency of the interval containing n · (.50); and (3) the width of the _____ _____ .

median
asymmetrical
unknown

25. As an alternative to the mean, the _____ can best be used when the shape of a distribution is known to be _____ or when its shape is otherwise _____ .

mode
lowest
highest

26. The _____ is simply the score that occurs most frequently. It is the weakest measure of central tendency because, in some cases, it may be the _____ or _____ value in a distribution.

tie
twice
nominal

27. The mode could represent more than one data value if (1) there is a _____ and (2) each value occurs at least _____ . The mode is restricted to _____ data.

unimodal
bimodal
nominal
central tendency

28. A distribution having one mode is called _____ , whereas a distribution having two modes is called _____ . The use of the mode is restricted to _____ scales of measurement and is seldom reported except in association with other measures of _____ _____ .

law of errors
normally
bell

29. In the nineteenth century, the German mathematician Carl Gauss formulated the _____ _____ _____ , which holds that the majority of repeated measurements made on the same subject _____ cluster about the center of distribution to form a _____ -shaped curve.

homogeneous
variability

30. If measurements are made on a number of individuals, they can be said to constitute a _____ group provided there is little _____ among scores.

31. The range is the _____ between the lowest and highest values in a distribution. Like the mode, the range is extremely sensitive to _____ in a data set.

difference
fluctuations

32. Mathematically, the measure of variance must calculate the _____ and the _____ of the deviations of a data set.

deviation
mean

33. The rule of zero-sum deviation confirms the fact that "the _____ spread-out the distribution, the larger the _____ _____ from the mean."

more
mean deviation

$$\frac{\Sigma(X-\mu)^2}{N}$$

34. The population mean squared deviation from the mean is symbolically expressed as _____ , or the _____ .

variance

35. The disadvantage of using variance as a measure of _____ can be repaired by simply taking the _____ _____ . The resulting value is called the standard deviation.

dispersion
square root

36. The standard deviation is useful for indicating the _____ of data values that are this _____ _____ away from the _____ .

position
mean distance
mean

37. The most practical use of the standard deviation can be observed in relation to what is called a _____ _____ curve that has a characteristic bell _____ .

normal distribution
shape

38. In a normal distribution, approximately _____ % of the data values lie within one standard deviation from the mean, _____ % of the data values lie within two standard deviations from the mean, and _____ of the data values lie within three standard deviations from the mean.

68.26
95.44
99.74

39. The standard deviation is a key measure of _____ that can be used to determine the _____ _____ of an individual's score in relation to other group members'.

dispersion
percentile rank

40. According to Chebyshev's theorem, at least _____ % of the data values normally lie within 1.5 standard deviations from the mean.

55.6

41. The coefficient of variation of the set and $\overline{X} = 20$ s = 5 is _____ %, suggesting that the data set is relatively _____ .

25
varied

42. The standard score, denoted by _____ , expresses the number of _____ _____ units away from the mean.

z
standard deviation

43. A percentile rank is a number on a particular measurement

at
below
percentage

scale _____ or _____ which a given _____ of the remaining distribution of scores can be found.

symmetrical
100

44. The normal distribution curve is _____ around the center and the entire area under the curve is _____ %.

28.98
87.4

45. The percentage of all PPVT-R scores falling between 76 and 94 is approximately _____ %. The cut-off score for the bottom 20% of the test scores obtained on the PPVT-R is _____ (calculate by referring to text).

criterion
predictor

46. In correlational studies, the variable Y is called the dependent or _____ variable and X is called the independent or _____ variable.

mutually dependent
related

47. Correlational problems pertain to observations made under conditions in which an observed change in one variable appears to be associated with a concomitant change in another. Such variables form a joint distribution of data sets that are said to be _____ _____ or _____ .

r
linear
two
0.80
0.40

48. The correlation coefficient, denoted by _____ , describes a _____ relationship between _____ variables. If the absolute value of r, denoted by $|r|$, is greater than _____ , it is said to be a strong correlation. If $|r|$ is less than _____ , it is said to be a weak correlation.

variability
predicted

49. When r is squared (r^2), it can be interpreted as the proportion of _____ in Y that can be _____ based on a knowledge of X.

slope
y intercept
predicted

50. The general equation for a regression line consists of the following major components, namely (1) _____ , sometimes called the "average rate of change;" (2) _____ , defined as the value of Y when X = 0; and (3) _____ score of Y for a given value of X.

logistic
probability
dichotomous

51. Generally, it can be said that _____ regression is useful in estimating the _____ that an event will occur when the independent variables in an experiment include both quantitative and nonquantitative measures and the criterion or outcome variable is _____ .

Clinical Application

Suppose a clinician or researcher is interested in examining the relationship between some measure of receptive language ability (X) and a measure of reading achievement (Y). Some hypothetical results for such a study are given on the next page:

X	Y
100	110
95	85
105	105
125	111
90	107
118	99

For the receptive language ability scores, the mean $\overline{X}$ is _____, the median is _____, the mode is _____, the variance s^2 is _____, and the standard deviation s is _____ .

The Pearson Product-Moment correlation coefficient r between X and Y is calculated as _____ and the coefficient of determination r^2 is _____ . Therefore, the actual percentage of variance in Y accounted for by X is _____ %.

If the Spearman rank correlation technique was used for this hypothetical study, then the correlation coefficient ρ is _____.

The linear regression equation for predicting Y from X yields the slope of _____ and the Y intercept of _____ . The predicted Y score for a given X score of 110 is _____ .

105.5
102.5
none
183.5
13.5

.29
.084
8.4

0.31

.21
80.68
103.78

7. Probability: The Basis for Decision Making

In previous chapters, we introduced the concept of probability, which underlies the theory and methods of drawing statistical inferences in scientific research. The purpose of this chapter is to develop further the elementary rules for calculating probability as a basis for the principles of statistical inference discussed in the next chapter.

DEFINITION OF PROBABILITY

The word probability is an elusive concept that is difficult to define. In the common vernacular, we use the term "probably" to express the notion that some event is likely to happen or that a particular observation is likely to be true. Indeed, the manner in which we make most routine decisions throughout the day is predicated on the likelihood for certain outcomes. For example, we either carry an umbrella or leave it at home based on our personal reactions to the weather forecast. Some might make the decision to carry the umbrella only if the likelihood for rain is 90%. Based on a more conservative view, a 50% probability of rain might lead some individuals to take it along "just in case."

In a clinical sense, the term probability is akin to the concept of **prognosis.** According to Emerick and Hatten (1979), prognosis involves:

> . . . a prediction of the outcome of a proposed course of treatment . . . how effective treatment will be . . . accurate prognosis can help establish our credibility . . . the ability to predict with reasonable precision is the highest form of scientific achievement. (pp. 67–68)

Like clinicians, researchers attempt to make good decisions based on the findings of their studies. From a statistical perspective, there are several meanings of probability. Perhaps the best known of these is the classical view, also called the "frequentist," "objectivist," or

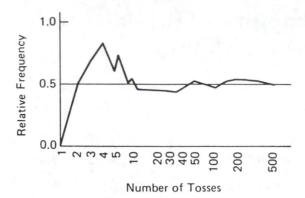

Figure 7.1. Given any number of coin tosses, the relative frequency of heads may differ from one-half but will approach this value in the long-run. Reprinted with permission from Leaverton, P.E. (1991). *A review of biostatics: A program for self-instruction.* (4th ed.) Boston: Little Brown and Company.

"a posteriori" view of probability. The **classical view** is based on a principle first developed by James Bernoulli in the eighteenth century. According to the so-called **Bernoulli theorem,** the relative frequency of an observed event will approximate its probable frequency of future occurrence if observed over an indefinitely long series of trials.

To understand the Bernoulli theorem in more concrete terms, imagine that you are asked to determine the probability of a tossed coin turning up "heads." In theory, provided that the coin is fair (unbiased), the probability of it turning up heads is 50%. Furthermore, the mathematical likelihood of the coin turning up heads will get closer and closer to 50% as the number of tosses increases. Thus, five tosses will typically yield results that conform with the expected outcome more often than one toss, 10 tosses will conform more often than five tosses, etc. (Figure 7.1). Nevertheless, it is important to understand that such outcomes can be predicted with only relative degrees of confidence. Although improbable, it is still possible that 100 tosses may yield a more equal distribution of heads and tails than, say, 500 or more tosses of the same coin.

PROBABILITY THEORY AND STATISTICAL INFERENCE

Just as chance can account for why a coin does not turn up heads or tails exactly 50% of the time when tossed, random variation must be considered when assessing the truth of our clinical observations and research findings. The fact that the future occurrence of an event can only be stated in relative terms is the basis for statistical inference.

Typically, the researcher begins with a theoretical proposition or hypothesis about the expected relative frequency of a particular observation or event as it might exist in a sample drawn from a population. For example, we might hypothesize about the degree to which an observed sample mean ($\overline{X}$) is representative of the population mean (μ) based on the probability of comparable findings in a long sequence of repeated trials or experiments. In fact, the sample mean might be greater or smaller than the population mean; it may be almost equal to, or quite different from, the population mean.

To determine the fairness of a coin in absolute mathematical terms, it would have to be tossed an infinite number of times—an obvious impossibility. Because of the same constraints, a theory or hypothesis can never be proved to be true in absolute terms. Nevertheless, the confidence that we can place in our data increases in proportion to sample size or the number (n) of observations made by the experimenter. The larger the sample n, the more confidence we can have in the credibility of our findings.

Table 7.1.
Common Qualifying Probabilities and Levels of Confidence

Qualifying Probability	Probability of Chance Error (Chance Differences)	Level of Non-chance Confidence (Non-chance Differences)
$P \leq .05$	5% or less	95.0%
$P \leq .025$	2.5% or less	97.5%
$P \leq .01$	1% or less	99.0%
$P \leq .001$	.1% or less	99.9%

PROBABILITIES AND LEVEL OF CONFIDENCE

As noted above, data can never be interpreted as having "proved" a hypothesis. For this reason, decisions about the statistical significance of data are most commonly formulated as probability statements like those found in Table 7.1. As the table shows, there is an inverse relationship between the probability for a chance error owing to random factors and the level of confidence that can be placed in a systematic experimental effect. More specifically, one can see that relatively small alpha (α) values such as $P \leq .001$ are interpreted as statements of greater confidence in the data (less chance for error) than are relatively large α values such as $p \leq .05$ (more chance for error). As statements of probability, the intermediate α values in the table reflect moderate positions relative to acceptable risks for error versus the levels of confidence in experimental findings based on statistical outcomes.

THE BAYESIAN VIEW OF PROBABILITY

Although the most popular view of probability is founded on the classical school of statistical inference, as developed by Sir Ronald Fisher and E. S. Pearson in the early 1900s, not all researchers and statisticians believe that frequentist methods are suitable for all problems. Indeed, some might say that in clinical practice, as in our assessment of everyday events, we rarely attempt to forecast the future by sampling the relative frequency of its past occurrence. In other words, we do not actually state a null hypothesis that the population percentage equals, say 50%, then use sample data to decide whether or not to reject the hypothesis based on the probability of achieving similar results over a long sequence of trials. Instead, we typically cast our predictions based on experiential beliefs or personal opinions. This so-called **subjective view** of probability, based on the "degree of belief" that one happens to hold, is summarized well by Good (1950):

> . . . subjective probability judgments . . . should be given a recognized place from the start . . . it is helpful if something is stated about the subjective initial probability of the hypothesis . . . To omit such a statement gives only the superficial appearance of objectivity. (p. 28)

A mathematical basis for assessing probability in terms of the subjective views of individuals was first introduced by a Presbyterian minister, **Thomas Bayes,** in 1763. Classical statisticians have often criticized the **Bayesian view,** as it has come to be known, based on the fact that subjective probabilities for a particular event may vary widely among individuals. The rejoinder of Bayesian statisticians has been that the ability to take such individual differences into account and to assess changes in subjective views as new information emerges is a strength rather than a weakness of the Bayesian approach. To the extent that this is true, Bayesian methods have obvious application to many clinical situations in which we must depend on personal experience or "intuition" to guide our decision making.

The clinical utility of Bayesian methods for inferring the consequences of certain diagnostic and management decisions (a priori) and for evaluating the validity of a clinicians' views given new data (a posteriori) is increasingly recognized in the field of medicine. Such methods have not yet been used extensively in the behavioral fields even though they would appear to have numerous applications. We will return to a discussion of **Bayes' rule** (theorem) later in this chapter.

In general, we can say that statistical inference, regardless of the point of view held by the researcher, requires an extrapolation from the given sample (explained portion) to the larger unknown population (unexplained portion). Because we are extrapolating in this manner, uncertainty always exists about our conclusions. This uncertainty may be dealt with using probabilities such as significance level (α), confidence interval, or Bayesian subjective probabilities.

LOGICAL AND MATHEMATICAL BASIS OF PROBABILITY

The New York Yankees' catcher, Yogi Berra, once said, "Baseball is 90% mental. The other half is physical." Although Yogi's pronouncement is humorous, his knowledge of the laws of probability is, at the same time, highly suspect. The term "probability" is correctly interpreted as asking, "How probable is it that a particular event will occur?" or "How credible is this particular research hypothesis?" The minimum confidence that can be placed in some observation is exactly 0%, and the maximum confidence is exactly 100%—nothing more, nothing less. If Yogi is right, baseball can be played with 140% confidence (90% mental plus 50% physical)!

In the language of mathematics, the calculation of the probability of an event E, denoted by P(E), must satisfy (1) $0 \leq P(E) \leq 1$ and (2) the total sum of probabilities of all possible outcomes is equal to 1, or $\Sigma \, P(E) = 1$. This is to say that probabilities can range from zero (0.00) to one (1.00). A value of 0.00 (0%) can be interpreted to mean that there is no chance for a particular event occurring, whereas a value of 1.00 (100%) expresses certainty for the future occurrence of an event. Given the truth of the adage that "the only human certainties are birth and death," a probability of 1.00 would be assigned to both of these events. On the other hand, most people would say that the chance of a human flying to the moon just by waving his or her arms equals 0.00. Typically, probability values fall somewhere within these extremes and are expressed as decimals. The larger the decimal, the greater is the probability for the occurrence of the event in question.

The underlying logic of probability provides a mathematical framework for predicting future outcomes in experiments. The probability in an experiment can be derived through the ratio of the number of outcomes in an **event** to the number of outcomes in a **sample space** in general. The sample space is the set of all possible outcomes, and an event is the set of particular outcomes of a researcher's particular interest. For example, the sample space of a single trial of rolling die is {1, 2, 3, 4, 5, 6}. If a researcher's particular interest is specified as "even face values," the event consists of outcomes such as {2, 4, 6}. In general, the probability of an event E in a sample space S, denoted by **P(E),** is expressed in the form of the following fraction:

$$P(E) = \frac{\text{Number of outcomes in E}}{\text{Total number of outcomes}}$$

DIFFERENT KINDS OF EVENTS

Two events are said to be mutually exclusive if when one event occurs, the other cannot. As an example, consider two events, A and B. Event A consists of even numbers and event

B consists of odd numbers. One randomly chosen number from a large set of integers must be even or odd, but not both at the same time. Therefore, no number belongs to the two events A and B simultaneously. Hence, two events A and B can be said to be **mutually exclusive.** Similarly, a child or adult with a hearing loss may be classified as having a mild, moderate, or severe hearing loss. These three severity levels are mutually exclusive because a single individual would be assigned only one of the ratings at a particular time. A set of events, say, E_1, E_2, . . ., E_K, are said to be **mutually exclusive and exhaustive** if one of them must occur at one time but with only one event in a single trial. Obviously, not all communication disorders are mutually exclusive—i.e., a client may possess several disorders of speech, language, and hearing simultaneously. Such instances as these constitute **nonexclusive events.**

Another important distinction to keep in mind is the difference between mutually exclusive and **equally likely** events. Whereas mutually exclusive events may also constitute equally likely outcomes, this is by no means a necessity. Using our previous example, we would expect to find many more people in the general population with a mild rather than moderate or severe loss of hearing acuity.

Still another distinction that we can make pertains to **independent events (unconditional)** and **nonindependent (conditional)** events. Different events can be said to be independent of one another provided that the occurrence of the first event does not influence subsequent events. Using the hearing example just cited, the gender of the client—"female versus male events"—should be independent of the severity of hearing loss. A person's gender should have no bearing on the level of hearing loss, and vice versa. On the other hand, if the probability of an event is influenced by the occurrence of another event, then the event thus influenced is said to be conditional on the other. Thus, the severity of one's hearing loss might be **conditional** on such other events as noise exposure, ear infections, genetic inheritance, etc.

TYPES AND RULES OF PROBABILITY

Professionals in the field of communication disorders spend a great deal of their professional careers collecting and interpreting data for the purpose of exercising "good judgment" in selecting among alternative courses of actions in servicing the needs of their clients. Most often, decisions are made on the basis of a constellation of findings, including information derived from case histories, interviews, formal and informal test instruments, the oral peripheral examination, laboratory studies, etc. No matter how broad our experience or depth of understanding, we must ultimately make decisions about problems when the final outcome is unknown. In effect, we must often guess what is most likely to happen given the results of certain diagnostic findings and therapeutic interventions.

Because of the ambiguity surrounding much of our professional work, it is best viewed as involving imperfect processes in which there are probabilities for making correct as well as incorrect decisions. An understanding of probability theory will not resolve all of our uncertainties but, hopefully, will allow us to make better and more informed choices.

Let us now review several types of probability and some of the rules that govern their calculation. For illustrative purposes, we will use the sample data compiled by Jerger et al., (1993) pertaining to the accuracy of acoustic reflex threshold measures in predicting audiometric hearing status. In the original study, the authors presented their results in the form of several matrices that compared predictions of audiometric status with actual au-

Table 7.2.
Two-by-Two Contingency Table for Predicting Audiometric Outcomes Based on Acoustic Reflex Thresholds

			(N=1043)
	Predicted Audiometric Outcome		
Actual Audiometric Outcome	Normal (T−)	Abnormal (T+)	Row Total
Normal (D−)	349	241	590
Abnormal (D+)	81	372	453
Column Total	430	613	1043

− sign represents "normality"
+ sign represents "abnormality"

diometric findings for a total of 1043 normal and abnormal ears. We have adapted and cross tabulated the finding of their investigation in the form of a two-by-two (2 × 2) contingency table (Table 7.2). Given these data, we can now proceed to discuss three types of probabilities that are important to both research and clinical decision making. These are (1) joint probability; (2) conditional probability; and (3) unconditional probability.

Types of Probability

Joint Probability

The joint probability of two or more events is the probability that such events will occur simultaneously or in succession. Symbolically, this can be expressed as **P(A and B).** Referring to Table 7.2, we can therefore ask, "What is is the probability that a randomly chosen ear will have a normal audiogram result (D−) that was previously found to illustrate a normal acoustic reflex (T−)?" By consulting the cross cells, we can observe that 349 of the 1043 ears satisfy two conditions of D− and T− simultaneously. Thus, (D− and T−) = 349/1043 = .33, or 33%.

Conditional Probability

Conditional probability also can be defined as the probability of an event, B, occurring given that another event, A, has already occurred. This is expressed as **P(B|A)**. Referring once again to Table 7.2, we can ask, "What is the probability of a randomly chosen ear yielding a normal audiogram (D−) given the finding of abnormal acoustic reflex threshold (T−)?" Symbolically, the probability that we wish to determine can be written as $P(D^-|T^-)$. The direct method of accomplishing this is to use our two-by-two contingency table to find the population of interest (i.e., the number of ears predicted to show normal audiometric results on the basis of normal acoustic reflex thresholds (T−) and the number of ears actually shown to have normal audiograms (D−).

More specifically, it can be seen that there were 349 D− ears out of 430 T− ears. Therefore, the probability (D− |T−) is equal to 349/430, or 81%.

Another way to determine the conditional probability is to calculate $P(D^-|T^-)$ by means of the conditional probability formula, where P(B|A) is given by

$$P(B|A) = \frac{P(A \text{ and } B)}{P(A)}$$

Therefore, $P(D^- | T^-)$ is written as

$$P(D^- | T^-) = \frac{P(T^- \text{ and } D^-)}{P(T^-)}$$

$$= \frac{349/1043}{430/1043}$$

$$= \frac{349}{430} \text{ or } 81\%$$

The conditional probability is also known as the **posterior probability** because it calculates the probability of a second event (B) occurring as the consequence of a first event (A).

Unconditional Probability

The probability of an event B occurring independent of the occurrence of event A is called an **unconditional probability.** Symbolically, this is denoted by $P(B)$, meaning that no prior knowledge of event A exists. This is also termed the **prior probability** because it calculates the probability of a second event (B) that is not contingent on the occurrence of a first event (A).

Using the data provided in Table 7.2, we can ask about the probability for any randomly selected ear illustrating a normal audiogram independent of the results of prior testing. Such a probability can be written as $P(D^-)$. To find the proportion of normal audiograms (D^-) out of the entire population, independent of the results of acoustic reflex testing, we can use the following the equation:

$$P(D^-) = \frac{\text{the number of ears labeled } D^-}{\text{total number of ears}}$$

$$= \frac{590}{1043} \text{ or } 57\%$$

Thus, the unconditional probability of a randomly chosen ear being audiometrically normal is 57%.

Rules of Probability

Two major probability rules have important application for research and clinical decision making. These are the (1) multiplication rule and (2) Bayes' rule. The following section discusses each of these rules in relation to the example data provided in Table 7.2.

Multiplication Rule

In some situations, we are interested in determining the probability of the joint or successive occurrence of two or more events based on more than one observation. Referring to Table 7.2, let us calculate the probability of randomly choosing an audiometrically normal ear that was also predicted to be normal on the basis of acoustic reflex threshold testing. This probability can be symbolically expressed as **$P(D^- \text{ and } T^-)$**. The mathematical calculation for this probability is given by

$$P(D^- \text{ and } T^-) = P(T^-) \cdot P(D^- | T^-)$$

$$= \frac{430}{1043} \cdot \frac{349}{430}$$

$$= \frac{349}{1043} \text{ or } 33\%$$

Bayes' Rule (Theorem)

A mathematical means of calculating the predictive value of a diagnostic test is through the application of **Bayes' rule** or **Bayes' theorem,** as it is also called. This rule describes the relations that exist among various conditional probabilities. As we noted previously in this chapter, Bayes' rule is useful in determining the accuracy of a diagnostic test.

Let us first examine this rule as it applies to the derivation of three general probabilities, including a prior probability, a data probability, and a posterior probability. Subsequently, we will relate these probabilities to the determination of what is termed the **predictive value** of a diagnostic test.

Previously, we discussed the prior and posterior probabilities. It will be recalled that the first of these, also called the unconditional probability, is based on a researcher's or clinician's prior knowledge of how probable various values of a test result are (i.e., actual audiometric results as shown in Table 7.2) before new data become available. Also, it will be recalled that the second of these probabilities, the posterior or conditional probability, is an updated probability of a prior probability of a test result after new data becomes available. In order to derive the posterior probability, an intermediate mathematical calculation is necessary that involves determining the *exact* probability of new data. The result of this calculation is called the **data probability.**

We will now discuss Bayes' rule as it incorporates the product of each of the three probabilities as briefly described above. Recall that the probability of two events, A and B, occurring simultaneously is calculated through the multiplication rule as previously discussed. The multiplication rule is an integral part of Bayes' rule as it is used for calculating the posterior probability of an event.

Suppose event A occurs when the results of a test are used to predict a particular disorder, and event B occurs when the disorder actually has been found to exist. According to the multiplication rule, the probability of satisfying both event A and B is symbolically expressed as

$$P(A \text{ and } B) = P(A) \cdot P(B|A)$$

From an algebraic standpoint, it does not matter if the labeling of the events A and B had been reversed in the above formula—i.e., $P(B \text{ and } A) = P(A \text{ and } B)$. From the multiplication rule, it follows that

$$P(A) \cdot P(B|A) = P(B) \cdot P(A|B)$$

This calculation leads to **Bayes' rule,** as given by

$$P(B|A) = \frac{P(B) \cdot P(A|B)}{P(A)} = \frac{P(A \text{ and } B)}{P(A)}$$

ACCURACY OF DIAGNOSTIC TESTING

The purpose of any diagnostic test is to detect a disorder or disease when present so that an appropriate intervention can be recommended. Because diagnostic tests are not perfect, some degree of error is to be expected in classifying people according to whether or not they have a particular disorder or disease. Three different ways to evaluate the accuracy of a diagnostic test are (1) test sensitivity; (2) test specificity; and (3) predictive value. As a means of illustrating each of these indices, we will again use the data in Table 7.2 and Bayes' rule.

Test Sensitivity

Generally speaking, test sensitivity can be defined as the probability that the test result is positive given that the disorder actually exists. Symbolically, it is written

$$P(T^+|D^+) = \frac{P(T^+ \text{ and } D^+)}{P(D^+)}$$

If a test has high sensitivity, it will have a low **false negative rate,** denoted by $P(T^-|D^+)$. In such a case, the test result will seldom indicate that the disorder is not present when in fact it is present. For example, it can be seen in Table 7.2 that of the 453 ears that actually demonstrated abnormal audiometric results, 372 ears were predicted to be abnormal. Hence, the test sensitivity of acoustic reflex threshold testing, as defined in this study, was equal to 372/453, or approximately 82%.

Test Specificity

Test specificity can be defined as the probability that the test result is negative given that the disorder actually does not exist. Symbolically, this is written

$$P(T^-|D^-) = \frac{P(T^- \text{ and } D^-)}{P(D^-)}$$

A test that has high specificity is one that has a low **false positive rate,** denoted by $P(T^+|D^-)$, meaning that it will seldom predict the presence of a disorder that does not exist. As we can observe in Table 7.2, the specificity of the test was such that, of the 590 ears that illustrated normal audiograms, 349 ears were predicted to be normal. Therefore, the test specificity is 349/590, or approximately 59%. Thus, the acoustic reflex threshold measure employed by Jerger et al. (1993) is more accurate in identifying individuals who are more likely to have an actual audiometric hearing loss than individuals without such a loss. In other words, the test has greater sensitivity than specificity.

Predictive Value of a Test

Although test sensitivity and specificity are important preliminary steps in constructing a diagnostic test, these indices alone have limited application to actual diagnosis and clinical decision making. More specifically, although these values may be used to estimate the accuracy of a particular diagnostic test, it is the **predictive value** of a test that is actually used in clinical decision making.

There are two major components of predictive value of a diagnostic test. The first of these is **predictive value positive,** which refers to the probability that a disorder exists when the test result is positive. Symbolically, this is expressed as

$$PV^+ = P(D^+|T^+) = \frac{P(D^+ \text{ and } T^+)}{P(T^+)}$$

By consulting Table 7.2, we can see that there were 613 ears that were predicted to have abnormal audiograms. Of this number, 372 ears were actually diagnosed as abnormal. Therefore, the predictive value positive of the test is 372/613, or approximately 61%.

The second component of the predictive value of a diagnostic test is called **predictive value negative,** which refers to the probability that a disorder does not exist when the test result is negative. This can be represented as

$$PV^- = P(D^-|T^-) = \frac{P(D^- \text{ and } T^-)}{P(T^-)}$$

In Table 7.2, it can be seen that of the 430 ears that were predicted to be normal, 349 ears actually were found to be normal. Hence, the predictive value negative of the test is 349/430, or approximately 81%. Thus, this value more accurately predicted audiometric hearing status than did the attribute of predictive value positive.

In summary, based on the results of the study by Jerger and his colleagues, it can be seen that certain "trade offs" exist between test sensitivity and test specificity. The ultimate purpose of a diagnostic test, however, is to maximize sensitivity, specificity, and predictive value to the fullest extent possible. In reality, as test sensitivity increases, test specificity decreases. Based on the results of their study, Jerger et al. concluded: "We think that the predictive accuracy of this technique is amazingly good." (p. 351) Despite this conclusion, we have illustrated through our calculations that although test sensitivity of the acoustic reflex measure was shown to be high (82%), the test specificity was relatively low (59%). Therefore, although the test is likely to identify a large number of individuals who actually have an audiometric hearing loss, it is considerably less accurate in identifying individuals who do not have such a hearing loss. This raises an important issue in evaluating the accuracy of any diagnostic test. Both test sensitivity and specificity must be taken into account in determining the ultimate predictive value of the test. Based on the study by Jerger et al., we have seen that those ears that were predicted to be audiometrically normal, given the results of acoustic reflex testing (Predictive value negative), tended to be identified more accurately than those ears that were predicted to be abnormal (Predictive value positive). Nevertheless, in terms of clinical considerations, it might be contended that it is more important for a diagnostic test to identify abnormality more accurately than normality because the former condition is necessary for implementing appropriate treatment for the disorder or disease in question.

In this chapter, we have outlined the theory and application of the principles of probability. The "probabilistic approach" is increasingly used as a basis for decision making in a number of clinical science fields. We believe that this approach is also highly relevant to problems found in the field of communication disorders. It should prove useful in the future as clinicians attempt to determine the accuracy of their clinical hypotheses and decisions and to update their views based on new information as it emerges from a variety of sources.

SELF-LEARNING REVIEW

1. In the vernacular of everyday language, we commonly use the term _____ to express the likelihood of a future event.

2. Clinically speaking, the term probability is akin to the concept of _____ .

3. According to the _____ theorem, the relative frequency of an observed event will approximate its _____ frequency of occurrence if observed over indefinitely _____ series of trials or experiments.

4. The mathematical likelihood of a coin turning up heads will get closer and closer to _____ % as the number of tosses _____ .

5. The classical view of probability is also called the _____ , _____ , or _____ view.

6. In a typical experiment, the researcher begins with a theoretical proposition or hypothesis about the _____ relative frequency of a particular observation or event. For example, we might hypothesize about the degree to which an observed sample _____ is representative of the _____ mean.

7. Relatively small _____ values such as $p \leq .001$ are interpreted with _____ confidence than are larger α values such as $p \leq .05$.

8. A mathematical basis for assessing probability in terms of the subjective views of individuals was introduced by Thomas _____ in 1763.

9. In the language of mathematics, the probability of an event E is denoted by _____ .

10. A probability value of 0.00 can be interpreted to mean that there is _____ _____ for an event occurring. A probability value of _____ expresses certainty for the future occurrence of an event.

11. The underlying logic of probability provides a _____ basis for predicting _____ outcomes.

12. $_____ = \dfrac{\text{Number of outcomes in E}}{\text{Total number of outcomes}}$

probably

prognosis

Bernoulli
probable
long

50
increases

frequentist,
objectivist, a
posteriori

expected

mean
population

alpha
greater

Bayes

P(E)

no chance
1.00

mathematical
future

P(E)

mutually exclusive

13. If one event occurs and the other cannot, they are said to be _____ _____ events.

equally likely

14. The fact that two or more events are mutually exclusive does not mean they are _____ _____ .

independent

15. An _____ event is one whose occurrence is not conditional on the occurrence of another event.

independent

conditional

16. A person's gender should be _____ of the severity of one's hearing loss. On the other hand, the severity of one's hearing loss may be dependent or _____ on noise exposure, ear infections, etc.

imperfect

probabilities

17. The work of professionals in the field of communication disorders is best viewed as involving _____ processes in which there are certain _____ for making correct and incorrect decisions.

joint

multiplication

18. The probability that two or more events will occur simultaneously is called a _____ probability. Such a probability is calculated by means of the _____ rule.

Conditional

B

P(B|A)

posterior

prior

19. _____ probability can be defined as the probability of event _____ occurring given that another event A has already occurred. Symbolically, this probability is denoted _____ . This is also termed the _____ probability. On the other hand, the probability of the first event A is called the _____ probability.

unconditional

prior

A

20. The probability of an event B occurring independent of the occurrence of event A is called an _____ probability, meaning that no _____ knowledge of event _____ exists.

multiplication

P(A and B)

product

P(B|A)

21. In order to calculate the probability of the joint occurrence of two events A and B, we use the _____ rule. This rule is symbolically denoted by _____ . The mathematical calculation for this probability is given by the _____ of P(A) and _____ .

prior

data

posterior

22. Bayes' rule consists of three general probabilities, including a _____ probability, a _____ probability, and a _____ probability.

posterior

prior

data

23. The _____ probability is an updated probability of a _____ probability of a test result after new data become available. The result of the calculation that involves determining the exact probability of new data is called the _____ probability.

Clinical Application

The next exercise involves an application of probability theory in predicting the diagnostic outcomes for 150 hypothetical cases suspected of having a particular type of communication disorder—i.e., stuttering, aphasia, sensorineural hearing loss, etc. A summary of some fictitious results for this study are shown below in a 2×2 contingency table:

		Diagnostic Outcomes		
		D^+	D^-	Row Total
Diagnostic Test Results	T^+	30	40	70
	T^-	10	70	80
	Column Total	40	110	150

Referring to the table above, it can be seen that the probability of having a hypothetical disorder and a positive diagnostic test result, denoted by $P(D^+$ and $T^+)$, is _____ or _____ %.

The sensitivity of the test, denoted by _____, is _____ or _____% . The specificity of the test, denoted by _____ , is _____ or _____ %. If a test has high sensitivity, it will have a low _____ _____ rate. If a test has high specificity, it will have a low _____ _____ rate. The predictive value positive of the test, denoted by _____ , is _____ or _____ %. The predictive value negative of the test, denoted by _____, is _____ or _____ %.

In summary, the diagnostic test in our example is more likely to identify those individuals who actually _____ the hypothetical disorder than those who do _____ the disorder. Also, based on the results of diagnostic testing, those individuals who illustrated a _____ test result tended to be identified more accurately than those who illustrated a _____ test result. Thus, on the basis of the results of our example, the test was found to have greater _____ than _____ . It will be recalled that the goal of diagnostic testing is to _____ both of these attributes to the fullest extent possible.

30/150
20
$P(T^+|D^+)$
30/40
75
$P(T^-|D^-)$
70/110
64
false negative
false positive
$P(D^+|T^+)$
30/70
43
$P(D^-|T^-)$
70/80
88

have
not have

negative
positive
sensitivity
specificity
maximize

8. Inferential Statistics: Estimating the Significance of Outcomes

Sampling Variability	Analysis of Variance (ANOVA)
Confidence Intervals	—*Logic of ANOVA*
One-Sample Case: Testing Hypotheses for a Single Group	—*Calculation of ANOVA*
	—*Two-Way ANOVA*
Errors and Power in Statistical Inference	**Multiple Comparison Methods**
	Other ANOVA Designs and Methods
Two-Sample Case: Testing Hypotheses for Two Groups	Randomized-Blocks Analysis of Variance (RBANOVA)
Unpaired t Test for Independent Samples	Analysis of Covariance (ANCOVA)
Paired t Test for Dependent Samples	Nonparametric Tests for Multigroup Designs
Nonparametric Alternative to Parametric Statistics	Meta-Analysis
Chi-Square Test	**Complex Statistical Methods**
Nonparametric Rank-Order Methods	Multivariate Analysis of Variance (MANOVA)
Multigroup Designs: Testing Hypotheses for Three or More Groups	Discriminant Analysis
	Factor Analysis
	Computer Applications in Statistics

In previous chapters, we discussed the concept of the normal curve and the calculation of standard scores. These can be useful in estimating the probability that the measured performance of a randomly sampled individual from a normally distributed population will be above or below a certain value. However, most research studies are concerned with the opposite problem of making inferences about a larger group or population based on representative sample cases drawn from that population. Quantities used to describe characteristics of populations are termed **parameters.** On the other hand, quantities derived from samples that are used in estimating population parameters are called **statistics.** This chapter discusses several methods for making inferences about the **significance** of sample statistics in conjunction with hypothesis testing.

SAMPLING VARIABILITY

Fundamental to the understanding of statistical inference is the notion that the amount of trust that can be placed in any measure obtained from a sample is directly dependent on its reliability as an estimate of the true measure of the population. Whether it be the sample mean, the standard deviation, or some other measure, all such measures should be stable—i.e., they should express little **variability.** A highly useful measure of the degree of variability in a sampling distribution is called the **standard error of the mean,** variously denoted as $\sigma_{\bar{x}}$, **SEM,** or **SE.** The SE is an estimate of the expected amount of deviation of sample means from the true population mean that is a result of chance or measurement errors. Stated more simply, SE is the standard deviation of a set of sample means. However, it is important to distinguish between the SE and the standard deviation (σ or **SD**). Whereas the SD is a measure of the degree of variability that *currently* exists among individuals in a population, the SE is an estimate of how much variability to expect in the means of *future* samples when the complete population parameter is unknown. On practical grounds, the SE has great value because it eliminates the need for repeatedly sampling the same distribution, thereby relieving investigators of what might otherwise be a highly onerous burden.

Consider a population of three individuals with the following raw scores on a digit span test: 5, 9, and 7. We consider two parameters, the mean and the standard deviation, from this population. Suppose we select two scores randomly from the population. With this sampling procedure, there are three equally likely possible samples of two raw scores that can be drawn from the population. They are as follows:

Sample	$\overline{X}$
(5, 9)	7
(5, 7)	6
(9, 7)	8

where $\overline{X}$ represents the sample mean of each outcome.

The mean of all possible sample means from the original population is referred to as the **sampling distribution of the mean of samples of size n.** Two parameters for sampling distributions are:

(a) **The mean = Mean of sample means =** $\mu_{\bar{x}}$
(b) **The standard deviation = Standard deviation of sample means =** $\sigma_{\bar{x}}$

In the original population ($N = 3$), we find μ (the population mean) to be 7. Let us calculate $\mu_{\bar{x}}$ given by the arithmetic average of three sample means 7, 6, and 8:

$$\mu_{\bar{x}} = \frac{7 + 6 + 8}{3} = 7 \text{ as well. Therefore, keep in mind that:}$$

(a) **The mean of the sampling distribution for the sample mean is ALWAYS the population mean** $\mu_{\bar{x}} = \mu$

By using the same mathematical procedure, we can compare the standard deviations for the original population $\overline{X}$ and the sampling distributions for the mean ($\sigma_{\bar{x}}$) in the sample above. Because the mathematical derivation for accomplishing this is relatively complex, only the result is given below. Furthermore, the standard deviation, as we already know, is sensitive to sample size so that the value of $\sigma_{\bar{x}}$ changes as n changes. Thus, it can be said that:

(b) **For random samples from a large population, the standard deviation of the sampling distribution for the mean of sample size n approaches** $\sigma_{\bar{x}} = \sigma/\sqrt{n}$ **as n increases.**

Combining the results of (a) and (b) above, we can state the characteristics of the sampling distribution for the mean of sample size n. More specifically, if the original population of the distribution of the raw scores is normal, then the sampling distribution for $\overline{X}$ will yield the following properties:

1. **normality**
2. $\mu_{\bar{x}} = \mu$
3. $\sigma_{\bar{x}} = \sigma / \sqrt{n}$
4. $Z = (\overline{X} - \mu_{\bar{x}}) / \sigma_{\bar{x}}$ for a large n (n > 30)

The combined properties as noted above are often referred to as the **Central Limit Theorem,** which provides the foundation for much of modern statistical inference. This theorem makes possible the ability to calculate the standard error as an estimate of the degree of dispersion present in any group of sampling means provided that the sample is random.

Confidence Intervals

As noted in earlier chapters, investigators are ultimately interested in determining the **significance** of their research findings. The statistical meaning of significance pertains to the probability that an observed result is truly the consequence of a systematic influence under investigation rather than the unlikely consequence of chance alone. Typically, in determining the significance of a single sample mean, its probable position in relation to the population mean is estimated to lie within the boundaries of certain **confidence intervals** or **confidence limits,** as they are sometimes called.

To illustrate the role of the standard error in statistical inference, suppose that we wish to estimate the probable mean intelligence of the current population of graduate students in the field of communication disorders. Using appropriate random sampling techniques, we first select a sample of 144 students for our study. Assume further that the mean IQ of this sample ($\overline{X}$) is determined to be 110, with a standard deviation (σ) of 12. What can be inferred about the probable position of the true population mean within one standard deviation from the mean? To answer this question, we must first calculate the standard error accordingly:

$$ SE = \frac{12}{\sqrt{144}} = \frac{12}{12} = 1.0 $$

Based on a standard error of this size, the true mean of graduate student IQ can be estimated to lie between $\overline{X} - 1 \cdot SE(109)$ and $\overline{X} + 1 \cdot SE(111)$. This assertion can be made with a limited degree of confidence. More specifically, if we were to randomly select numerous repeated samples from the same population, we could expect the same or highly similar findings about 68% of the time (see Figure 6.7). Should we wish to take a conservative position, we could assert that the true mean lies between $\overline{X} - 2 \cdot SE(108)$ and $\overline{X} + 2 \cdot SE(112)$ about 95% of the time. An ultraconservative assertion might be that μ is located between the limits $\overline{X} - 3 \cdot SE(107)$ and $\overline{X} + 3 \cdot SE(113)$. In the latter case, we could be confident of the relative truth of our assertion in about 99 cases out of one hundred.

Remember that the larger the confidence interval, the more confident one can be that the population mean is included within that interval. The resultant "tradeoff" is less precise information about the exact value of the population mean.

In general, there are two different types of questions that researchers ask. The first type of question determines whether or not a *single sample* belongs to some defined population. The second question asks whether *two or more different samples* come from the same population.

The general steps in performing hypothesis testing are as follows:

1. Form the hypothesis in statistical terms
2. Select an appropriate statistical test
3. Choose a significance level and criterion for rejecting H_0
4. Calculate the test statistic by computing what is variously termed the *observed* or *calculated* value.
5. Draw conclusions

ONE-SAMPLE CASE: TESTING HYPOTHESES FOR A SINGLE GROUP

The simplest type of hypothesis testing involves the one-sample case, also known as the **single-group design.** In essence, it asks if the mean of a single sample is comparable to the population mean.

In order to understand the application of this test, imagine that we are interested in investigating the intelligence of school-age children born with clefts of the palate. To do so, we will randomly select a hypothetical group of 36 subjects from the population of children with this type of cleft who are being followed by a number of craniofacial clinics. Assume that we administer the Wechsler Intelligence Scale for Children (WISC-III) to our sample with the following results:

$$\overline{X} = 89, \sigma = 15, \mu = 100, \mu_{\bar{x}} = 100, \text{ and } SE = \frac{15}{\sqrt{36}} = 2.5$$

The steps necessary for hypothesis testing are outlined below:

Step 1. Form the hypothesis in statistical terms:

Null Hypothesis: (H_0): $\mu = 100$
Alternative Hypothesis (H_1): $\mu \neq 100$

If the null hypothesis is rejected, the alternative hypothesis is supported. In the absence of a significant finding, the null hypothesis is retained pending the outcome of future experiments. Remember that the null hypothesis cannot be accepted because it is always possible that it will be disproved in some future investigation.

The alternative hypothesis as stated above signifies that the result will be evaluated by means of a **two-tailed test.** Such a test is selected when the **direction** of the difference cannot be predicted on the basis of preexisting knowledge. In the case of our example, the research findings from previous studies that bear on this problem are equivocal leading to the selection of a two-tailed test. If we had wished to predict the research outcome on the basis of prior knowledge, the alternative hypothesis would have been directional—i.e., would have been stated as $\mu > 100$ or $\mu < 100$. A **one-tailed test** of this kind is said to be "less stringent" than a two-tailed test because a smaller amount of variance between mean scores is needed to be considered a significant finding.

The direction of the sign contained in H_1 identifies the area within the normal curve for rejecting H_0. More specifically, the basis for deciding where to look within the curve for a significant difference is summarized below:

If H_1 contains	$\neq$	$<$	$>$
Perform	two-tail	one-tail (left-sided)	one-tail (right-sided)

Step 2. Select an appropriate statistical test.

Given our hypothetical problem, the appropriate test for evaluating the null hypothesis is based on the **Z** distribution. The major criterion for using the **Z** test is that the population standard deviation (σ) must be known. In studies of intelligence based on the WISC III, the population mean is known to be 100 with a σ of 15.

When the population standard deviation (σ) is unknown, the appropriate statistical test for evaluating the null hypothesis is the **t test.** Furthermore, a t distribution is designed for testing hypotheses when the sample size is small (n $\leq$ 30).

Step 3. Choose the significance level and criterion for rejecting H_0.

A two-tailed test will be performed at **α=.05** because the alternative hypothesis (H_1) is nondirectional ($\mu \neq 100$). Recall that the significance level must be established *before* the study is conducted. The decision rule for a two-tailed test at α = .05 involves the following considerations:

1. Reject H_0 if the magnitude of the observed value is greater than or equal to a critical value of 1.96

$$(|Z(observed) \geq Z(critical)| = 1.96).$$

2. Do not reject H_0 otherwise.

Step 4. Calculate the test statistic.

Given the data provided in our hypothetical study, we will now calculate the test statistic. The formula for calculating Z is as follows: $Z = \dfrac{X - \mu}{SE}$

Entering the appropriate values into the formula above, we find that:

$$Z = \frac{89 - 100}{2.5} = -4.4$$

Step 5. Draw conclusions on the basis of critical value(s):

Because the magnitude of the observed Z value exceeded the critical value of 1.96 (Figure 8.1), a decision is made to reject the null hypothesis. More specifically, even though the mean IQ of the sample (89) was in the range of low average intelligence, our fictitious data indicate that the children's scores on the WISC III were significantly different from (lower than) the population mean IQ of 100.

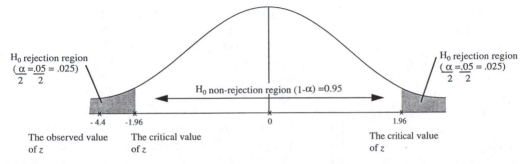

Figure 8.1. The critical Z values ($\pm$1.96) associated with α/2=.025 and a nondirectional, two-tailed test of the null hypothesis.

Although the Z test is highly useful in testing hypotheses when the population mean is known, in reality, this is rarely the case. In most research studies, the standard error must be estimated based on the sample data alone. In place of Z scores, t scores are used to make estimates about the values of sample means in relation to their population values.

The distribution for t scores was first described by the English statistician William Gossett in 1908. As an employee of the Guinness Brewery, he was required to publish his findings anonymously in order to protect the secrets of a beer-making process. Because he chose to sign his name merely as "A Student," Gossett's statistical distribution subsequently became widely known as the **Student t Test.**

The formula for t is:

$$t = \frac{\overline{X} - \mu}{SE}, \text{ where}$$

$\overline{X}$ = mean of sampling distribution

μ = population mean

SE = standard error of the mean = $\dfrac{s}{\sqrt{n}}$

As can be seen in this formula, the t test is actually a ratio wherein the numerator is the difference between two means. The denominator (standard error) is an estimate of the degree of variance between the means. Generally, a t value of approximately 2 corresponds to a probability value of p>.05, which means that the difference between two means resulting from chance is less than 5% (1 chance in twenty). A t value of 3 would be considered significant beyond the .01 level.

As noted previously, in addition to the relevance of the t test in cases in which σ is unknown, its use is also applicable to circumstances in which the sample size n<30. We will now demonstrate the application of this test based on the previous example. However, in testing H_0, the sample size in this case will be 9 instead of 36. Furthermore, assuming the σ is unknown, we will replace it by the estimated sample standard deviation (s).

Based on our example, the following values are given:

$$\overline{X} = 89, S = 16, \mu = 100, \text{ and } SE = \frac{16}{\sqrt{9}} = 5.33$$

Substituting these values into the appropriate formula below, we find the value of t:

$$t = \frac{\overline{X} - \mu}{SE} = \frac{89 - 100}{5.33} = -2.064$$

The decision rule for a two-tailed t test at α = .05 involves the same considerations as stated previously for a two-tailed Z test. However, the critical value of t in the former case depends in part on the **number of degrees of freedom (df)** allowed. Df is best viewed as an "index number" for the purpose of identifying the appropriate distribution to be used given a specific sample size. The value of df for a one-sample t test is n − 1. Referring to the table for t values found in Appendix C.2, it can be seen that the critical value for our hypothetical study is 2.306 for df=9−1=8.

Because the magnitude of the observed t value does not exceed the critical value (Figure 8.2), the decision is made to retain the null hypothesis. More specifically, in contrast to the significant finding for the Z test based on the same example, the nonsignificant t test result indicates that the IQ scores of children with cleft palates are equivalent to the population mean.

The reader may wonder why the Z and t tests in this example produced disparate out-

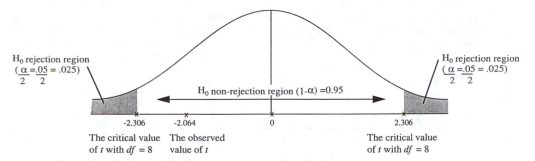

Figure 8.2. The critical t values (±2.306) associated with $\alpha/2 = .025$, 8 *df*, and a nondirectional, two-tailed test of the null hypothesis.

comes so that the first value was associated with a statistically significant result in contrast to the second value. Generally, researchers can expect the results of Z and t tests to reflect comparable results because their distributions are highly similar. However, our hypothetical t test results are predicated on an n of only nine subjects. For small n's of this size, t values may differ significantly from Z values based on larger n's. On the other hand, with successive increments in sample size, the obtained t value becomes closer to the obtained Z value.

Errors and Power in Statistical Inference

As discussed in previous chapters, there are two major types of errors a researcher can commit when making statistical inferences. The first type of error is called a **type I error** (denoted by α). Recall that this error is the result of rejecting the null hypothesis when it is true. The second type of error, called a **type II error** (denoted by β), is the consequence of retaining the null hypothesis when it is false.

Ideally, the goal of research is to avoid or minimize the probability of both type I and type II errors. However, the unfortunate reality is that these errors are interactive to the degree that when one type decreases, the other type increases. In most cases, researchers are more concerned about making a type II error than a type I error because the former type primarily determines the power of a statistical test, denoted by $1-\beta$.

The **power of the test** can be defined as the probability of rejecting a *false* null hypothesis, i.e., the probability of reaching a correct decision. Determining the power of the test is an important goal in research because an investigator wishes to make valid conclusions based on *true* differences rather than on chance occurrences.

The calculation of the power of a statistical test is beyond the present aim of this chapter. Nevertheless, for the more mathematically inclined reader, we have included the steps involved in this calculation in Appendix B. A summary of statistical errors in relation to the power of the test is illustrated in Table 8.1.

TWO-SAMPLE CASE: TESTING HYPOTHESES FOR TWO GROUPS

In the behavioral sciences, researchers frequently are interested in testing the significance of difference between two means reflecting the scores of two randomly assigned groups. One of these groups receives an experimental treatment (experimental group) and another group is given no treatment or a different form of treatment (control group). The mean scores of the two groups are then compared to determine the probability that a particular finding is statistically significant.

We noted earlier that in cases where the standard deviation of a population is un-

Table 8.1.
Possible Correct and Incorrect Decisions in Hypothesis Testing.

	H_0 is True	H_0 is false
Do not reject H_0	Correct decision $(1 - \alpha)$	Type II error (β)
Reject H_0	Type I error (α)	Correct decision power $(1 - \beta)$

known, Z scores cannot be calculated. Thus, the standard error must be estimated based on the sample data alone. In place of Z scores, **t scores** are used to make estimates about the values of sample means in relation to their population values regardless of sample size.

The calculation of t is similar to that of Z except that t is calculated by *estimating* the number of standard errors that a sample mean lies above or below the population mean. On the other hand, Z is derived by finding the *actual* population parameter. As noted previously, for large samples (n>30), the values of t and Z scores become increasingly comparable.

In order to determine whether two or more means come from the same population, researchers employ the strategy of testing the statistical significance of the null hypothesis, which is a proposition that no significant difference between mean scores will be found. If the results of such testing reveal that the probability for the sample means to reflect a common mean is less than 5% (P<.05), the null hypothesis is usually rejected in favor of a significant finding.

In testing the differences between two means, several methods may be used depending on the type of research design employed by the investigator. Two common statistics used for this purpose are (1) the unpaired t test for independent samples and (2) the paired t test for dependent samples.

Unpaired t Test for Independent Samples

In cases in which the data arising from separate and unrelated groups of subjects are independent of one another, the unpaired t test is an appropriate statistic to use.

Suppose we are interested in evaluating the effectiveness of "therapy approach X" as compared to "therapy approach Y." Assume further that, from a common pool of available subjects, 14 subjects are randomly assigned to group X and 11 subjects to group Y. We wish to know whether the performance of group X will differ from that of group Y under two different sets of treatment circumstances. More specifically, we wish to determine whether the true population mean score of group X (μ_X) will differ from the true population mean score of group Y (μ_Y) based on the results of statistical testing. Assume further that there is no basis for predicting, prior to the experiment, whether one therapy approach is more effective than the other.

The actual steps involved in testing the significance of the difference between the means using the unpaired t test are outline below:

Step 1. Form the hypothesis in statistical terms:

Null Hypothesis (H_0): $\mu_X = \mu_Y$
Alternative Hypothesis (H_1): $\mu_X \neq \mu_Y$

Stating the null hypothesis as $\mu_X = \mu_Y$ is the same as saying that μ_X and μ_Y will be assumed not to differ unless a difference is found in a subsequent experiment. If the null hypothesis is rejected, the alternative hypothesis is supported. In the absence of a significant finding, the null hypothesis is retained pending the outcome of future experiments. Remember that the null hypothesis cannot be accepted because it is always possible that it will be disproved in some future investigation.

The alternative hypothesis as previously stated signifies that the result will be evaluated by a **two-tailed test.** Such a test is selected when the **direction** of the difference is not predicted because no prior expectation is held by the investigator about the outcome. If the investigator had expected that one treatment would be more effective than the other treatment, the alternative hypothesis would have been stated as either $\mu_X > \mu_Y$ or $\mu_X < \mu_Y$. A one-tailed test is said to be "less stringent" than a two-tailed test because a smaller amount of variance between mean scores is needed to be considered a significant finding.

Step 2. Select an appropriate statistical test.

As noted previously, the most commonly selected statistics used for evaluating the significance of difference between two means are the Z and t tests. The Z test may be used in cases in which the conditions of the central limit theorem are satisfied, i.e., the distributions are presumed to be normal and the population standard deviation is known. However, in the field of communication disorders, research often involves the use of small samples of individuals having relatively unique problems so that the population standard deviation is unknown. Given such limitations, as in the case of our experiment, the t test often is the more appropriate choice for the statistical analysis of data.

Step 3. Select the level of significance.

In order to evaluate a null hypothesis, it must be decided *before* the investigation begins the point at which a difference between the means will be considered significant, i.e., not a result of chance as the null hypothesis claims. This decision requires the establishment of an alpha value (α) as the criterion for rejecting the null hypothesis. In conjunction with this decision, the alpha is typically set at .05 as the highest cutoff value for rejecting the null hypothesis. Although lower alpha values (e.g., .01 or .001) may be used for determining statistical significance, they rarely are set higher than the .05 level.

Step 4. Calculate the test statistic.

The calculation of the t test for independent samples is illustrated here as follows:

a. First, calculate the means for the two distributions. These are given here as: $\overline{X} = 100$, $\overline{Y} = 88$

b. Calculate the standard deviations for the two distributions. These are given as: $Sx = 12$, $Sy = 15$

c. Calculate the pooled standard deviation of the means. In order to do this, the values of n for each mean are also needed. They are given here as:

$$Sp = \sqrt{\frac{(n_x - 1)Sx^2 + (n_y - 1)Sy^2}{n_x + n_y - 2}}$$

$$= \sqrt{\frac{(14 - 1)(12)^2 + (11 - 1)(15)^2}{14 + 11 - 2}}$$

$$= \sqrt{\frac{4122}{23}}$$

$$= 13.39$$

d. Calculate the standard error of the mean difference:

$$SE(\bar{x} - \bar{y}) = Sp \sqrt{\frac{1}{n_x} + \frac{1}{n_y}}$$

$$= 13.39 \sqrt{\frac{1}{14} + \frac{1}{11}}$$

$$= 5.39$$

e. Determine the value of t. This score constitutes the ratio of the difference between two means to the standard error of the difference. In our investigation, it is given by

$$t = \frac{\overline{X} - \overline{Y}}{SE(\bar{x} - \bar{y})}$$

$$= \frac{100 - 88}{5.39}$$

$$= 2.23$$

Step 5. Draw conclusions on the basis of critical value(s).

Having completed the t test, the next step is to determine the probability that a t score as large or larger than the value obtained might have resulted as the consequence of chance. This can be accomplished by consulting a probability table, like that in Appendix C.2, that lists the **critical values for the t distribution.** Determining the significance of a critical value is possible by examining the areas for acceptance and rejection under the normal curve. The t distribution conforms closely to the shape of the normal curve for large sample sizes (n>30).

The critical value of t depends in part on the **number of degrees of freedom (df)** allowed. In the case of testing the difference between two means, as in the above study, the df is defined as $n_x + n_y - 2$. The critical value of t also depends on whether the test is one-tailed or two-tailed and on the significance level selected (.05, .01, etc.).

Referring to the table for t in Appendix C.2, we note that the calculated value of t (2.23) for 23 degrees of freedom exceeds the critical value of t (2.069) located under the column designating the 0.05 significance level for a two-tailed test. These results are shown graphically in Figure 8.3.

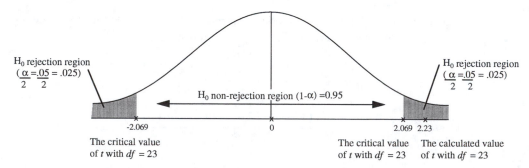

Figure 8.3. The critical t values (±2.069) associated with $\alpha/2=.025$, 23 *df*, and a nondirectional, two-tailed test of the null hypothesis.

Thus, we are able to reject the null hypothesis in favor of the alternative hypothesis. More specifically, we are able to conclude that there was a significant difference between the two therapy approaches, with therapy approach X appearing to have been more effective than therapy approach Y. Had the calculated t score exceeded the critical value of 2.807 listed in the table under the area of the upper tail of the curve, the result would have reached an even higher level of significance (p<.01). However, recall from our previous discussion that the choice of a particular alpha value should be made before the test is performed. The actual probability value (p) or calculated t value is determined on the basis of statistical testing. If the observed t value is greater than the critical value shown in the table, the null hypothesis is rejected.

To say that p<.01 is *more* significant than p<.05 may be statistically correct but has little substantive importance in evaluating possible outcomes of an experiment. Based on the statistical evidence, the null hypothesis is either rejected, indicating a significant outcome, or retained, indicating a nonsignificant outcome. In the former case, the significant difference is considered to result from the systematic influence of the independent variable rather than from chance alone. On the other hand, in the instance of a nonsignificant finding, the amount of difference found is considered to be the result of chance factors rather than the consequence of systematic influences known to the investigator.

Paired t Test for Dependent Samples

In our discussion above, we outlined the steps required for testing the significance of difference between the means of two independent random samples. However, certain hypotheses can be better evaluated using what are variously called *dependent, correlated,* or *related* samples. Such samples can result from certain matching procedures to form **matched pairs,** or the same group can be measured twice in a **pairing-design** in which each subject is used in both conditions. Sampling procedures that entail matching subjects on factors that might influence the outcome of an experiment, other than the independent variable, were considered in Chapter 5. The so-called pairing design involves the use of subjects as their own control. This type of design is also known as a *within-subject, self-control,* or *repeated measurements* design.

The formula for the paired t test is given by

$$t = \frac{\bar{d}}{s_d/\sqrt{n}} \text{ with df} = n - 1$$

in which

$\bar{d}$ = **The mean of the difference scores for the sample pair**
s_d = **The standard deviation of the sample difference calculated by**

$$s_d = \sqrt{\frac{\Sigma d^2 - \dfrac{(\Sigma d)^2}{n}}{n - 1}}$$

n = **The number of pairs in the sample**

Let us now illustrate the use of the paired t test as it might be applied to a clinical problem in the area of stuttering. There is evidence that the adrenergic blocking agent propranolol is useful in controlling certain neuromotor disorders such as essential tremor and tardive dyskinesia. Hypothetically, assume that we want to investigate the potential effect of the minimal therapeutic dose of this drug against a placebo on self-ratings of stuttering severity using a Likert-type scale in which 1 = least severe and 5 = most severe. For purposes for our study, a **cross-over design** is selected for use in which half of ten subjects initially will be treated with propranolol and the other half treated with placebo for a two-week period, at the end of which they will provide self ratings of stuttering severity. A six-week "wash-out period" will separate the two treatments before crossing over to the alternate form. At the end of the second two-week treatment period, self ratings of stuttering severity will be made again.

The actual steps involved in testing the significance of the difference between the means of the drug and placebo conditions using the paired t test are outlined below:

Step 1. Form the hypothesis in statistical terms.

The null hypothesis that we wish to evaluate statistically is

$$H_0 : \mu_d = 0 \text{ (The mean difference in the paired observations is zero.)}$$

The alternative hypothesis can be stated as

$$H_1 : \mu_d < 0 \text{ (The mean difference in the paired observations is less than zero).}$$

Step 2. Select an appropriate statistical test.

The statistical test for comparing the differences between two means of dependent samples is the t test for paired observations, or the **paired t test.** This test statistic is comparable to the previously discussed test for unpaired samples. However, the calculations for the means and the standard deviations are replaced by difference scores (ds).

Step 3. Choose the significance level.

In order to evaluate the null hypothesis, the significance level will be set at .05 for a one-tailed test. More specifically, because we are predicting that stuttering will be rated as less severe under the propranolol condition than under the placebo condition, we will look for a significant difference in the left tail of the curve.

Step 4. Construct a table to include n, d, d^2, Σd, $\bar{d}$, Σd^2, and $(\Sigma d)^2$, and calculate the test statistic. (See Table 8.2.)

Table 8.2.
Paired t Test Results for the Self Rating of Stuttering Under Two Treatment Conditions (1 = least severe and 5 = most severe).

Subject	Propranolol	Placebo	Difference d	Difference Squared d^2
1.	4	5	−1	1
2.	0	1	−1	1
3.	0	0	0	0
4.	2	4	−2	4
5.	1	4	−3	9
6.	3	5	−2	4
7.	3	3	0	0
8.	1	3	−2	4
9.	2	2	0	0
10.	1	4	−3	9
Σ(sum)			−14	32

n=10, Σd=−14, $\bar{d}$=−1.4, Σd^2=32, $(\Sigma d)^2$=196

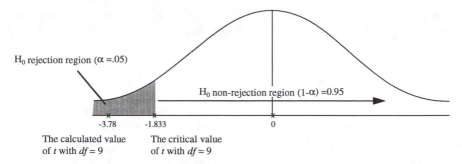

Figure 8.4. The critical t value (-1.833) associated with $\alpha = .05$, 9 *df*, and a directional, one-tailed test of the null hypothesis.

The calculation of the paired t test proceeds as follows:

    a. Calculate s_d: Based on the data in Table 8.2, it is equal to 1.17.

    b. Calculate the observed t value: $t = \dfrac{-1.4}{1.17/\sqrt{10}} = -3.78$

    Step 5. Draw conclusions on the basis of critical value(s):

Referring to Appendix C.2, we can determine the critical value of t for df=9, which is -1.833. The observed value of t, -3.78, falls into the H_0 rejection region ($\alpha=.05$). These results are shown graphically in Figure 8.4. Hence, the null hypothesis that the two treatments are equivalent can be rejected in favor of a significant finding in support of H_1. In other words, we can conclude on the basis of our hypothetical results that the self-rating of stuttering severity was lower under the propranolol condition than under the control condition.

NONPARAMETRIC ALTERNATIVES TO PARAMETRIC STATISTICS

Thus far, our discussion of statistical inference has focused on the use of parametric tests of significance, which generally include the following assumptions:

1. The population distribution is normal. (**Normality**)
2. When two populations are being compared, especially in the case of independent observations, their distribution values should have relatively equal variances. (**Homogeneity**)
3. Subjects should be chosen randomly. (**Randomness**)
4. The data should be quantifiable on a numerical scale when common arithmetic is appropriate. (**Interval/Ratio Data**)

When these assumptions cannot be met, the use of such parametric statistics as the mean, standard deviation, and t test may be inappropriate and may lead to invalid conclusions. Three **nonparametric statistics** that do not make these assumptions are discussed below.

Chi-Square Test (χ^2)

A test that is useful in evaluating hypotheses about the relationship between nominal variables having two or more independent categories is the χ^2 statistic, or chi-(pronounced kai) square. The inventor of this test, Karl Pearson, also developed a well-known method for computing correlation coefficients as discussed in Chapter 6. Throughout his career, this acknowledged founder of modern statistics was interested in studying the relations among variables. One of the most modern thinkers of his time, Pearson rejected the search for causality in favor of studying the association or *contingency* of phenomenon. Pearson's fervent interest in the topic of association also extended into the social realm, to such matters as the relations between the sexes. In 1885 he founded a "Men and Women's Club" in England to promote the discussion of such relations, where he met his future wife (Peters, 1987). Apparently, their interests were indeed contingent—i.e., a "good fit!"

In essence, the chi-square test provides a means of determining the **independence** between two or more nominal variables by calculating the discrepancy between the **observed frequencies** (actual counts) for a set of categories and the **expected frequencies** for the same categories (probability estimates). Suppose we wish to determine whether graduate students preparing for clinical careers in either speech-language pathology *or* audiology have different preferences for the type of setting in which they might choose to work—e.g., a medical versus a nonmedical setting. Imagine further that our two-sample case is based on the job preferences expressed by 50 students who wish to be certified as speech-language pathologists and an equal number who desire certification in audiology. Let us now illustrate the steps involved in testing to see whether the variables of interest are independent or in some way associated.

Step 1. Form the hypothesis in statistical terms:

H_0: The proportion of subjects from each sample selecting a particular preference category will be independent (unrelated).

H_1: The proportion of subjects from each sample selecting a particular preference category will *not* be independent (somehow related).

Step 2. Select an appropriate statistical test.

The chi-square test is appropriate for our problem because two samples of subjects are being compared on a nominal variable that has two categories.

Step 3. Choose the significance level.

We will set the significance level (α) at .05 for a one-tailed test. A one-tailed test is employed for interpreting the statistical significance of χ^2 because the result is used to evaluate whether the discrepancy between the observed and expected frequencies is *greater* than can be accounted for by chance.

Step 4. Organize the data in a 2 x 2 contingency table and calculate the test statistic.

The data are organized into a contingency table, like that shown in Table 8.3, in order to compare the frequency of responses in each cell that *actually* occurred (observed frequency) with the number of responses *estimated* to occur (expected frequency). The latter proportion can be calculated with the following formula:

$$E = \frac{\text{Row Total} \times \text{Column Total}}{\text{Grand Total}}$$

Table 8.3.
Hypothetical Survey of Work Preferences Among Speech-Language Pathology Students and Audiology Students.

	Medical	WORK PREFERENCE Nonmedical	Row Sum	N=100
Sp-lang. path.	18	32	50	
Audiology	31	19	50	
Column sum	49	51	100	

For example, the expected frequency of speech-language pathology students preferring to work in a medical setting is the computational result of 50 (first row sum) times 49 (first column sum) divided by 100 (grand sum), which is equal to 24.5. The same computation is performed for the remaining cells to yield an expected frequency for each category.

Once the observed values have been entered into a 2x2 contingency table, we can perform the chi-square test in accordance with one of the following formulas, depending on the number of degrees of freedom:

1. $\chi^2 = \Sigma \dfrac{(0 - E)^2}{E}$ for degrees of freedom greater than 1,

2. $\chi^2 = \dfrac{N(ad - bc)^2}{(a + b)(c + d)(a + c)(b + d)}$ for degrees of freedom $= 1$, where

N = the total number of subjects
a = the observed frequency of the first row and first column
b = the observed frequency of the first row and second column
c = the observed frequency of the second row and first column
d = the observed frequency of the second row and second column

For degrees of freedom equal to 1, the second formula, called **Yates' Correction for Continuity,** should be used instead of the first formula. Generally, Yates' formula deals with the inconsistency between the theoretical chi-square distribution and the actual sampling distribution having 1 df. Based on our example, it can be seen that Yates' correction must be used because df$=(r-1)(c-1)=(2-1)(2-1)=1$, where r represents the total number of rows and c represents the total number of columns. Next, enter the appropriate values into the formula to calculate the χ^2 value.

$$\chi^2(\text{observed}) = \frac{100(18 \cdot 19 - 32 \cdot 31)^2}{(18+32)(31+19)(18+31)(32+19)} = 6.76$$

Step 5. Draw conclusions on the basis of critical value(s).

For a 2x2 contingency table like the one in our example, there are two rows and two columns so that the degrees of freedom (df) = $(2-1) \cdot (2-1) = 1$. Chi-square tables have been constructed that allow the statistical significance of χ^2 to be assessed directly. By referring to such a table, as that found in Appendix C.3, we note that with 1 df, the critical value that must be exceeded to achieve a .05 level of significance is 3.841 for a one-tailed test. Because the observed (calculated) value of χ^2 obtained from our table exceeds the critical value of 3.841, we can reject the null hypothesis of independence. Given the fictitious results of our example, we are able to conclude that there is a significant relationship between emphasis in graduate training and preferences for future employment. More specifically, it appears that there is a difference in job setting preferences between students of speech-language pathology and students of audiology. Whereas the majority of the former group in our sample preferred a nonmedical as opposed to medical work setting, the opposite was true for the latter group.

Because of its wide range of applications, the chi-square test is useful for many problems involving the comparison of proportions. The example we used involved only two groups and two categories of variables. However, the number of rows and columns can be extended for the study of relationships among multiple groups and variables depending on the nature of the research question.

The chi-square test is often referred to as a **"goodness-of-fit"** test when the question pertains to whether distributions of scores fall equally into certain categories. Other uses include testing to see whether an obtained distribution drawn by random sampling reflects a normally distributed population. A nonsignificant chi-square would indicate that the shape of the obtained distribution fits the shape of the normal curve. On the other hand, a significant chi-square would be interpreted as a lack of fit between the obtained and normal distribution.

Unfortunately, the chi-square test is often applied inappropriately to statistical problems for which it is not intended. Remember that it is most suited for categorical data in which each case falling within a category or cell is independent of every other case. This is necessary to determine the true relationship between column and row variables—i.e., whether they are indeed independent of one another. In the case of our example, had we inadvertently mixed among our categories graduate students pursuing certification in *both* speech-language pathology and audiology, such a linkage would have violated the assumption of independence. In the use of the chi-square, the best policy is to have only one frequency count per subject and to have the subjects be as unrelated to one another as possible.

Nonparametric Rank-Order Methods

There are two highly useful alternative methods to the t test developed by Wilcoxon that are said to be **"distribution free"** for two reasons. First, like the chi-square, they are free of assumptions about the shape of the underlying population distribution. Second, they both entail *transforming* scores to ranks. Such tests are well suited for ordinal scales of measurement when the scores in a distribution can be logically arranged from most to least frequent but the intervals between the data points are either unknown or skewed.

The Wilcoxon Matched-Pairs Signed-Ranks Test is a commonly used nonparametric analog of the paired t test that utilizes information about both the *magnitude* and *direction* of differences for pairs of scores. Within the behavioral sciences, it is the most commonly used nonparametric test of the significance of difference between dependent samples. This test is appropriate for studies involving repeated measures, as in pretest-posttest designs in which the same subjects serve as their own control or in cases that use matched pairs of subjects. The ranking procedures used by the Wilcoxon test allow for (1) determining which member of a pair of scores is larger or smaller than the other, as denoted by the sign of the difference (+ or −, respectively) and (2) the ranking of such size differences. The null hypothesis under this test is that the median difference among pairs of ranked scores is zero.

Let us illustrate the steps in hypothesis testing using the Wilcoxon test in conjunction with some hypothetical data that might be generated in a study of the relationship between grammatical complexity and phonologic production. More specifically, suppose we wish to determine whether preschool children with impairments in both grammar and phonology will make more speech sound errors when imitating grammatically complex sentences than when imitating relatively simple sentences that are comparable in length. We can proceed as follows:

Step 1. Form the hypothesis in statistical terms:

H_0: There is no difference in the occurrence of phonologic errors when subjects imitate complex and simple sentences of the same length.

H_1: Phonologic errors will occur more often in the production of complex sentences than in that of simple sentences of the same length.

Step 2. Select an appropriate statistical test.

As an alternative to the paired t test, the Wilcoxon test has been selected because it also is an appropriate test for the analysis of dependent or correlated samples. With respect to its overall **power** (probability for rejecting a false null hypothesis), the Wilcoxon test closely approximates the efficiency of the parametric t for large ns. For small ns, the power efficiency of the Wilcoxon test is approximately 95% of its counterpart (Siegel, 1956). For data that are not normally distributed, the Wilcoxon test is more powerful than the t test. The likelihood of skewness increases as n becomes small as in the case of our sample.

Step 3. Choose the significance level.

The significance level (α) is set at .05 in a one-tailed test. We have chosen a one-tailed test in view of some preexisting evidence that phonologic errors occur more often in the production of complex sentences than simple sentences (Menyuk and Looney, 1972; Panagos and Prelock, 1982).

Step 4. Organize the paired-scores into a table and calculate the test statistic (Table 8.4.)

The difference score is positive if the first number of a pair is larger than the second or, conversely, carries a negative sign if the second number is larger than the first. The sign of a number has no real mathematical significance in the Wilcoxon test, but serves to mark the direction of difference between the pairs of scores. The next step is to rank the difference scores according to their relative magnitude, assigning an average rank score to each tie irrespective of whether the sign is positive or negative. Zero difference scores between pairs (d=0) are dropped from the analysis. Therefore, the *total number of signed ranks* (n) in determining the criterion for rejecting H_0 is 9. For the final step, in the last column of the table, sum the absolute value of the ranked difference scores having the *least* frequent sign. This last operation yields **T:** the smaller sum of the least frequent ranks.

Step 5. Draw conclusions on the basis of critical value(s):

Critical values for one-tailed and two-tailed tests have been developed for T, which has its own sampling distribution developed by Wilcoxon. Recall that in the case of the parametric t, values of t *larger* than the critical values listed in the probability table under the

Table 8.4.
Hypothetical Study of Speech Sound Errors for Preschool Children During Imitation of Complex and Simple Sentences.

Subject	Complex	Simple	d	Rank	Less frequent rank
1.	17	18	−1	−1.5	1.5
2.	14	11	3	4.5	
3.	16	13	3	4.5	
4.	11	11	0	0	
5.	13	7	6	8	
6.	31	29	2	3	
7.	12	7	5	6.5	
8.	29	21	8	9	
9.	17	12	5	6.5	
10.	9	10	−1	−1.5	1.5
					$\overline{T=3}$
					n=9

chosen significance level serve as the basis for rejecting the null hypothesis in favor of a significant finding. However, in the case of the Wilcoxon T, values *smaller* than the listed table values under a particular α for the total number of signed ranks (n) is the basis for rejecting the null hypothesis. Turning to Appendix C.5, we find that the critical value for an n of 9 is 6. Because our observed T value is less than the critical value of 6, we can reject H_0 in favor of H_1. More specifically, we can conclude that the complexity of imitated sentences seems to have a direct bearing on phonologic productions. Thus, the outcome of our hypothetical study is consistent with the results of previous investigations that have found more phonologic errors in children occurring during imitation of complex sentences than of simple sentences.

The **Mann-Whitney U Test** is a highly useful test for determining the probability that two independent samples came from the same population. It is variously called the Mann-Whitney U or Wilcoxon-rank sum test. In contrast to its parametric equivalent, the unpaired t test for independent sample, the Mann-Whitney U test is concerned with the equality of medians rather than means.

Suppose we are interested in knowing whether the physical status of newborns is related to their subsequent development of receptive language. For this purpose, we conduct a prospective study in which Apgar scores are collected on a random sample. Such scores are used to denote the general condition of an infant shortly after birth based on five physical indices including skin color, heart rate, respiratory effort, muscle tone, and reflex irritability. The maximum score of 10 is indicative of excellent physical condition. Using these numerical values as our independent variable, we divide our sample into two groups: (1) 10 children with high Apgar scores (greater than 6) and (2) 8 children with low Apgar scores (less than 4). Composite receptive language scores, obtained for these same children at ages 3 to 3.5 years on the appropriate subtests of the Clinical Evaluation of Language Functions-Preschool (CELF-P) (Wigg, et al., 1992), serve as the dependent variable.

We will now use some fictitious data in order to illustrate an application of the Mann-Whitney U test. The steps for calculating the Mann-Whitney U statistic are shown below:

Step 1. Form the hypothesis in statistical terms:

H_0: There is no difference in the receptive language ability of children who scored high on the Apgar scale versus those who scored low.

H_1: There is a difference in the receptive language ability of children who scored high on the Apgar scale versus those who scored low.

Step 2. Select an appropriate statistical test.

As an alternative to the unpaired t test, the Mann-Whitney U is chosen because it is an appropriate test for detecting differences between two independent groups. It is commonly used when the parametric t test's assumptions of normality and homogeneity of variance are violated.

Step 3. Choose the significance level.

The significance level (α) is set at .05 in a two-tailed test. In the case of our problem, a two-tailed test is appropriate because we are assuming that no prior knowledge is available that can be used as a basis for predicting the outcome of our study.

Step 4. Organize a table to include test scores, their ranks, and the sum of their ranks, and calculate the test statistic (Table 8.5):

Table 8.5.
Receptive Language Scores for Children with High and Low Apgars (Fabricated Data).

Language Scores (High Apgar Group)	Rank	Language Scores (Low Apgar Group)	Rank
37	14.5	22	1
32	11.5	23	2
34	13	30	9.5
28	6.5	37	14.5
32	11.5	24	3
47	18	27	5
29	8	30	9.5
45	17	28	6.5
39	16		
26	4		
	Sum=120		Sum=51

T_L=Larger sum of the ranks=120
n_L=number of subjects in the group with the larger sum of ranks=10
n_S=number of subjects in the other group=8

Table 8.5 shows the results for our hypothetical study, including CELF-P scores for the two groups, their corresponding ranks, and the sum of their ranks. The Mann-Whitney U is calculated as the smaller of U_1 and U_2, where

$$U_1 = (n_L)(n_S) + \frac{n_L(n_L + 1)}{2} - T_L$$

$$U_2 = (n_L)(n_S) - U_1$$

where n_L = the number of subjects in the group with the larger sum of ranks (denoted by n_1 in Appendix C.6), and n_S = the number of subjects in the other group (denoted by n_2 in Appendix C.6). Given our hypothetical data, U_1 and U_2 are found to be 15 and 65, respectively. Thus, the value of the Mann-Whitney U is 15.

Step 5. Draw conclusions on the basis of the critical value(s):

By consulting a special table for Mann-Whitney critical values like that found in Appendix C.6, we can observe that the obtained U of 15 is less than the table value of 17(n_L=10, n_S=8 for a two-tailed test at α=.05). In the table shown, n_L is labeled as n_1, and n_S is labeled as n_2. The criterion rule for rejecting the null hypothesis (H_0) indicates that we reject H_0 when the observed value of U *is less than or equal to* the critical value of U. Therefore, because the observed value of U is less than the critical value, we conclude that the receptive language abilities of the two groups, as distinguished on the basis of their Apgar scores, are significantly different.

MULTIGROUP DESIGNS: TESTING HYPOTHESES FOR THREE OR MORE GROUPS

In previous sections of this chapter, we discussed a variety of parametric and nonparametric tests for analyzing data from two different experimental conditions or from two different groups of subjects in order to test hypotheses. However, researchers often wish to set up experiments in which a single independent variable (factor) may be represented by more than two treatments (levels), and/or two or more factors may be manipulated consecutively.

Analysis of Variance (ANOVA)

More **complex designs** than the t test are often necessary for answering questions that go beyond the two sample case—e.g., "Is treatment **A** more effective than treatment **B**?" In some cases we might want to compare the treatment effectiveness of approaches **(A, B, C, etc.)** or the performance of *several* groups on a particular dependent variable. It is also possible to study combined treatment effects as might result from the interactions of treatment **(A×B, A×C, B×C, etc.).**

One could ask, "Why not perform a single t test for each statistical comparison of mean scores that might need to be made?" There are two main answers to this question. First, if no significant differences exist among any of the comparisons, then conducting numerous t tests in order to make this "dry gulch" determination is a needless waste of time. If this could be achieved by a single **omnibus** test, the goal of research efficiency is better served. Such a test, called the **Analysis of Variance (ANOVA),** invented by the British Statistician Sir Ronald Fisher, accomplishes this very goal. Although the ANOVA can be used for the analysis of two means, its greater utility lies in testing variation among three or more means.

A second problem relating to the use of multiple t tests is the probability that one or more of them will reach significance merely by chance. Because multiple t tests typically are not independent of one another, the probability of a type I error becomes greater with the number of tests performed. For example, assuming that three t tests are performed where $\alpha = .05$, the actual probability of obtaining a significant result by chance from any of the three tests is not .05. Rather, the true probability is given by:

P(type I error) $= 1-(1-\alpha)^n$, where n represents the number of the tests performed.

Thus, the true probability is $1-(1-.05)^3 = .14$, not .05.

Logic of ANOVA

The use of ANOVA for hypothesis testing is somewhat analogous to a familiar problem encountered in studies involving the electronic transmission of signals, called the "signal-to-noise ratio." For example, a "good" tape recorder is one that allows for the input of signals at high sound pressure levels with as little as possible distortion owing to extraneous noise. No doubt, we have all experienced the unpleasant "hum" that occurs on playback when the capacity of the recording unit has been exceeded. Thus, a good recording device is one in which the ratio of the signal to the noise is large—i.e, one that is able to maximize the transmission of salient information (the signal) while minimizing the transmission of artifacts (noise). In designing instrumentation, an oscilloscope can be helpful to electronic engineers in the computation of the signal-to-noise ratio. Similarly, the main goal in using the ANOVA is to "scope the data" in an effort to isolate systematic treatment effects intended by the experimenter (the signal) from sources of error (noise).

Chapter 3 discussed the conceptual basis of systematic variance versus error variance in accounting for the results of an experiment. The main goal of the ANOVA is to compute the ratio of systematic variance (the amount of variation owing to a treatment effect) to the degree of error variance that may involve both sampling errors and measurement errors. Recall that a statistical term for systematic variance is **between-group variance,** whereas the statistical moniker for error variance is **within-group variance.** As was also noted, the difference between these types of variance can be expressed symbolically as an *F* ratio, or

$$F = \frac{V_b}{V_e}$$

where the denominator in the equation is error variance and the numerator is systematic variance.

In reality, the degree of systematic variance in any experiment is the consequence of not only treatment effects but some chance fluctuations as well. Therefore, the *total variability* in data sets can also be expressed as:

S^2 **within groups = error variance**
S^2 **between groups = error variance + treatment effects**

The ANOVA provides a convenient method of calculating whether the variability between group means is greater than the variability within group means. This is accomplished by dividing up sources of variance into two major components: (1) the variation of the score of each subject from the mean of their group and (2) the variation between each group mean and the grand mean for the sample. If there are large differences between the group means, the variation between them and the grand mean will be large compared to the amount of variation within each group. If this is found to be true on the basis of an **F test,** then the null hypothesis of equivalence between groups is rejected. On the other hand, if the group means are similar in size, their variation from the grand mean should not differ substantially from the variation among the subjects within each group beyond chance expectations. In such a case, the null hypothesis is retained.

Calculation of ANOVA

In order to illustrate the use of ANOVA in hypothesis testing, let us examine its application in estimating the significance of difference among three independent means. For this purpose, the simplest of the ANOVA designs involving the analysis of a single factor will be used. This method, called a **one-way ANOVA,** may be viewed as an extension of the unpaired t test for two independent means discussed previously in this chapter.

Suppose we are interested in exploring the relationship between auditory processing abilities and phonologic disorders. We will model our hypothetical study, in part, after the investigation of Thyer and Dodd (1996), who evaluated the auditory perceptual abilities of children whose speech sound errors consisted of either *delayed* phonologic acquisition or *disordered* phonology against a control group.

For purposes of our example, we will fabricate some data for three groups of children: Control group (A), Consistent group (B), and Delayed group (C). The Consistent group is made up of children who display consistent phonologic errors that are atypical of normal phonologic development. On the other hand, the Delayed group is constituted of those subjects whose speech sound errors are inappropriate for age but typical of earlier stages of phonologic development. Assume that there are 10 children in each of the three groups. As in the study by Thayer and Dodd, the Paediatric Speech Intelligibility (PSI) Test will be used for the assessment of the subjects' auditory processing abilities. This test involves assessment of the ability to process messages in the presence of competing but semantically related sentences presented either contralaterally (one sentence to each ear) or ipsilaterally (both sentences to the same ear). For purposes of simplifying the analysis, we will limit our discussion to some hypothetical outcomes for the right ear results under contralateral testing conditions.

Let us now illustrate the steps in testing the hypotheses associated with this problem and the procedures necessary for their evaluation based on a one-way ANOVA.

Step 1. Form the hypothesis in statistical terms:

H_0: There is no difference in the auditory processing ability among the three groups. Symbolically, we can also state that $\mu_A = \mu_B = \mu_C$.

H_1: There is a difference in the auditory processing ability among the three groups. Symbolically, we can also state that at least one μ is different from other μs.

Step 2. Select an appropriate statistical test.

The use of one-way ANOVA is predicated on the following three assumptions: (1) there is independence among the groups; (2) the sampling distribution of the groups follow a normal curve; and (3) the variances of the scores in each group are equal. Symbolically, we can state that the σs of all groups are equal (homogeneity of variance). The first two assumptions are also necessary for the use of the t test for two independent groups, as previously described. However, the third assumption is an additional component underlying the use of any parametric ANOVA. In cases in which the homogeneity of variance among groups is questionable, the **Bartlett test** should be used for making this determination. An application of this test as it is used as a prerequisite to the ANOVA is illustrated in Appendix A.

As long as each group is constituted by an equal number of subjects or scores, the assumption of homogeneity of variance will not be violated. Thus, the one-way ANOVA design is appropriate for hypothesis testing given our hypothetical research problem.

Step 3. Organize a table to include the necessary numerical values and calculate the test statistic (Table 8.6):

The mathematical formula for the one-way ANOVA F value is given by

$$F = \frac{[\Sigma n_j(\bar{Y}_j - \bar{Y})^2] \div (J - 1)}{[\Sigma(Y_{ij} - \bar{Y}_j)^2] \div (N - J)}$$

$$= \frac{\text{Between-group variance}}{\text{Within-group variance}}$$

with df (between)$=J-1$ and df within$=N-J$

The actual calculation of an observed F value involves the following substeps:

a. Calculate the between-group variance (numerator):

$$\textbf{between-group} = \frac{10[(2.33)^2 + (0.33)^2 + (-2.67)^2]}{3 - 1} = 63.34$$

b. Calculate the within-group variance (denominator):

$$\textbf{within-group} = \frac{628 + 850 + 888}{30 - 3} = 87.63$$

c. Calculate the observed F value:

$$F = \frac{63.34}{87.63} = 0.73 \text{ with df (numerator)} = 2 \text{ and df (denominator)} = 27$$

Step 4. Draw conclusions on the basis of critical value(s):

By consulting the table for F in Appendix C.4, we can observe that the critical value of the test statistic at $\alpha = .05$ for df(numerator) = 2 and df(denominator) = 27 is 3.35. Be-

Table 8.6.

PSI Scores for the Right Ear Under Contralateral Testing Conditions for Three Groups of Children Classified According to Pattern of Phonologic Development (Fabricated Data).

Control (A)	Consistent (B)	Delayed (C)
73	74	86
98	100	76
100	100	90
99	100	88
99	96	99
100	78	74
100	100	100
98	95	98
100	97	100
93	100	99

$n_A = 10$	$n_B = 10$	$n_C = 10$
$\tilde{Y}_A = 96$	$\tilde{Y}_B = 94$	$\tilde{Y}_C = 91$
$\Sigma(Y_{ij} - \tilde{Y}_A)^2 = 628$	$\Sigma(Y_{ij} - \tilde{Y}_B)^2 = 850$	$\Sigma(Y_{ij} - \tilde{Y}_C)^2 = 888$
$\tilde{Y}_A - \tilde{Y} = 2.33$	$\tilde{Y}_b - \tilde{Y} = .33$	$\tilde{Y}_C - \tilde{Y} = -2.67$

where $\tilde{Y}$ = Overall mean = $\dfrac{96 + 94 + 91}{3}$ = 93.67

J = Total number of groups=3

N = Total number of subjects in all groups combined=30

j = Group identification where j=A, B, C

nj = Number of subjects in each group where n_A=10, n_B=10, and n_C=10

$\tilde{Y}_j$ = Sample mean of each group such as $\tilde{Y}_A$ = 96, $\tilde{Y}_B$ = 94, $\tilde{Y}_C$ = 91

Y_{ij} = Sample scores in rows (i) by group (j), e.g., Y_{1A} is the score of the first row in the control group (A) or 73

$\Sigma(Y_{ij} - \tilde{Y}_j)^2$ = Sum of the squares of between-group differences

$\tilde{Y}_j - \tilde{Y}$ = Between-group differences

cause the observed F value does not exceed the critical F value, we must retain H_o. More specifically, as in the case of the actual study by Thayer and Dodd, our hypothetical findings indicate that the consistent and delayed groups did not perform differently from one another nor from the control group. Therefore, we can conclude that auditory processing abilities as operationally defined in our investigation do not appear to provide a basis for determining the risk for phonologic disorders.

Two-Way ANOVA

In cases in which an investigator is interested in the effect of two independent variables on one dependent variable involving two or more groups, a two-way analysis of variance (two-way ANOVA) may be performed. For example, if we are interested in comparing the effect of individual therapy (factor 1) versus group therapy (factor 2) on some specific measure of language performance (dependent variable), this statistical method would be suitable for data analysis. Based on a hypothetical problem of this kind, there are three different ways to measure the relative effect of the individual variables under investigation. These are (1) the main effect owing to factor 1; (2) the main effect owing to factor 2; and (3) the interaction effect owing to factors 1 and 2 (denoted by factor 1 × 2). The **main effect** can be defined as the average effect of an independent variable across levels of the dependent variable—e.g., how each *separate* therapy factor will contribute to the outcome measure of language performance. The **interaction effect** can be defined as the *joint* effect of the two independent variables—e.g., how the two therapies combine or interact to influence measured language performance. The latter effect is extremely important in many clinical studies because clinicians often combine treatment modalities instead of using a single treatment approach. The conceptual basis for computing the two-way ANOVA is illustrated below:

Total variability of effects = variability owing to main effect of factor 1
                        + variability owing to main effect of factor 2
                        + variability owing to interaction effect (1×2)
                        + variability within groups (error variance)

A clinical example from an actual research study and the mathematical calculations associated with performing a two-way ANOVA is illustrated in Appendix A.

MULTIPLE COMPARISON METHODS

As noted previously, in cases in which three or more group comparisons are to be made, ANOVA is typically performed as the first step in statistical testing. If the result of the F test indicates that the null hypothesis should be rejected, we conclude that at least one of the group means is different from other group means. However, we are unable to know on the basis of the F test alone which *specific* group means among the various comparisons are significantly different from others. In order to make this determination, several so-called post hoc multiple comparison tests are available, such as **Scheffé's method** or **Tukey's method.**

In the case of an unequal sample size among the comparison groups, Scheffé's test is highly useful for calculating the significance of the observed F and t values for each combination of two group means. For instance, having found a significant F value among three groups (say groups A, B, C) based on calculation of an ANOVA, the null hypothesis for Scheffé's test can be stated as:

H_0: $\mu_A = \mu_B$, $\mu_A = \mu_C$, $\mu_B = \mu_C$

In a statistical sense, this procedures is considered to be somewhat conservative, i.e., the Scheffé method increases the critical value for determining significance. Therefore, the α level is generally set at .10 if the α level of the ANOVA was previously set at .05. Scheffé's method is used to control for a type I error, entailing the rejection of the null hypothesis when it is correct.

When the sample sizes among comparison groups are equal, the **Tukey test** (sometimes called HSD—Honestly Significant Difference) may be performed instead of the Scheffé test. The latter method is less conservative than Scheffé's test and is designed to make all possible pairwise comparisons among group means while maintaining the type I error rate at the same α as set in the ANOVA. The null hypothesis is identical to that of the Sheffé test.

Finally, we will briefly mention three **planned** or **a priori comparison procedures** used in cases in which an investigator wishes to accomplish the analysis of a limited number of pairwise comparisons in lieu of performing a more comprehensive and time-consuming ANOVA. Such procedures are used when prior theory leads to specific hypotheses about where significant differences between means might be found. For this purpose, we might use a **revised version of the t test.** The revised t procedure is accomplished by means of the following formula:

$$t = \frac{(\overline{X}_i - \overline{X}_j)}{\sqrt{2\,MS_E/n}} \text{ with df} = N - J \text{ as defined above}$$

where subscripts $_i$ and $_j$ represent group identifications and

$$MS_E = \sqrt{(\frac{s_i^2}{n_i} + \frac{s_j^2}{n_j})}$$

Thus, rather than using the pooled standard deviation in the denominator, we use MS_E (the error mean square) instead.

Another planned comparison method designed to reduce the probability of making a type I error is to shift the **α** (significance level) downward. For example, given the probability that approximately one t test in four will be significant as the consequence of chance alone ($4 \times .05 = .20$), an option is to shift the **α** downward by dividing it by the number of comparisons to be made. Thus, $.05/4 = .0125$—a more stringent significance level.

Another approach to making an a priori pairwise comparison of group means is called the **Bonferroni t procedure,** also termed Dunn's multiple-comparison procedure. This method increases the critical value (table value) of an *F* needed for reaching statistical significance, depending on the number of comparisons to be made and the sample size. It is used in cases in which the researcher wishes to avoid a type I error (rejecting the null hypothesis when it is true).

OTHER ANOVA DESIGNS AND METHODS

Numerous variations of ANOVA designs and methods are available for special types of research applications. The following sections will summarize some of the more widely used techniques.

Randomized-Blocks Analysis of Variance (RBANOVA)

This test is especially appropriate for within-subject designs in which the data comes from repeated measures on the same subject. According to Shavelson (1988), "the RBANOVA is to the t test for dependent samples what the one-way ANOVA is to the t test for two independent samples." (p. 487) Its primary purpose is to determine whether or not the differences between two or more groups may be due to chance or to systematic differences among the groups. Although RBANOVA is similar to ANOVA, the former method also takes into account the fact that two or more observations can be made on the same subject as opposed to a single observation as in the case of the latter. This is accomplished by (1) partitioning subjects into homogeneous blocks and (2) randomly assigning subjects to different levels within each treatment. For example, this design would be appropriate if we were interested in studying the relative influence of three treatment conditions (A, B, C) as these interact with three different severity levels (1, 2, 3) on some element of measured performance.

In many research studies, a **latin square** is used in conjunction with a block design when order effects may otherwise confound the influence of two or more treatment conditions. To control for the unwanted influence of confounding factors, a contingency table can be used to form a latin square, in which the confounding factors are assigned to rows and columns and the cells within the table are used to denote the observations (treatments) of interest. The objective of this procedure is to arrange the order of treatment conditions so that each condition precedes and follows each treatment condition. The number of ordinal arrangements should equal the number of treatment conditions, and each treatment (letter) should appear only once within a cell of each column and row. For example, in a study of treatment efficacy in aphasia, suppose we wish to control for the possible confounding influences of *language severity* and *time postonset*, as these nuisance variables might interact with three levels of an independent variable, e.g., the number of therapy sessions per week. In accordance with the **blocking principle** of the latin square, the levels of the confounding factors could be assigned to columns and rows of a square, with the cells of the square then used to identify the levels of treatment. Given this arrangement, there are three blocks of severity, three blocks of time postonset, and three treatment levels (A, B, C) forming a latin square consisting of nine cells for analysis. This hypothetical design is illustrated below.

		Time Postonset (in months)		
		1	2	3
Severity	≤35	A	B	C
Based on	36–55	B	C	A
Percentile Rank	>55	C	A	B

An example of a clinical research study that used a RBANOVA in conjunction with a latin square design can be found in Appendix A.

Analysis of Covariance (ANCOVA)

The major purpose of the analysis of covariance is to allow for an adjustment in factors that might potentially influence the results of an experiment *before* the experiment begins. More specifically, this test, abbreviated **ANCOVA,** allows for the statistical adjustment of data values of a dependent variable in accordance with known quantities of a variable that the investigator might wish to control (control variable). In effect, this adjustment removes from a dependent variable the degree of variability that otherwise could be attributed to the control variable.

Mathematically, the calculation of such variance is made possible by the use of the linear regression line, discussed in Chapter 6, to specify the slope of the relationship between a dependent variable and a control variable. By using the regression line, scores on the dependent variable can be predicted based on a knowledge of corresponding scores on the control variable. Residual deviation scores are used to specify the degree of variability in the dependent variable that is not associated with the control variable.

Suppose we wish to measure the maintenance of clinical gains in response to some treatment for three groups of subjects following the termination of therapy. Group A will be evaluated 6 months after therapy, Group B after 12 months, and Group C after 18 months. There are several within-group and between-group variables besides the independent variable that might potentially influence the outcome of such a study. For example, the researcher may wish to control for the degree of improvement that occurred during the course of therapy. It is possible that subjects who made more progress in therapy will be the same individuals who best maintain clinical gains through time. Although this is an interesting question in its own right, it is not the purpose of our study, which seeks only to determine the degree of maintenance across different spans of time. Thus, we might wish to control for within- and between-group differences for the *degree* of progress that occurred during therapy by factoring these *gain scores* into the analysis of the dependent variable. The intelligence and motivation of the subjects are examples of other control variables that might need to be considered. Because the mathematical calculation of ANCOVA is highly complex, we refer the reader to Appendix A, where the necessary computational steps are outlined in relation to an actual research study along with a discussion of the relative advantages and disadvantages of ANCOVA as compared to ANOVA.

Nonparametric Tests for Multigroup Designs

There are several nonparametric tests that can serve as alternative methods to ANOVA for testing hypotheses for multigroup designs. As an alternative to the two-way ANOVA, one of the most commonly used of these is the **Friedman Two-Way Analysis of Variance by Ranks.** Remember that nonparametric tests of this kind should be chosen when the assumption of homogeneity of variance is questionable or has been violated.

Just as the Wilcoxon-Matched Pairs Signed-Ranks Test is a useful distribution-free method for detecting a significant difference between two matched or related groups, the Friedman Two-Way Analysis of Variance by Ranks test is also useful with a randomized block design when a block consists of three or more repeated measures obtained from the same subject. As an example application of the Friedman test, let us consider a question in the aural rehabilitation of profoundly hearing-impaired children related to the effectiveness of various communication methods in facilitating the accuracy of speech reception. More specifically, imagine that we wish to evaluate the use of a training system known as Cued Speech in association with other training modalities. Cued speech involves the use of a set of hand cues to reduce or resolve ambiguities in speech reception (Cornett, 1967). In our hypothetical study, this system will be examined as it might be used in conjunction with three other conditions, namely: (1) audition (AC); (2) lip reading (LC); and (3) audition and lip reading (ALC). For this purpose, a group of 10 profoundly hearing-impaired adolescents will serve as subjects. Assume that a speech recognition task is designed that requires subjects in each of the groups to identify key words embedded in sentences. Subjects' responses to the stimulus items are recorded in terms of the percentage of correct identifications made. Let us now illustrate the steps in conducting the Friedman test in the context of our example:

Step 1. Form the hypothesis in statistical terms:

H_0: There is no difference in the subjects' speech recognition scores under the three conditions.

H_1: There is a difference in the subjects' speech recognition scores under the three conditions.

Step 2. Select an appropriate statistical test.

As noted above, the Friedman test is an appropriate statistic for data involving repeated measures of subjects tested in three or more conditions when scores are to be ranked. The specific goal of the test is to determine whether the sums of the ranks for the various conditions differ significantly.

Step 3. Choose the significance level.

An α level of .05 will be used to test the null hypothesis in a one-tailed test. A one-tailed test is always applied in testing the significance of three or more treatment conditions or groups.

Step 4. Organize a table to include test scores, their ranks, and the sum of their ranks, and calculate the test statistic (Table 8.7)

The test scores for the subjects in the three conditions of our hypothetical experiment are cast in a two-way table of n rows (subjects) and k columns (conditions). It can be seen that:

n=total number of subjects=10
k=total number of conditions=3
ΣR=a column sum of ranks such as 10(AC), 26 (LC), and 24 (ALC)

Table 8.7.
Hypothetical Results for a Study of Cued Speech Training in Association with Audition, Lip-reading, and Audition and Lip-reading.

Subjects	AC	LC	ALC	Ranks (R) AC	Ranks (R) LC	Ranks (R) ALC
1.	31	83	63	1	3	2
2.	42	77	81	1	2	3
3.	44	81	76	1	3	2
4.	33	69	65	1	3	2
5.	37	69	74	1	2	3
6.	32	70	72	1	2	3
7.	35	87	82	1	3	2
8.	39	86	73	1	3	2
9.	45	95	96	1	2	3
10.	35	81	79	1	3	2
N=10				Sum=10	26	24

The observed value of the Friedman test statistic approximates the chi-square distribution with df=k−1. Therefore, the general formula for the Friedman test statistic is given by:

$$\chi^2 = \frac{12(\Sigma R^2)}{nk(k + 1)} - 3n(k + 1) \text{ with df} = k-1$$

Entering the appropriate values into the formula above,

$$\chi^2 = \frac{12[10^2 + 26^2 + 24^2]}{10 \cdot 3 \cdot (3 + 1)} - 3 \cdot 10 \cdot (3 + 1) = 15.2$$

Step 5. Draw conclusions on the basis of critical value(s).

Appendix C.3 lists critical values of the chi-square distribution. For a critical value of 5.991, where $\alpha = .05$ and df=3−1=2, it can be seen that the observed value of χ^2 is greater than the critical value of 5.991 listed in the table. Thus, we can reject the null hypothesis and conclude that there was a difference in the speech recognition abilities of subjects among the three conditions. Our hypothetical results are compatible with the findings of an actual experiment concerned with a similar problem (Nicholls and Ling, 1982).

Another nonparametric alternative to the ANOVA is the **Kruskal-Wallis One-Way Analysis of Variance by Ranks (KWANOVA).** This test, a nonparametric version of the one-way ANOVA and an extension of the Mann-Whitney U test, is useful for deciding whether the distributions of scores in the populations underlying each group are identical. Instead of using actual test scores, ranks are substituted in order to represent the dependent variable. As in the case of the Friedman, scores are entered into a table and rank ordered from lowest to highest without regard to group membership. After summing the ranks of each group, if their respective sums are similar, the null hypothesis is retained. Otherwise, H_0 is rejected. An application of KWANOVA-based data from an actual research study is included in Appendix A.

Meta-Analysis

An increasingly popular methodology for statistically combining the results from two or more independent studies is called **meta-analysis**—a term introduced by Glass (1977) to describe a kind of higher-order level of data synthesis. Meta-analytic techniques should not be confused with traditional reviews of literature in which the findings of separate but related studies are summarized in an effort to "make sense out of the data." However, the underlying concern of meta-analysis is focused on the same problem, namely, the tendency of many research studies, designed to answer the same or a highly similar question, to yield conflicting results.

According to Sachs et al. (1987), meta-analysis has four main objectives:

1. Increasing statistical power by enlarging the size of the sample
2. Resolving the uncertainty associated with conflicting results
3. Improving estimates of effect size
4. Answering questions not posed at the beginning of the study

Among these aims, number 3, relating to effect size, is a key concept underlying the application of many meta-analysis techniques. **Effect size** is an index of the degree to which the phenomenon of interest exists in the population (Cohen, 1977). There are several methods of determining effect size, depending on the unit of analysis. In the case of mean scores, effect size is the difference between the means divided by the averaged standard deviations between the groups.

As noted above, effect size relates to the **power of the test** to yield a significant finding if the research hypothesis is true. The greater the difference between means, and the smaller the population variance, the larger will be the effect size. Criteria for interpreting effect sizes have been established by Cohen (1977). An effect size of .2 (interpreted as small) indicates that the means of two groups are separated by .2 standard deviations. Effect sizes of .5 (moderate) and .8 (large) indicate that the means are separated by .5 and .8 standard deviations, respectively. Meta-analytic technique can be used to combine effect sizes from independent studies into an overall average effect size and probability value based on the pooled results.

As an example of the use of effect size in conjunction with meta-analysis, a study by Nye and Turner (1990) is noteworthy. Using a data base of 65 studies to evaluate the effectiveness of articulation therapy, the authors reported a mean effect size (ES) of .892, "indicating that articulation treated subjects moved from the 50th to the 81st percentile as a result of intervention . . ." Several variables were sorted out that appeared to have the greatest influence on articulation improvement.

In the field of communication disorders, some researchers have held that statistical significance testing has been overly emphasized (Attansio, 1994; Maxwell and Satake, 1993) or should be supplemented by additional tests (Young, 1993; Maxwell and Satake; 1993; Attansio, 1994). Although the authors of this text firmly believe that statistical significance testing has value, the calculation of effect size can be of equal importance, particularly in the context of applied research as demonstrated in studies like those of Nye and Turner and others as completed by Andrews et al. (1980) in assessing the effects of stuttering treatment. In discussing the future role of meta-analysis, Attanasio (1994) noted that its importance lies in providing " . . . an estimate of the practical importance of statistical significance testing." For a more detailed discussion of meta-analysis, see Pillimer and Light, 1983; Cooper & Lemke, 1991; and Wolf, 1986, as well as many advanced statistical textbooks that provide a review of the subject.

COMPLEX STATISTICAL METHODS

Several other complex statistical techniques are frequently encountered in the reading of research literature. Although demonstrating the steps involved in calculating these statistics exceeds the purpose of this textbook, we will briefly mention three of the more commonly used multivariate methods that involve the analysis of more than one dependent variable, including: (1) multivariate analysis of variance (**MANOVA**); (2) discriminant analysis; and (3) factor analysis.

Multivariate Analysis of Variance (MANOVA)

This method is designed for problems in which there is more than one dependent variable under investigation. In general, two or more different measures of approximately the same characteristic (related variables) are taken, and a question is asked regarding the degree to which these dependent variables serve to separate two or more groups. Hypothetically, suppose we wish to determine whether or not children classified according to three levels of socioeconomic strata (low, mid, high) show different profiles on three types of language processing measures (phonologic, syntactic, semantic). In this case, our independent variables are constituted of the three levels of random group assignment, whereas our dependent variables consists of the three language measures. One option would be to conduct a univariate ANOVA for each of the dependent variables and calculate the significance of three separate F tests. However, this would be akin to conducting three separate experiments. As an alternative, we can use the MANOVA to accomplish the same goal more efficiently and in a manner in which the main effects and their interactions on the combinations of all the dependent variables can be evaluated simultaneously. Just as performing an ANOVA often eliminates the need for numerous t tests, so too can the MANOVA eliminate the need for numerous ANOVAs, thereby reducing the likelihood of a type I error. In cases in which the value of F for MANOVA is significant, leading to a rejection of the null hypothesis of no differences, post hoc ANOVAs are performed to determine where such differences can be found. The same statistical assumptions for performing ANOVA apply to MANOVA as well.

Discriminant Analysis

A statistical procedure whose purpose is somewhat similar to MANOVA is called **discriminant analysis.** The name of the test is appropriate because it is often employed to identify which dependent variables in a set of such variables are *most* responsible for discriminating among groups. Thus, whereas both MANOVA and discriminant analysis are concerned with identifying which variables contribute to group separation, only the latter evaluates the *magnitude* of the contribution of each variable toward this end. Discriminant function analysis can be useful in identifying factors that distinguish among subtypes of communication disorders such as stuttering—e.g., Van Riper's (1982) four developmental tracks that he distinguished on the basis of different combinations of factors including age of stuttering onset, manner of onset, symptoms, and general speech skills. Whereas Van Riper's approach to subtyping of developmental stutterers was largely based on the methods of clinical observation and description, discriminant analysis has obvious applications to problems of this kind.

Although mathematically complex, the method essentially involves identifying which variables or combination of variables are most powerful in discriminating among groups. In addition to its primary use in studies concerned with describing or identifying factors that discriminate groups, the method also has utility in predicting group membership of an individual. For example, based on a prior knowledge of certain factors in a client's history, we might calculate the probability that he or she belongs to a particular category or subtype of disorder within the population of stutterers. The accuracy of discriminant analysis is based on the percentage of cases that are classified correctly. Some of the basic assumptions of the discriminant analysis are that (1) there are two or more groups; (2) there are at least two cases per group; and (3) discriminating variables have nominal characteristics for dependent variables and continuous characteristics for independent variables.

Factor Analysis

A major goal of scientific research is to organize data in such a way that existing relationships among variables can be more readily comprehended. An important statistical method for accomplishing this goal is termed **factor analysis.** Some of the earliest work on factor analysis was carried out by Thurstone (1947) who believed it to be a powerful tool for exploring "vectors of the mind." Its primary aim is to reduce or condense a large number of observations into a small number of key indicators of underlying constructs (factors). Over the years, factor analysis has found many theoretical and practical applications. It is especially useful in the development of clinical tests and rating scales by summarizing the relationships among variables in a concise way.

Suppose we are interested in uncovering some of the principle dimensions of intelligence in children. Assume further that we do not know what these dimensions are and therefore decide to collect several types of measures on a large number of subjects. We select our measures given the presumption that some of them ought to be related to intelligence, but we are unsure how or to what degree this is true. After administering a large array of tests as shown in Table 8.8, the second step is to calculate correlations among each and every one of them. The result of correlating each test item with all other test items in the list results in a very large number of **intercorrelations.** The third step is to see how the measures tend to **cluster** or condense based on their intercorrelations. This can be done by constructing a matrix that displays the correlations between each possible variable or more conveniently by the use of a computer. Some measures will be correlated with each other but not with other measures. Measures that are found to be correlated are called **factors.** The fourth step is to determine the **factor loadings** for the various measures. The mathematical basis for such loading is beyond the scope of this book. Generally, this is done by determining the degree to which the measure correlates with a certain factor. Like other correlations, factor loads can range from −1 to +1. Although a measure may load onto more than one factor, it is generally the case that it will load *highly* on only one. The fifth step in factor analysis is to name or label the factors based on our theoretical understanding of their nature.

Table 8.8.
Test Items Used in a Factor Analysis Study of Intelligence.

1.	Picture completion
2.	Information
3.	Coding
4.	Similarities
5.	Picture arrangement
6.	Arithmetic
7.	Block design
8.	Vocabulary
9.	Object assembly
10.	Comprehension
11.	Symbol search
12.	Digit span
13.	Mazes

Table 8.9.
Subtest Composition for Four Named Factors.

Factor 1 Verbal Comprehension	Factor II Perceptual Organization	Factor III Freedom from Distractibility	Factor IV Processing Speed
Information Similarities Vocabulary Comprehension	Picture completion Picture arrangement Block design Object assembly Mazes	Arithmetic Digit span	Coding Symbol search

The results of the factor analysis are displayed in Table 8.9. As can be seen from such an analysis, four factors emerged, which have been named (1) Verbal comprehension; (2) Perceptual organization; (3) Freedom from distractibility; and (4) Processing speed. Of course, the knowledgeable reader will recognize that the factors named and their associated test measures constitute a well-known intelligence test—the Wechsler Intelligence Scale for Children-Third Edition (WISC-III) (Wechsler, 1991).

Although we have illustrated the use of factor analysis based on 13 subtests of a standardized test instrument, it is common for dozens or even hundreds of measures to be included at the outset of factor analytic studies. Over the years, factor analysis has led to the refinement of the theoretical foundations of the WISC as it has gone through several revisions. A major strength of factor analysis is that it advances conceptualization of the quality being studied. On the other hand, in the absence of some theoretical approach designed to integrate data toward a meaningful end, it probably should not be done. Such "fishing expeditions" rarely advance our conceptual understanding of complex phenomena. For additional information on the theory and methods of factor analysis, the reader is referred to Gorsuch (1983).

COMPUTER APPLICATIONS IN STATISTICS

Before the development of modern computer systems for data analysis, statistics were performed by hand or with the aid of a calculator. Such calculations were extremely time-consuming and often fraught with human error. Because of this fact, many researchers and statisticians expended much effort in devising short-cut formulas for analyzing data more efficiently. Nevertheless, until the computer became available, many of the complex designs that currently exist exceeded the statistical abilities of researchers to answer certain questions. Access to high-speed computers and the software that runs them presently allows researchers to expend their energies more creatively in designing and conducting scientific studies. A brief description of three commonly used software packages follows:

MINITAB is an easy to use software package often incorporated within the curriculum of introductory computer/statistics courses. It is especially appropriate for descriptive statistical applications such as calculations of measures of central tendency, variability, simple linear regression, and correlation. Some limited number of inferential statistics, such as the Z or t test for univariate calculations, can also be performed. This software stores the data values in rows and columns, like a spreadsheet, allowing for various types of elementary analyses. For example, after inputting the data into the appropriate cells, the computer can be instructed to perform the desired calculation. Although this is a good introductory program for students, it is unable to perform multivariate statistical calculations as required by many complex research designs.

Biomedical Computer Programs P-Series (BMDP) is one of the most sophisticated packages for statistical analysis. It is especially suitable for many applications in the medical and biological sciences, such as in clinical trial studies, pharmaceutical research, and prevalence/incidence studies. The data management programs contained within this software are well organized and flexible as to allow for different types of analyses on the same data to be performed with only minor changes in the coding operations. Among the operations that the BMDP can perform are data description, frequency tables, regression analysis, ANOVA, and MANOVA.

Statistical Package for the Social Sciences (SPSS) programs are widely used in the educational, social, and behavioral sciences because of their simplicity and the complete labeling of statistical analyses on data printouts.

We use the printout from SPSS computer program to illustrate the calculation of a one-way ANOVA (Figure 8.5). This example from the SPSS reference guide (1990) is based on the study of 500 sample cases concerning their sense of well-being, termed **WELL** (dependent variable) with respect to educational level, termed **EDUC** (independent variable). WELL was computed based on measures of happiness, health, life, helpfulness to others, etc. EDUC constituted six different levels of educational attainment.

As shown on the example page of the 1990 SPSS reference guide, three steps are required to perform the calculation.

1. Get and input data into file
2. Create and define each variable by coding (X1, X2, . . . 1, 2, etc.)
3. Calculate data values using appropriate commands/subcommands (oneway well . . ., etc.; and polynomial = 2 . . ., etc.)

Shown at the bottom of the page is the output of the one-way ANOVA, based on the example provided, which includes between-group and within-group variances, degrees of freedom, sum of squares, mean squares, F ratio, and F PROB. The latter value represents the statistical significance under the null hypothesis. The outputs for corresponding subcommands, also provided in the SPSS reference guide, are not shown.

The SPSS program is capable of performing a wide range of graphical and data analysis operations as appropriate for descriptive statistics, categorical analysis, univariate and multivariate ANOVA, correlation/regression, discriminant analysis, log-linear models, factor analysis, etc. Among the three software packages that we have mentioned, SPSS is the most comprehensive. Another system, called **Statistical Analysis System (SAS),** performs statistical functions in a manner comparable to SPSS.

One or more of the programs described in the previous paragraph are on the mainframes of academic computing services in colleges and universities so that data management operations can occur on-line from the desk top or laboratory through links to one's own personal computer. Although fluency in a computer language such as **BASIC** (Beginner's All-purpose Symbolic Instruction Code) may prove useful, this is no longer a requirement for using the technology successfully for a myriad of research applications. Software packages have detailed instructional manuals and many have "tutorials" that help the user find and correct errors as they occur. Programming assistance is typically available in academic computer centers to help the researcher to design an operation for a specialized need. For more limited graphic and data analysis applications, there are many commercial software packages for personal computers available through computer stores.

In this example we determine the degree to which sense of well-being differs across educational levels. The SPSS commands are

```
GET FILE GSS80/KEEP EDUC HAPPY HEALTH LIFE HELPFUL TRUST
                      SATCITY SATHOBBY SATFAM SATFRND.
COUNT  X1=HAPPY HEALTH LIFE HELPFUL TRUST SATCITY SATHOBBY
              SATFAM SATFRND(1).
COUNT  X2=HAPPY HEALTH SATCITY SATHOBBY SATFAM SATFRND(2).
COUNT  X3=HEALTH HELPFUL TRUST (3).
COUNT  X4=SATCITY SATHOBBY SATFAM SATFRND(6).
COUNT  X5=HAPPY LIFE (3).
COUNT  X6=SATCITY SATHOBBY SATFAM SATFRND(7).
COMPUTE WELL=X1 + X2*.5 - X3*.5 - X4*.5 - X5 - X6.
VAR LABELS  WELL 'SENSE OF WELL-BEING'.
RECODE  EDUC (0 THRU 8=1)(9,10,11=2)(12=3)(13,14,15=4)
             (16=5)(17,18,19,20=6) INTO EDUC6.
VAR LABELS  EDUC6 'EDUCATION IN 6 CATEGORIES'.
VALUE LABELS  EDUC6 1 'GRADE SCHOOL OR LESS'
              2 'SOME HIGH SCHOOL' 3 'HIGH SCH GRAD'
              4 'SOME COLLEGE' 5 'COLLEGE GRAD'
              6 'GRAD SCH'.
ONEWAY  WELL BY EDUC6(1,6)
    /POLYNOMIAL = 2
    /CONTRAST = 2*-1, 2*1
    /CONTRAST = 2*0, 2*-1, 2*1
    /CONTRAST = 2*-1, 2*0, 2*1
    /RANGES = SNK
    /RANGES = SCHEFFE (.01)
    /STATISTICS  ALL.
```

- The GET command defines the data to SPSS and selects the variables needed for analysis.
- The COUNT and COMPUTE commands create variable WELL by counting the number of "satisfied" responses for each variable on the scale and computing a weighted sum of these responses.
- The RECODE command creates the variable EDUC6 which contains the recoded six categories of education.
- The VAR LABELS and VALUE LABELS commands assign labels to the new variables, WELL and EDUC6.
- The ONEWAY command names WELL as the dependent variable and EDUC6 as the independent variable. The minimum and maximum values for EDUC6 are 1 and 6 (see Figure 1).
- The POLYNOMIAL subcommand specifies second-order polynomial contrasts. The sum of squares using the unweighted polynomial contrasts is calculated because the analysis design is unbalanced (see Figure 2).
- The CONTRAST subcommands request three different contrasts (see Figure 3).
- The RANGES subcommands calculate multiple comparisons between means using the Student-Newman-Keuls and Scheffe tests. (see Figures 4 and 5).
- The STATISTICS subcommand requests all the optional statistics (see Figure 6).

Figure 1 Analysis of variance table from ONEWAY

```
- - - - - - - - - - - - - - - - - - - - - - - - -  O N E W A Y - - - - - - - - - - - - - - - - - - - - - - - - -

       Variable  WELL      SENSE OF WELL-BEING SCALE
    By Variable  EDUC6     EDUCATION IN 6 CATEGORIES

                            ANALYSIS OF VARIANCE


                              SUM OF        MEAN         F      F
           SOURCE      D.F.   SQUARES      SQUARES     RATIO  PROB.

BETWEEN GROUPS          5     361.3217     72.2643    11.5255  .0000

WITHIN GROUPS         494    3097.3463      6.2699

TOTAL                 499    3458.6680
```

Figure 8.5. Printout from SPSS computer program showing calculation of a one-way ANOVA.

SELF-LEARNING REVIEW

1. Quantities used to describe characteristics of populations are termed _____ . On the other hand, quantities derived from samples that are used in estimating population parameters are called _____ .

parameters
statistics

2. A highly useful measure of the degree of variability in a sampling distribution is called the _____ error of the _____ , denoted by $\sigma\bar{x}$ or SE. The SE is an estimate of the expected amount of _____ of sample means from the true population mean as a result of chance or _____ errors.

standard
mean
deviation
measurement

3. Whereas the SD is a measure of the degree of _____ that exists among individuals in a population, the SE is an estimate of the amount of _____ in the means of _____ samples when the complete population parameter is unknown.

variability
variability
future

4. The Central Limit Theorem states that (a) the mean of the sampling distribution for the sample mean is always equal to the _____ mean and (b) the standard deviation of the sampling deviation of the sampling distribution for the mean of sample size n approaches _____ as n increases.

population
$\sigma/\sqrt{n}$

5. The statistical meaning of significance pertains to the _____ that an observed result is truly the consequence of a _____ influence under investigation.

probability
systematic

6. Assuming that the mean IQ score is 100 with a standard deviation of 15, the true mean for a sample of 225 subjects can be estimated to lie between _____ and _____ about 95% of the time.

98
102

7. The simplest type of hypothesis testing involves the one-sample case, also known as a _____-group design. In essence, we are asking if the sample mean of one group is comparable to the _____ mean.

single
population

8. An alternative hypothesis containing an unequal sign will be evaluated by means of a _____-tailed test. Such a test is selected when the _____ of the difference cannot be predicted on the basis of preexisting knowledge.

two
direction

9. An alternative hypothesis containing either > or < is called a _____-tailed test. Such a test is said to be _____ stringent than a _____-tailed test because a smaller amount of _____ between mean scores is needed to be considered a significant finding.

one
less
two
variance

t

30

rejected
greater
1.96

$$\frac{\overline{X} - \mu}{SE}$$

$s/\sqrt{n}$

freedom
n−1

α
rejecting
true

β
retaining
false

II
power

unpaired

$n_1 + n_2 - 2$

paired
n−1

matched
pairing

within
repeated

10. When **σ** is unknown, the appropriate statistical test for evaluating H₀ is the _____ test. Furthermore, such a distribution is designed for testing hypotheses when the sample size is less than or equal to _____ .

11. When a two-tailed test Z test is performed at **α**=.05, H₀ will be _____ if the magnitude of the observed value is _____ or equal to a critical value of _____ .

12. In a sampling distribution, the formula for calculating a Z score can be written symbolically as Z=_____ .

13. In a t distribution, the standard error of the mean (SE) is equal to _____ .

14. The critical value of t depends on the number of degrees of _____ allowed. The value of df for a one-sample t test is _____ .

15. A type I error, denoted by _____ , is the result of _____ the null hypothesis when it is _____ .

16. A type II error, denoted by _____ , is the consequence of _____ the null hypothesis when it is _____ .

17. In most cases, researchers are more concerned about making a type _____ error because it is the one that primarily determines the _____ of a statistical test.

18. In cases in which the data arising from separate and unrelated groups of subjects are independent of one another, the _____ t test is an appropriate statistic to use.

19. In testing the difference between two independent group means (**μ**₁ and **μ**₂), the number of degrees of freedom is defined as _____ .

20. When we test the significance between the means of two dependent groups, the _____ t test is used with df= _____ .

21. Dependent samples can result from certain correlating procedures to form _____ pairs, or the same group can be measured twice in a _____ design.

22. A pairing design is also called a _____- subject, self-control, or _____ measures design.

23. The formula for the paired t test is written symbolically as

$t = \dfrac{\bar{d}}{s_d/\sqrt{n}}$, in which $\bar{d}$ represents the mean of the _____ scores for the sample pair, Sd represents the _____ _____ of the sample difference, and n represents the number of _____ in the sample.

difference
standard deviations
pairs

24. The four basic assumptions underlying the use of parametric tests of significance include _____ of variance; _____ or _____ data; a _____ curve; and _____ .

homogeneity
interval
ratio
normal
randomness

25. If one or more of these assumptions are violated or remain questionable, a _____ statistic should be used.

nonparametric

26. A test that is useful in evaluating hypotheses about the relationship between nominal variables having two or more independent categories is the _____ -square test, denoted symbolically as _____ . This test calculates the discrepancy between observed frequencies and _____ frequencies.

chi
χ^2
expected

27. The chi-square test is most suited for _____ data in which each case falling within a cell is _____ of every other case. When the question pertains to whether distributions of scores fall equally into certain categories, χ^2 is called the "goodness of _____ " test.

categoric
independent

fit

28. The Wilcoxon Matched-Pairs Signed-Ranks test is a nonparametric version of the _____ t test.

paired

29. For small n, the power efficiency of the Wilcoxon test is approximately _____ of its parametric equivalent.

95%

30. The Mann-Whitney U test, as a nonparametric equivalent of the _____ t test, is concerned with the equality of _____ .

unpaired
medians

31. The use of multiple t tests increases the probability of a type _____ error.

I

32. The main goal of ANOVA is to find the ratio of systematic variance, also called _____-group variance, and the degree of error variance, also termed _____-group variance.

between
within

33. The two-way ANOVA consists of main effect and _____ effect.

interaction

34. In the case of an unequal sample size among comparison groups, _____ test is highly useful for post hoc multiple comparisons. On the other hand, if the sample sizes are equal, the _____ test may be performed.

Scheffé's
Tukey

increases

I

within

systematic

before

χ^2

ANOVA
U

meta-analysis

one

group

intercorrelations
factors

MINITAB

coding

SPSS

35. The Bonferroni t procedure _____ the critical value of an *F* needed for reaching statistical significance. This procedure is used in cases in which the researcher wishes to decrease a type _____ error.

36. RBANOVA is appropriate for _____-subject designs in which the data come from repeated measures on the same subject. The primary purpose of this method is to determine whether or not the differences between two or more groups may be due to chance or to _____ differences among the groups.

37. ANCOVA allows for an adjustment in factors that might potentially influence the results of an experiment _____ the experiment begins.

38. The observed value of the Friedman test statistic approximates the _____ distribution.

39. The KWANOVA test is a nonparametric equivalent of the one-way _____ and is an extension of the Mann-Whitney _____ test.

40. An increasingly popular methodology for statistically combining the results from two or more independent studies is called _____-_____.

41. MANOVA is designed for problems in which there is more than _____ dependent variable under investigation.

42. Discriminant analysis has utility in predicting _____ membership of an individual.

43. In performing factor analysis, researchers must see how the measures tend to cluster based on the test items' _____ . Measures that are found to be correlated are called _____ .

44. _____ is an introductory computer software package that stores the data values in columns and rows like a spreadsheet.

45. BMDP is used in medical sciences and allows for different types of analyses on the same data to be performed with only minor changes in the _____ operations.

46. _____ is suitable for the behavioral and social sciences and widely used because of its simplicity and complete labeling of statistical analyses on data printouts.

Application # 1

Referring to our previously cited hypothetical study of the effect of propranolol on self ratings of stuttering severity, perform a paired t test to evaluate the significance of the difference between the mean scores for the drug and placebo conditions at $\alpha=.05$. Use the data below to perform your calculations.

SELF-RATINGS OF SEVERITY

Subject	Propranolol	Placebo
1.	3	5
2.	0	1
3.	2	4
4.	1	3
5.	3	3
6.	1	4
7.	2	3
8.	4	5

The null hypothesis stated as: H_0: The mean difference is _____ . The formula for the paired t test is given by $t= \dfrac{\bar{d}}{s_d/n}$ with df= _____ , where $\bar{d}$ represents the mean _____ , s_d represents the standard deviation of the sample difference, and n represents the number of _____ in the sample.

In order to calculate $\bar{d}$ and s_d, we must first find the sum of d, denoted by _____ , and the sum of the square of d, denoted by _____ . The sum of d is _____ , and the sum of the square of d is _____ . Similarly, $\bar{d}$ = _____ and s_d= _____ . Finally, the observed value of t is _____ with df = _____ . The absolute critical value of t at $\alpha = .05$ for a two-tailed test is _____ . Therefore, the null hypothesis is _____ .

zero
n−1
difference
pairs
Σd
Σd²
−12
24
−1.5
.94
−4.52
7
2.365
rejected

Application # 2

Based on our previously cited study of work preferences among speech-language pathology versus audiology students, conduct a chi-square test at $\alpha=.05$ to determine whether or not the membership of the two groups and their work preference are independent. Use the hypothetical data given below:

WORK PREFERENCE   N=100

	Medical	Non-Medical	Row Sum
Sp/Lang. Path	16	34	50
Audiology	32	18	50
Column Sum	48	52	100

independent
one
Yates'
1
10.26
3.841
rejected

The null hypothesis can be stated as: H_0: The two categories are _____. For this study, a _____-tailed test will be used and _____ Correction for Continuity should be used because df = _____.

The observed chi-square value is found to be _____ , and the critical χ^2 is found to be _____. Hence, the null hypothesis is _____.

Application #3

Recalling our hypothetical study concerning the auditory processing abilities of three groups of children with different phonologic skills: Control Group (A), Consistent Group (B), and Delayed Group (C), perform a one-way ANOVA to determine the significance of difference among them.

The table shown below summarizes the data you need to complete the calculations.

Control (A)	Consistent (B)	Delayed (C)
78	72	88
98	100	78
100	98	91
97	99	87
96	94	100
100	85	76
100	90	98
94	100	96
95	100	100
92	92	96

null hypothesis

The _____ _____ can be symbolically stated as $\mu_A = \mu_B = \mu_C$.

independence
normal
variance
homogeneity

The three basic assumptions of the one-way ANOVA are (1) _____ among the groups; (2) the sampling distribution of the group follows a _____ curve; and (3) the _____ of the scores in each group are equal. This assumption is also referred to as _____ of variance.

Assuming these assumptions have been met, calculate the necessary numerical values to obtain the F value for the above scores. These values are found to be as follows:

10 10
10 95
93 91
93 3
30
40
66.37

n_a = _____ , n_B = _____

n_C = _____ , $\overline{Y}_A$ = _____

$\overline{Y}_B$ = _____ , $\overline{Y}_C$ = _____

$\overline{Y}$ = _____ , J = _____

N = _____ ,

Between-group variance = _____

Within-group variance = _____

df(between) = _____ ,   2
df(within) = _____   27

Finally, the observed F value is _____ . By consulting   0.60
the F table in Appendix C.4, the critical F value at $\alpha = .05$ is found   3.35
to be _____ . Therefore, we must _____ H_0.   retain

9. Reading, Writing, and Presenting Research

The Value of Critical Thinking	Institutional Funds
Catabolic Thinking in Reading Research	NIH Grants and Contracts
—*Research Article Questionnaire*	Foundation and Corporate Grants
Anabolic Thinking in Writing Research	**Theses and Dissertations**
—*Research Proposal Outline*	**Writing Well**
Funding Research	**Professional Presentations**

According to one dictionary definition, a profession is the " . . . faith in which one is professed." To a large degree, "faith" in any scientific discipline is based on the quality of its research and the manner in which new knowledge is communicated. Good reading, writing, and oral communication skills are essential tools for interpreting and professing thoughts, opinions, ideas, and conclusions about new findings as they emerge.

THE VALUE OF CRITICAL THINKING

In earlier chapters, the point was made that different people may differ widely in their perceptions of truth based on a wealth of accumulated information. The same can be said for those professionals working in scientific fields who are frequently critical of the research of their colleagues. Among scientists, **critical thinking** is a highly regarded means of exercising judgment in the search for truth. Evidence of this fact can be found in the "letters to the editor" section of many scientific journals where space is provided for thoughtful analyses and commentaries by the readers of articles. Such letters are often geared toward uncovering methodological problems in a research study or providing alternative interpretations of the data. Sometimes, letters may include brief summaries of other research findings that bear on the problem. Authors of articles are typically given the opportunity to reply to criticisms of their work. This frequently results in a lively and useful interchange of opinion about the validity and implications of the research outcome. Much can be learned from a careful review of the articles that initially stimulated such commentaries as well as from the debate subsequently highlighted in letters written to the editor. Of course, we must keep in mind that critical thinking is not only usefully applied in the analysis of the work of others but also in the design and evaluation of one's own work.

By being critical in the course of reading and writing research literature, we ultimately build a rational foundation for decision making, or **"quasi-faith,"** in what is professed. In essence, we construct a kind of temporary reality by seeking and finding empirical evidence for hypotheses, knowing that their ultimate proof will always remain questionable to some degree. Because critical reading and writing are the best tools available for evaluating and communicating such evidence, these skills are important to learn.

Catabolic Thinking In Reading Research

As an integral part of a course in research and statistical methods, the authors of this text require that students engage in two kinds of critical thinking exercises that are akin to two well-known processes in the field of biochemistry. The first of these exercises is designed to foster what we choose to call **catabolic thinking.** Catabolism is actually a metabolic process of breaking food particles down into smaller parts to facilitate digestion. Therefore, in a figurative sense, we ask that students thoroughly "digest" the various components of a research article by critically evaluating each of its subcomponents. To guide this process, the students are asked to provide a detailed evaluation of a selected research article according to the following Research Article Questionnaire.

Research Article Questionnaire

I. Title and Abstract

    A. Did the title of the article clearly and accurately represent the topic or overall purpose of the study? Were words used that should have been omitted or substituted for by better words? Could the words in the title be readily adopted as "key words" in reference guides and computer-based information services to accurately identify the content of the article? Was the title condensed and abbreviated appropriately as to provide a running header at the top of the article's pages?

    B. Did the abstract provide a concise yet adequate description of the problem? Generally, were the questions or hypotheses investigated, the methods employed, the statistical analyses obtained, and the conclusions drawn clarified?

II. Introduction

    A. Did the introduction provide an objective and balanced survey of the literature that progressed smoothly and logically to culminate in a summary statement of the problem?

    B. Was the rationale (need) for the study firmly established based on a paucity of previous research or observed limitations in other studies—i.e., inadequacies in sampling, design errors, inappropriate choice of statistics, mistakes in the analysis, or interpretation of data, etc.?

    C. Was the theoretical and practical importance of the findings adequately addressed?

    D. What specific research questions or hypotheses were raised? What independent and dependent variables were incorporated within these questions or hypotheses?

III. Methods

    A. Were the characteristics of the sample fully described in terms of the population to which the results were generalized; the number of subjects used; the criteria for the subjects' inclusion or exclusion; their physical, psychosocial, and educational attributes; the manner of their selection and assignment to various treatment conditions; and the attrition of subjects from the control and experimental groups during the course of the experiment?

    B. Were all known variables in the study specified and their validity established? Could these be replicated in future research? What instruments, test measures, or recording devices were used to operationally define the parameters of the dependent and independent variables? Were specific brand names, model numbers, or other kinds of identifying information listed? If a noncommercial specialized apparatus was used, were descriptive diagrams or sketches provided to explain its various components, their electrical/mechanical operations, and the manner of calibration and reliability?

C. What type of design was used in the study? Was a rational basis for its selection made known? Were the controls (e.g., randomization, counterbalancing, blinding, etc.) appropriate for eliminating threats to internal and external validity? Were the test environment and testing conditions adequately described? What instructions were given to the subjects? Were the procedures for manipulating the independent variable and recording the dependent variable clearly specified, and was their reliability established?

IV. Results

A. Were the data qualitative or quantitative in nature? What types of statistical methods were selected to test the research questions or hypotheses? Were the methods chosen appropriate for this task? Were all relevant results reported, including those running counter to the hypotheses? Were any findings presented that seemed tangential to the stated goals of the investigation?

B. Were the data well organized and logically presented using suitable tables and figures? Were clear legends and captions provided? Were averages and standard deviation reported in addition to probability values, the degrees of freedom, and the direction of the effect? Did the data appear to come from a normal distribution, or did the distribution appear skewed (e.g., containing an inordinate number of scores higher or lower than the mean)? Was the power of the test evaluated in relation to the likelihood for a type II error? How many statistical comparisons were made on the groups? Was the probability that some of these tests might yield statistically significant findings as a result of chance alone taken into account?

C. Were the data assessed in an objective and straightforward manner while avoiding theoretical speculation?

V. Discussion

A. Did the discussion provide a brief summary of the study in view of the questions or hypotheses posed in the introduction and the data presented in the results section? If hypotheses were stated in the introduction, was every one of them evaluated and its validity interpreted based on the results of the present study as well as the findings of similar investigations? If new hypotheses were advanced, were these consistent with the present findings, or did the authors extrapolate beyond the limits of their statistical analyses?

B. Were the strengths and weaknesses of the study thoroughly evaluated? To what degree did possible design problems or the failure to control for extraneous or confounding influences hamper the generalization of findings?

C. Were both positive and negative results discussed in view of their theoretical or practical implications? What suggestions were offered for future research, and did the suggestions appear to be logical and justifiable given the results of the current study?

VI. References and Appendices

A. Were all references used in the text of the article included in an alphabetical list at the end of the article? Was an appropriate bibliographic style used? In the case of journal publications of the American Speech-Language-Hearing Association, the style of reference should conform with the format recommended in the current *Publication Manual of the American Psychological Association* (APA).[1]

---

[1] Available through the American Psychological Association: Order Department, P.O. Box 2710, Hyattsville, MD 20784.

B. Was any supplementary information included in alphabetically arranged appendices, such as additional statistical data, questionnaires, technical notes or equipment diagrams, instructions for subjects, and details of clinical treatments or training programs? Did this material facilitate understanding? Was certain material omitted that should have been included, particularly in reference to its judged importance for replication of the study?

VII. Overall Assessment. Imagine that as an editorial consultant for a journal you had been asked to peer review and evaluate the publication merit of the same article you selected for this exercise. Would you have judged the article acceptable for publication, perhaps with some revisions, or recommended that it be rejected? Provide a concise rationale for your decision in either case. If revisions had been recommended, what constructive advice might you have offered? If the investigation was so flawed as to have been rejected, what practical steps might be taken in future studies to correct the problems you identified?

A research article questionnaire of the kind just described can help to make the reading of scientific literature an important scientific activity in its own right. In essence, it serves as an analytic tool for *investigating an investigation* in order to judge its worth. Although no questionnaire should be expected to provide universal coverage for all types of research problems, we have found ours to be a useful guide for the systematic dissection of most articles, as one of our students said, "right down to the bones."

Anabolic Thinking in Writing Research

Earlier, we noted that the term catabolism is a useful metaphor for describing the process of breaking down the separate elements of a research article so that the validity of its contents can be digested and logically appraised. Of equal importance to the development of critical thinking skills is the notion of **anabolism**—a process that entails building up or assembling complex structures from more elementary components. That which we call anabolic thinking is reflected in the type of scientific work that culminates in a written research proposal. Such a proposal requires not only a critical review of the separate elements of many previous studies, but also a well-crafted and integrated plan for addressing current deficiencies in knowledge uncovered in the literature review.

The format for writing a research proposal will vary depending on its use. Students enrolled in the course we teach are asked at the beginning of the semester to form a designated number of "research teams." Each team is required to develop a research proposal as outlined below. A well-written proposal shares many of the same features as a good research article. In addition, it must address important administrative, ethical, and financial concerns if the project is to succeed.

Research Proposal Outline

I. Title. The **title** should be effective in conveying what the study is about. Avoid the use of unnecessary words that lead to cumbersome and confusing titles such as, "A *Study to Investigate* Physiological *Measures of* Anxiety and *Their Relation to* Stuttering Adaptation *During Oral Reading Trials* Under Two Levels of Audience Complexity." A shorter, neater version of this title would be: "Physiological Anxiety and Stuttering Adaptation Under Two Levels of Audience Complexity." The improved version is achieved by simply omitting the italicized words. Paring down verbiage in the titles of articles generally achieves the dual goals of brevity and increased clarity. Of course, a title that is too short may also cause ambiguity. For example, the following title meets the criterion of brevity but conveys little information: "Stuttering and Anxiety." A good rule to follow in constructing titles is to include **key words** that *concisely* identify the variables under investigation and the conditions used for testing their relationships.

The title page should also include the following identifying information under the title:

- The first name, middle initial, and last name of each investigator, their highest academic degree, and their institutional affiliation(s).
- The name of the institutional unit, review board, or agency to whom the proposal is being submitted.
- The name, address, and telephone number of the individual who is to serve as the principal investigator or coordinator of the project.

II. Abstract. As a comprehensive summary of the content of the proposed research study, an abstract should be approximately 100 to 150 words in length. Because the abstract provides a succinct summary of the problem, the subjects and methods to be used, and the importance of the findings, it should be written after the components of the proposal are assembled in final form. According to the APA's publication manual, a good abstract is one that is accurate, self-contained, concise and specific, nonevaluative, coherent, and readable.

III. Table of Contents. A table of contents should be included on a separate page to provide a convenient means of locating specific information contained in the proposal by page number. Pages preceding the table of contents are typically paginated using lower case roman numerals (i.e., i, ii, iii, etc.). Consecutive Arabic numbers are used for pagination following the table of contents.

IV. Budget. A budget should be included to cover anticipated expenses over the time frame of the study. A detailed budget should be provided for the first year and a summary budget for each subsequent year. Such costs might be incurred because of the need to

- purchase, fabricate, or maintain equipment and supplies
- compensate subjects for their participation
- pay salaries and fringe benefits of individual investigators and support staff based on the percentage of their time allocated to the project
- reimburse travel expenses
- cover consultant costs, the fee for service contracts, or expenses connected with physical alterations or renovations
- pay for administrative and overhead costs—e.g., telephone and utility bills, mailing, photocopying, computer use, rental fees

A good budget is realistic to the degree that it (1) *truly* reflects the estimated funds needed for completing the research study within a given time frame and (2) complies with the funding guidelines of the institution or granting agency from whom support will be requested. A rationale must be provided for each budget need accompanied by documented evidence for all estimated costs (manufacturer's quotes, catalog prices, etc.).

V. Other Support and Resources. Be sure to describe any other sources of funds, whether federal, nonfederal, or institutional that will be used to support the project. Such funds might include training grants, cooperative agreements, contracts, fellowships, gifts, prizes, or other awards specifically related to the study.

The available resources for completing the study are also important to describe. This might include a description of the space allocated for testing subjects, special laboratory equipment, and computer facilities. Formal agreements with other institutions to provide needed resources for the study and related administrative details are typically included in an appendix. Confirming letters of all institutional agreements must be included and signed by authorized officials. In the case of complex arrangements with other institutions or the need to coordinate the activities of multiple investigators, such documentation is important for clarifying the administrative authority and responsibility in overseeing various operations of the project.

VI. Biographical Sketches. Institutional review boards and funding agencies will want to know about the education and special abilities of the investigator(s) to complete the proposed investigation as well as those of all consultants. Therefore, a resume summarizing the academic training, academic degrees, and relevant professional accomplishments of each investigator should be included with the research proposal. It is especially important that the resumes of investigators highlight those pilot studies, completed investigations, or former grant support for projects most relevant to the proposed topic of research. This may not be necessary for certain types of **internal reviews**—e.g., reviews of Master's theses or Doctoral dissertations proposals. However, virtually all **external reviews** of research proposals conducted by outside institutions, government agencies, corporations, or foundations require an evaluation of the credentials of the applicant investigator(s).

VII. Research Protocol (Study Plan). A protocol is a detailed narrative of the research study that one wishes to perform. It should include the following elements: (1) Specific Aims; (2) Background and Significance; (3) Methods; and (4) Ethical Considerations.

A. Specific Aims

The objectives of the study, i.e., what the investigator intends to accomplish, should be stated clearly and include the rationale for the research questions or hypotheses upon which the study is based. An example of a specific aims statement, excerpted from a funded NIH proposal, that meets these requirements is quoted below:

> Many studies have shown a higher frequency of language impairments and reading disabilities in children with socially disadvantaged backgrounds . . . However, most definitions of language and reading disorders exclude socially disadvantaged children because of the *implicit* assumption that cultural and sociological deprivation "causes" the disability. Consistent with our emphasizes on validation of definitional criteria, we propose to study explicitly the influence of social disadvantage on language and reading disability. This study will permit clarification of the role of social disadvantage on disability definitions and the more general issue of the influence of social disadvantage on developmental reading disabilities. We hypothesize that language impairment and social disadvantage will exercise joint but independent influences on reading disability consistent with a main effects model (i.e., no interaction effect). (Aram, D., et al., 1994, p. 5–6)

The point at which the specific aims should be addressed within the sequence of the various sections of a research proposal is a matter for debate. Logically, it might be contended that a statement of the aims should follow a background review of the salient literature after establishing a well-grounded need for further investigation. On the other hand, an equal if not better argument is that the specific aims should be stated at the beginning of the protocol so that reviewers can determine from the outset just what the research is about. As noted by Colton (1974), " . . . effective critical appraisal hinges on the reader's initial understanding of the aim of the investigation." (p. 317) Ultimately, the "formula" for structuring a research proposal must be based on the requirements stipulated by the reviewers who will read and decide on its merit.

B. Background and Significance

The background and significance section of the protocol provides a critical review of the literature relevant to the problem to be investigated. In effect, it marshals the facts about what is presently known and unknown and states the importance of learning more. Any preliminary work by an investigator related to the proposed study should receive special emphasis because it may strengthen the investigator's credibility for continuing studies in a particular research area in which certain types or levels of expertise may be desirable or required. It is particularly important to state clearly the theoretical and practical importance of the findings. As much as possible, one should describe how the results of the study might alter understanding, influence clinical procedures, resolve theoretical debates, etc.

C. Methods

The methods section should be written to allow the reviewers to assess the appropriateness of your sampling techniques, measurements, experimental procedures, design for executing the study, and plans for data analysis. Any anticipated difficulties with proposed procedures along with alternative approaches to achieve the aims should likewise be discussed.

The organization and content of the narrative in the methods section is much like the format found in a research article (see Chapter 1). In essence, you should describe in specific terms:

- who you plan to use for subjects
- what you wish to do to them
- how it will be done
- the means for assessing outcomes

The methods section of the protocol is also a convenient place for the inclusion of a **timetable** that specifies when each stage of the investigation will start and be completed. The specification of such deadlines is important for assuring the accountability of the investigator(s) to the goals stated in the research proposal. Furthermore, institutional sponsors of research, review boards, and government agencies typically mandate adherence to certain calendar deadlines for submitting research applications, progress reports, and the renewal of funding for projects.

As noted in Chapter 1, the method section serves as the blueprint for conducting the investigation. If this section of a research protocol is flawed or written poorly, the study will likely be rejected.

D. Ethical Considerations

Ethical considerations *must* be addressed in protecting the rights and welfare of subjects. As discussed previously in Chapter 4, if human subjects are to participate in an investigation, the research proposal must be evaluated and given approval by an Institutional Review Board (IRB). Federal regulations pertaining to the composition and duties of an IRB have been specified in the *Federal Register*, June 18, 1991. The Department of Agriculture and Public Health Service has also published guidelines related to the use and care of laboratory animals in research. Institutions that use animals for such purposes must also have an Institutional Animal Care Committee (IAUCC) consisting of a veterinarian, a scientist, and an individual who is not a member of the institution. The American Speech-Language-Hearing Association has also established publication guidelines for approval of articles in its journals related to the use of humans and animals in research (Figure 9.1).

GUIDELINES FOR RESEARCH SUBJECTS

Humans in research: All research to be submitted for publication in journals of the American Speech-Language-Hearing Association in which human subjects are used must adhere to the basic ethical considerations for the protection of human subjects in research. The basis for these considerations can be found in The Belmont Report: Ethical Principles and Guidelines for the Protection of Human Subjects.[1] Where applicable by law or institutional affiliation, authors must provide assurance of approval by an appropriate Institutional Review Board or equivalent review process.

Animals in research: All research to be submitted for publication in journals of the American Speech-Language-Hearing Association in which animal subjects are used must adhere to the statement of the American Physiological Society regarding use and care of animals in research. The applicable portions follow:

> Animal experiments are to be undertaken only with the purpose of advancing knowledge. Consideration should be given to the appropriateness of experimental procedures, species of animals used, and number of animals required.
>
> Only animals that are lawfully acquired will be used in the laboratory, and their retention and use will be in every case in compliance with federal, state, and local laws and regulations in accordance with the NIH Guide.[2]

Animals in the laboratory must receive every consideration for their comfort; they must be properly housed, fed, and their surroundings kept in a sanitary condition.

Appropriate anesthetics must be used to eliminate sensibility to pain during all surgical procedures. Where recovery from anesthesia is necessary during the study, acceptable technique to minimize pain must be followed. Muscle relaxants or paralytics are not anesthetics and they should not be used alone for surgical restraint. They may be used for surgery in conjunction with drugs known to produce adequate analgesia. Where use of anesthetics would negate the results of the experiment, such procedures should be carried out in strict accordance with the NIH Guide. If the study requires the death of the animal, the animal must be killed in a humane manner at the conclusion of the observations.

The postoperative care of animals will be such as to minimize discomfort and pain, and in any case will be equivalent to accepted practices in schools of veterinary medicine.

---

[1]Office for Protection from Research Risks (1979). *The Belmont Report: Ethical Principles and Guidelines for the Protection of Human Subjects.* Bethesda, MD: U.S. Dept. of Health and Human Services.

[2]Office of Science and Health Reports (1980). *Guide for the Care and Use of Laboratory Animals* (DHEW Publication #80–23). Bethesda, MD: National Institutes of Health

Figure 9.1. ASHA's publication guidelines for research in which human or animal subjects are used.

Because IRB approval is necessary *prior* to implementing most research studies, it is wise to seek such approval early in the process of planning the investigation. This is particularly important if the **ratio of potential risks to potential benefits** is estimated to be high. Although the majority of studies in the field of communication disorders involve minimal risk of harm or discomfort to subjects, this is not always the case. The use of certain drugs, the surgical removal of tissue, the implantation of foreign devices or materials, radiographic imaging techniques, and aversive conditioning procedures are examples of the kinds of experimental methods that may carry a high level of risk.

An IRB will look carefully at the written consent form that subjects will be asked to sign as well as the research protocol. It is particularly important that the consent form is written in a manner that can be easily comprehended by the subjects or parents or legal guardians for whom its use is intended. An example of a well-written consent form is shown in Figure 9.2 (Barresi, 1996). An IRB protocol and consent form written in a precise and organized style will be of great help in gaining approval for your study and assuring its ultimate success.

VIII. References. All names cited in the proposal should be properly referenced. In the text of the proposal, names that are directly cited in the context of a sentence should be referenced by listing the last name of the author(s) followed by the date of the publication enclosed in parentheses: *"Boberg and Kully (1996) reported . . ."*

When there are multiple authors of a single research study, list all of their last names in the initial reference but only the name of the first author in subsequent references to the same study: *"The results of a study by Conture, Colton, & Gleason (1986) indicated . . .",* and subsequently, *"As the results of the study by Conture et al. indicated . . ."*

If an author's name is not directly used in the sentence but his or her work is cited, the following format is appropriate: *"In a review of the research literature on child language disorders . . ., it was noted that . . . (Miller, 1991).* Multiple references of this kind should be listed alphabetically and separated by a semi-colon: *(Green & Kuhl, 1989; MacDonald & McGurk, 1978; Massaro, 1987).*

Complete references also should be listed alphabetically in a "Reference" section at the end of the text. The following examples illustrate the style recommended by the APA for referencing several types of published and unpublished resources:

Book (single author):

Conture, E. G. (1990). *Stuttering.* 2nd ed. Englewood Cliffs, NJ: Prentice Hall.

Book (multiple authors):

Palmer, J. M. & Yantis, P. A. (1990). *Survey of communication disorders.* Baltimore: William & Wilkins.

Chapter in Edited Book:

Maxwell, S. E. & Wallach, G. P. (1984). The language-learning disabilities connection: Symptoms of early language disability change over time. In G. P. Wallach & K. G. Butler (Eds.), *Language learning disabilities in school-age children* (pp. 15–340). Baltimore: Williams & Wilkins.

Journal Article (multiple authors):

Grievink, E., Peters, S., van Bon, W., & Schilder, A. (1993). The effects of early bilateral otitis media with effusion on language ability: A prospective cohort study. *Journal of Speech and Hearing Research,* 36, 1004–1012.

Master's Thesis:

Diamond, K. M. *Non-verbal temporal order processing in adult dyslexia* (1989). Unpublished Master's thesis, Emerson College.

Conference Paper

Solomon, N. P., Robin, D. A., & Luschei, E. S. (1994, March). *Strength, endurance and sense of effort: Studies of the tongue and hand in people with Parkinson's disease and accompanying dysarthria.* Paper presented at the Conference on Motor Speech, Sedona, AZ.

Participant's Name _____ Date _____

Principal Investigator: (Name), (Institution), (Address)

Informed Consent

1. *Title of Study:* Proper Name Recall in Younger and Older Adults: The Contributions of Word Uniqueness and Reported Strategies.

2. *Purpose of the Study:* The purpose of this study is to investigate the effects of aging on the learning and retrieval of proper names and occupations assigned to pictures of unfamiliar faces.

3. *Procedures:* I will be asked to look at some pictures of people and learn their names and occupations so that I can recall them later. I will also be asked to complete a brief questionnaire related to my recall of these items and to complete a rating scale of the names and occupations. In addition, there will be some tests to test my memory and attention. The testing will take approximately 1 to 2 hours. All testing will be scheduled at my convenience.

4. *Risks and Discomforts:* There are no known medical risks or discomforts associated with this project, although I may experience fatigue and/or stress when taking these tests. I will be given as many breaks as I want during the testing session.

5. *Benefits:* I understand there are no known direct medical benefits to me for participating in this study. However, the results of the study may help researchers gain a better understanding of how we learn and recall information about other people.

6. *Participant's Rights:* I may withdraw from participating in the study at any time.

7. *Financial Compensation:* I will be reimbursed $ __ per hour for my participation and $ ___ or any travel expenses.

8. *Confidentiality:* In order to record exactly what I say in the tests, a tape recorder will be used. The tape will be listened to only by the Principal Investigator and authorized members of the research team at _____. I understand that the results of testing will be kept confidential unless I ask that they be released. The results of this study may be published in professional journals or presented at professional conferences, but my records or identity will not be revealed unless required by law.

9. If I have any questions or concerns, I can call _____at (000) 000-0000 at any time during the day or night.

I understand my rights as a research subject, and I voluntarily consent to participation in this study. I understand what the study is about and how and why it is being done. I will receive a signed copy of this consent form.

_____   _____

Subject's Signature   Date

_____

Signature of Investigator

Figure 9.2. Example of a written consent form.

IX. **Appendices.** Technical descriptions of instrumentation, photographs, test questionnaires, documentation of IRB approval if already obtained, and other relevant information that supplements the proposal is included within alphabetically arranged appendices (A, B, C, etc.).

FUNDING RESEARCH

Research proposals are often motivated by the need to obtain financial support for new or continuing research projects. Funds for such support are available through a variety of sources including department or institutional funds, government agencies, and foundations and corporations.

Institutional Funds

Many colleges and universities allocate "seed money" for getting new research projects started. At our own institution, applications for **intramural research funds,** as they are called, are made through the office of the Graduate Dean. A faculty research committee is appointed each year to evaluate the proposals, which must be structured and written according to uniform guidelines. The awards are made through a competitive process in which the merit of each proposal is evaluated according to well-defined criteria. As in many institutions, the amount of money available for the support of individual faculty projects is relatively small, consisting of a few thousand dollars. Nevertheless, these funds are often crucial for collecting preliminary data or laying the ground work for more extensive studies. The appeal of an **extramural grant application** (beyond the institution) often can be greatly enhanced by providing tangible evidence that an investigator is not only motivated but also competent to complete the proposed study. Intramural research awards can assist in marshaling such evidence, particularly for young faculty members at the start of their careers. Such awards to faculty can also serve the interests of graduate students who may receive stipends and gain experience as research assistants by working on such projects. Students might also be afforded data collection opportunities that facilitate their own plans for completing theses and dissertations in related areas of research.

NIH Grants and Contracts

A major source of research funds is through the federal government with the National Institutes of Health (NIH) serving as the primary agency for the support of projects in biomedical fields. The work involved in completing an NIH research grant application can be an arduous and time-consuming process requiring careful attention to each detail of the form. Research applications that are self-initiated by investigators are called **RO-1 proposals.** The proposal must be written strictly in accordance with the instructions provided in **Grant Application Form PHS 398.** NIH will mail this form to applicants on request or a copy can usually be obtained through the grants or development office of one's own institution.

The review of individual research grants by NIH is also a complex affair that generally involves three scheduled review cycles per year. Applications must by sent to the **Division of Research Grants (DRG)** before the stipulated deadline date for consideration within a certain review period. The DRG assigns applications to particular institutes or divisions within NIH. An institute whose funding policies are directly aligned with much research in the field of communication sciences and disorders is the **National Institute on Deafness and Other Communication Disorders (NIDCD).**

Applications received by DRG are assigned to one of several **Initial Review Groups**

(IRGs) or so-called **study sections** judged appropriate for reviewing particular research proposals. Research grant applications in communication disorders typically are reviewed by the Hearing Research, Sensory Disorders and Language, Human Development and Aging, or Biopsychology study sections. Such study sections are said to conduct **peer reviews** because working scientists review proposals in the research field of their own expertise. Although the DRG makes the final decision about which study group is most appropriate to review a particular application, the applicant may express her or his preference in a cover letter.

After deliberating the merits of a grant application, the study section members vote as to whether the proposal should be approved, disapproved, or deferred for final judgment pending the receipt of additional information. Approved applications are assigned a priority rating score on a scale of 100 (highest priority) to 500 (lowest priority). A summary of the review is forwarded to the applicant on the "pink sheet" notifying her or him of the rating score assigned to the proposal and the action taken by the study committee. The comments and criticisms of the reviewers can be quite useful in revising and resubmitting an application at a later time. The **advisory council** for the institute also reviews the results of the committee's actions and makes final decisions about which applications are funded or not funded. On the average, the minimum time from receipt of an application to making an award is approximately 10 months.

Not all approved applications receive funding. Indeed, of the new applications submitted to NIH, only 30% or less receive grant awards (Gartland, 1993). Generally, the period for these awards for successful applicants is between 2 and 5 years.

Many other categories of research awards are available through NIH. One of these, called a **FIRST** award (R29 application), is particularly well-suited for newly independent investigators who are at the beginning of their research careers. The criteria for the these awards are different than for the traditional RO-1 grants. Support must be requested for a five-year period, with at least 50% of the time devoted to the project.

NIH also makes efforts to stimulate and support research in various areas designated by its own advisory committees. Applications under this program, called **P0–1 applications,** are made either in response to a **Request for Proposals (RFP)** or a **Request for Application (RFA).** Essentially, investigators who respond to an RFP may be awarded a contract to conduct research as determined by NIH. On the other hand, although a grant awarded under an RFA also addresses a topic of interest to NIH, the research plan used for this purpose is the creation of the investigator. Program announcements **(PAs)** are published regularly in the **NIH *Guide for Grants and Contracts*** and the *Federal Register.*

Foundation and Corporate Grants

Thousands of nongovernmental, nonprofit foundations in the United States give money to assist worthy projects of special interest to them. Although the total giving of foundations amounts to billions of dollars each year, only a small percentage of this money is allocated for research in the behavioral, educational, and health science fields. Nevertheless, research projects that require a modest level of funding and that have goals closely related to the mission of a particular foundation are strong candidates for support.

An excellent resource that describes the goals and objectives of major foundations and the kinds of projects they fund is the *Foundation Grants Directory,* maintained by a national organization called the **Foundation Center.** The Foundation Center is an independent agency that gathers and disseminates factual information on the philanthropic foundations through programs of library service, publication, and research. It has organized a nationwide network of foundation reference collections in all 50 states. **The Centers for**

Cooperating Collections offer a number of free publications and provide a trained staff to assist patrons in locating resources on funding information. The Foundation Center also maintains a data base of more than 40,000 grantmaking foundations and direct corporate-giving programs. The center staff will provide assistance in searching its data base for foundations whose interests align with the individual or institution seeking support for a particular project, or it will recommend the best on-line and other sources of regional and national information.[2]

Once an appropriate foundation has been identified, a three- to five-page letter should be written to the grants officer describing the objectives of the research plan. The qualifications of the investigator(s) to carry out the research, the anticipated time period for the project, and the amount of money needed for its completion should also be described. Depending on the level of interest in the applicant's letter, the grants officer of the foundation may respond by requesting additional information. Some foundations will only make awards under certain cost-sharing arrangements with the applicant's own institution or in conjunction with another philanthropic organization.

Some businesses and corporations are also interested in funding research or providing needed equipment, particularly if the anticipated outcome is consistent with their own advertising and marketing objectives or is expected to enhance their public image. Manufacturers of hearing aids, augmentative communication devices, diagnostic equipment, or computer software are examples of the kinds of enterprises that may be interested in cooperative research ventures. In considering such partnerships, it is imperative that the researcher be able to conduct an independent and impartial research study untainted by the biasing influences of certain expectations that might otherwise operate, even in subtle ways. The use of blinding control procedures (see Chapter 5) in both the collection and analysis of data may be highly useful in assuring valid results.

THESES AND DISSERTATIONS

In numerous fields of graduate study, a written thesis (Master's level) or dissertation (doctoral level) is required to demonstrate mastery of the thinking processes and tools of research.

The majority of graduate programs in communication disorders no longer require the completion of a formal thesis project. The reasons underlying the lack of such a requirement are complex. Perhaps the most important of these are the market forces that have led to a rapidly expanding demand for trained clinicians. Such growth has placed great strain on the educational resources of many college and university programs. Furthermore, the corpus of knowledge pertaining to speech, language and hearing disorders has also grown immensely requiring additional course work and clinical training to meet the increased requirements for certification.

Whether or not all students who plan to work professionally in the field of communication disorders should have formal research training is a matter for debate. Some might argue, as Jerger (1963) did in an often-cited editorial that stirred up much debate in the field, that the practical realities of the profession are such that research cannot be done well by everyone and is best left to those who are trained to do it well. Research, Jerger said, "is the province of trained researchers, just as diagnosis and therapy are the province of trained clinicians." (p. 3) A counter argument to the Jerger position is that the mean-

---

[2]For the address and telephone number of a Cooperating Collection in a given location, write the Foundation Center at 79 Fifth Ave., New York, NY 10003–3076 or telephone 1-800-424-9836.

ing of the term "research" should not be restricted to carrying out a set of narrowly defined procedures. Research also should be thought of as those antecedent scientific thinking processes that *lead* to the application of certain methods in problem solving. In extending this line of logic, it could be said that the primary value of thesis and dissertation research is not so much in the research outcome but in the development of the scientific thinking processes that make the outcome possible.

Although a thesis may not be required, many academic programs often give students the option of pursuing this experience. Assuredly, the demands associated with writing a thesis will help prepare students for even a more rigorous level of advanced scholarship—the doctoral dissertation. To gain approval for either a thesis or dissertation, a **prospectus** must be written. Such a prospectus is a detailed outline of the plan for research. Although there is no universally acceptable format for writing a prospectus, it will share many of the same elements of any research proposal.

Prior to writing a prospectus, you should ask a professor to serve as your thesis or dissertation advisor. The choice of a particular advisor is usually based on her or his expertise in the area related to the topic that you would like to pursue. Based on a review of salient literature and discussions with your advisor, you will gradually refine the subject matter of your research into testable questions or hypotheses backed up by well-grounded rationales. Important considerations in selecting and defining a research problem were discussed previously in Chapter 4. The type of question or hypothesis that is finally selected for study may be a component of a larger ongoing research program being pursued by your advisor or may be of your own invention. In either case, the problem should be intellectually challenging and judged worthy of investigation by both you and your advisor. Working together, you will also decide on the methods to be employed in the investigation, and a plan for data analysis (see Chapter 5).

You should also ask your advisor to help you develop a realistic timetable for completing your thesis or dissertation. Despite unforeseen obstacles that might hinder your progress, such a timetable can serve as a highly useful plan for guiding and disciplining the course of your actions as you work toward the goal of successfully completing your project. While most colleges and universities stipulate that theses and dissertations *must* be completed within a specific time period, both you and your advisor will prefer adhering as closely as possible to a reasonable schedule for finishing the project well within the strictures of such deadlines.

Your advisor will also assist you in selecting and assembling a thesis or dissertation advisory committee. Such a committee typically consists of three or more faculty members. It is common practice to select at least one member of the committee from a related discipline outside one's major department who can represent and uphold the overall academic standards of the college or university in evaluating the proposed research.

When you have completed a clearly written and well-organized plan for your research, your advisor will distribute it to all members of the advisory committee who will critically evaluate its quality using the same standards as they would apply to any research protocol as previously discussed. Subsequently, your advisor will schedule a prospectus meeting during which time you will be asked to summarize your plans for the proposed research and answer all questions raised by the advisory committee. Changes in the prospectus may be recommended by one or more committee members. Sometimes, disputes about recommended changes will need to be reconciled by your research advisor. Once the prospectus has been formally approved, it serves as a kind of "contract of agreement" between all the involved parties that the study will be carried out precisely as stated. Any variance in the written plan of research must be reflected in a revised prospectus that meets with the approval of the advisory committee. Thus, in addition to providing an action plan for the proposed research, an approved prospectus safeguards against future criticisms of the research protocol by committee members *provided* that the research was conducted carefully and competently as originally proposed. This assurance is important because the content of a thesis or dissertation when completed must be approved by the advisory committee that reviewed the original plan. Generally, such approval is contingent on an evaluation of the written document in addition to a successful oral defense by the student. Although a well-written research prospectus is no guarantee of a successful outcome, one that is ambiguous or lacking in sufficient details can lead to shoddy results accompanied by a negative evaluation.

WRITING WELL

Whether writing a research proposal, a thesis or dissertation, or an article for publication, it is important to attend closely not only to the content but also to the mechanics of the written result. Unfortunately, this principle is often ignored by researchers. Indeed, as a study by Armstrong (1980) made clear, obscure, pedantic writing with a high frequency of polysyllabic sentences can sometimes be more highly esteemed by college professors than prose characterized by simple straightforward sentence structures. Commenting on the obscurity and awkwardness of prose in many medical science areas, Crichton (1975) noted that the preferred " . . . stance of authors seems designed to astound and mystify the reader with a dazzling display of knowledge and scientific acumen . . ." (p. 1297). This "stance" also commonly prevails in many applied behavioral science areas to the detriment of clarity in written communication.

In addition to conforming to grammatical rules, good writing possesses the properties of **efficiency** and **effectiveness.** Efficient writing is constituted of concise sentences that state the point directly. Don't say: *"On the basis of the results of this study, it is possible to form a tentative hypothesis of a possible relationship between anxiety and stuttering."* Instead, simply state, *"The results are indicative of a relationship between . . ."* or, better still, *"A relationship was found between . . ."* Efficient writing conveys meaning using a minimal number of words.

Effective writing also possesses the property of clarity. Imprecise or vague words should be avoided whenever possible. Consider the following:

> *The results of the study indicated that when faced with hyperactive children with short attention spans (AD-HD) who were clearly unmotivated and who eventually became unresponsive to test stimuli because of their distractibility, clinicians were prone to modify their instructional techniques by terminating reinforcement followed by the introduction of a "time out" phase, during which time the training program was suspended for a period of a few minutes or more.*

The above sentence not only contains superfluous words, but it creates unnecessary ambiguity by the use of many vague, abstract words and professional jargon. Clarity is achieved by the use of precise, concrete, specific words that convey quantitative meaning whenever possible. Thus, the above sentence might be improved by the following revision:

> *When the rate of the response being reinforced decreased by 10%, the clinicians suspended the training program for 5 to 10 minutes.*

The readers of scientific articles often complain of difficulty in comprehending the content of such articles. Most often, the fault lies in the obscure verbiage of the writer—not because of inadequacies in the readers' comprehension abilities. As the professional writer Michael Alley (1987) said, "In scientific writing, precision is the most important goal of the language. If your writing does not communicate exactly what you did, then you have changed your research." (p. 28)

Many manuals and handbooks are available to help writers improve the efficiency and effectiveness of their writing style. Some of the most useful of these aids to scientific writing include the previously mentioned *Publication Manual of the American Psychological Association*, the *MLA Handbook for Writers of Research Papers, Theses, and Dissertations*,[3] and Kate Turabian's *Manual for Writers of Term Papers, Theses, and Dissertations*. The latter publication is available from University of Chicago Press, which also publishes a comprehensive style manual appropriately entitled *The Chicago Manual of Style*.[4] Also, a small book that has become a classic reference on matters of style and is widely used by writers from all fields is entitled *The Elements of Style* (Strunk and White, 1979). In addition, a comprehensive reference for students and professionals in communication disorders and allied fields has been published by the faculty at California State University, Fresno (Shipley, 1982).

PROFESSIONAL PRESENTATIONS

An important channel for communicating current research findings is that of oral presentations. The conveyance of information to professional audiences "by word of mouth" allows the speaker to communicate directly with her or his peers and to receive immediate feedback. Such feedback can be particularly useful in exploratory studies or pilot investigations when refinements in one or more components of the research protocol may need to be made before submitting an article to a journal for peer review. Critical comments and constructive advice offered by audience members during question and answer periods, especially from those whose expertise is in the subject matter presented, may be highly useful in evaluating the validity of the findings and in uncovering potential pitfalls that might jeopardize publication of the work. In this sense, an oral presentation can sometimes serve as a kind of "testing ground" in considering the publication merit of a research study.

Generally, opportunities for orally presenting one's research findings exceed the prospects for a journal publication. Such opportunities can be found within the colloquia of colleges and universities, in the "grand rounds" of clinics and hospitals, and through the sponsored institutes or research seminars and the professional programs of state, regional, or national conferences of scholarly organizations.

Program committees for conferences will typically require that proposals for oral presentations be written in a standard format in accordance with the submission guidelines of the organization. In the case of conventions sponsored by ASHA, submission requirements include the completion of cover sheets, a narrative summary, and a proposal rating form. The cover sheets include the title of the proposal, the content area to be covered (fluency/fluency disorder, voice/voice disorder, language science, etc.), the session type requested (brief presentation, poster presentation, experimental seminar, etc.), any special equipment requests, the names and professional affiliations of the presenters, and a brief abstract.

The abstract serves two major purposes. First, it provides a basis for the program committee to determine the overall suitability of the research for the intended scholarly aims of the conference and the degree to which it is likely to align with the interest of the au-

---

[3]Order from Publication Center, Modern Language Association, 62 Fifth Ave., New York, NY 10011
[4]Order from University of Chicago Press, 5801 Ellis Ave., Chicago, IL 60637

dience. Second, because all abstracts of accepted presentations are usually published in a program bulletin of the conference proceedings, audience participants can quickly review the key elements of the research paper(s) to be presented within a particular session and decide whether or not they wish to attend. As in the case of abstracts prepared for journal publications, the abstract for an oral presentation should be well-written because it too may be selected for inclusion within certain indexing services and data bases. Because of space limitations in program bulletins, abstracts may have to be condensed to an even greater degree than required for article publications. Abstracts of research studies proposed for presentation at ASHA's convention currently are required not to exceed 75 words. The following is an example of an abstract that the first author of this text recently submitted to ASHA's program review committee in response to a "call for papers" for a forthcoming convention:

> The California Verbal Learning Test (CVLT) was used to investigate a number of interrelated components of verbal memory in a group of dyslexic readers and matched control subjects. Several between-group differences were observed on measures of verbal learning ability, immediate recall, and recognition measures. The CVLT was found to be a reliable instrument for differentiating several cognitive processes and mnemonic strategies used by impaired versus normal readers in learning and remembering verbal material.

In addition to a written abstract, the program committee often will require a narrative summary of the research paper that describes the background, methods, and results of the research study in greater detail. ASHA specifies that the summary should, in 1500 words or less, give the program committee a clear understanding of the proposal's content. The proposal should also describe learner outcomes. For the proposal described above, the following learner outcomes were appended to the summary:

> Session participants will learn about:

- The general utility of the California Verbal Learning Test as it is designed to assess multiple components of verbal memory.
- The way the CVLT was used in this particular study to assess memory operations in adult dyslexics as compared to normal readers.
- The predominant types of errors found in the recall and recognition measures based on a statistical analysis of within- and between-group differences.
- Theoretical and clinical implications of the results, particularly in reference to the finding that dyslexics appeared to rely more heavily on the semantic than phonologic memory route during word retrieval.

An increasingly popular medium for presenting research at professional conferences consists of **poster presentations.** As opposed to brief research papers, where the allotted time may be 30 minutes or less, poster sessions are usually allowed to run for 90 minutes or more. Poster sessions are typically much more informal and interactive than research paper sessions. Furthermore, specific aspects of the research study often can be addressed and debated in greater detail. Especially for students and young investigators, poster sessions provide an excellent opportunity for presenting research findings in a relaxed and nonthreatening atmosphere and for meeting other researchers in a similar field who may offer useful advice. Such educational "networking" not only affords opportunities for mutual learning experiences but may also lead to future research collaborations with other colleagues.

Whatever the type of proposed presentation, it must be in accordance with certain criteria used by the program review committee if it is be accepted. In a recent call for papers for its national convention, ASHA noted that it would be guided in the selection of such papers based on the following criteria:

1. Quality
2. Distribution of subject matter, timeliness, popular demand. Preference will be given to new and innovative issues, submissions that address the convention theme, and clinical application of research.
3. Program balance. The committee seeks to create a convention with balanced offerings of different session types, content areas, and instructional levels.
4. Other. Only unpublished papers or presentations may be submitted. Research submissions must be based on completed work; promissory proposals will not be considered . . . (etc.)

The program committee of ASHA to whom a proposal is submitted will use a rating form to evaluate its acceptability for presentation. A five-point rating scale is used for this purpose as follows:

0	1	2	3	4	5
Unacceptable		Consider		Highly recommend	

In summary, oral communication can be an efficient, effective, and powerful means of communicating research findings. ASHA publishes a useful pamphlet that helps presenters develop and deliver a successful presentation at ASHA's annual conventions and other education programs (See Appendix E).

SELF-LEARNING REVIEW

1. Among scientists, _____ _____ is a highly re-garded means of exercising judgments in the search for truth.

critical thinking

2. Evidence for the above fact can be found in the "_____ to the _____" section of scientific journals.

letters
editor

3. By being critical in reading and writing research literature, we ultimately build a rational foundation for _____ making or "_____-_____" in what is professed.

decision
quasi faith

4. _____ thinking is similar to a metabolic process that en-tails breaking particles down into smaller parts.

Catabolic

5. "Digesting" the various components of a research article by critically evaluating each of its subcomponents is akin to what the authors call _____ thinking.

catabolic

6. A research article questionnaire serves as a tool for evaluating an _____ .

investigation

7. A process that entails building up or assembling complex structures from small elementary components is called _____ .

anabolism

8. The type of scientific work that culminates in a written re-search proposal is representative of _____ thinking.

anabolic

9. A _____ should be effective in conveying what the study is about.

title

10. A good rule to follow in constructing titles is to include _____ _____ that concisely identify the variables un-der investigation and _____ for testing their relationships.

key words
conditions

11. According to the APA's publication manual, a good _____ is one that is accurate, self-contained, concise and specific, nonevaluative, coherent, and readable.

abstract

12. A detailed budget section of a proposal should be provided for the _____ year and thereafter a _____ budget for each _____ year.

first
summary
subsequent

13. A good budget is realistic to the degree that it (1) _____ reflects the estimated funds needed for the research study within a given time period and (2) complies with the fund-ing _____ of the institution from whom the funds are sought.

truly

guidelines

pilot
completed
grant

14. The biographical sketches of investigators submitted with a research proposal should highlight those _____ studies, _____ investigations, or former _____ support for projects most relevant to the proposed research.

specific aims

15. The _____ _____ , or objectives of the study, describe what the investigation intends to accomplish.

background
significance
known
unknown
more
who
what
how
means

16. The _____ and _____ section of the protocol provides a critical review of the literature. It also marshals the facts about what presently is _____ and _____ and states the case for learning _____ .

17. In the methods section, you should describe in specific terms _____ you plan to use for subjects, _____ you wish to do to them, _____ it will be done, and the _____ for assessing the outcome.

Institutional Review
Board

18. If human subjects are to participate in an investigation, the research proposal must be evaluated and given approval by an _____ _____ _____ .

consent form
protocol

19. An IRB will look carefully at the written _____ _____ that subjects will be asked to sign as well as the research _____ .

seed money
intramural

20. Many colleges and universities allocate "_____ _____" for new research projects. These are called _____ research funds.

competent
Intramural

21. The appeal of an extramural grant application can be greatly enhanced by proving that the investigator is not only motivated but also _____ to complete the proposed study. _____ research awards can assist in marshaling such evidence.

National Institutes
Health
PHS 398

22. The _____ _____ of _____ is the primary agency for supporting research in biomedical fields. To apply for such funds, Grant Application Form _____ _____ is used.

Division
Research Grants
review

23. Applications must be sent to the _____ of _____ _____ by a certain deadline date for consideration within a particular _____ period.

institutes
National Institute
Deafness
Communication
Disorders

24. DRG assigns applications to particular _____ or divisions within NIH. An institute whose funding policies are directly aligned with much research in the field of communication science and disorders is the _____ _____ on _____ and other _____ _____ .

25. Research applications undergo a _____ review by one of several Initial Review Groups or so-called _____ sections.

peer
study

26. Study section members vote as to whether a proposal should be _____ , _____ , or _____ for final judgment pending additional information.

approved
disapproved
deferred

27. The _____ _____ for the institute makes final decisions about whether applications are funded or not funded.

advisory council

28. NIH also makes efforts to stimulate and support research in various areas by issuing a _____ _____ _____ (RFP) or a _____ _____ _____ (RFA). These announcements appear in the NIH Guide for _____ and Contracts and the Federal _____ .

Request for Proposal
Request for
Application
Grants
Register

29. An excellent resource that describes the major foundations and the kinds of projects they fund is the _____ Grant Directory maintained by the _____ _____ .

Foundation
Foundation Center

30. In seeking research support from businesses and corporations, it is important that researchers be able to conduct an _____ and _____ research study. The use of _____ control procedures in the collection and analysis of data is recommended.

independent
impartial
blinding

31. It could be argued that the primary value of thesis and dissertation research is not so much in the research _____ but in the development of the scientific _____ processes that make the outcome possible.

outcome
thinking

32. To gain approval for a thesis or dissertation project, a _____ must be written. This is a detailed outline of the _____ for research.

prospectus
plan

33. In addition to providing an action plan for the proposed research, an approved prospectus safeguards against future criticism of the research _____ by the advisory committee, provided that the research was conducted _____ and _____ as originally proposed.

protocol
carefully
competently

34. In addition to conforming to grammatical rules, good writing possesses the properties of _____ and _____ .

efficiency
effectiveness

35. _____ writing conveys meaning using a minimal number of words. _____ writing also possesses the added property of _____ .

Efficient
Effective
clarity

obscure

*American
Psychological
Association*

*Elements of Style
Strunk
White*

36. When readers of scientific articles complain of the difficulty in comprehending the content of research, the fault often lies in the _____ verbiage of the writer.

37. ASHA journals follow the recommendations offered in the style manual of the _____ _____ _____ .

38. A small style manual for writers from all fields that has become a classic reference guide is entitled *The* _____ _____ _____ , written by _____ & _____.

Some Statistical Applications and Questions (Q) (Adapted from Published Literature)

Correlation Coefficient [Q1 (a)]	**Latin Square Design [Q5 (a)]**
Linear Regression [Q1 (b)]	**Randomized Blocked ANOVA [Q5 (b)]**
Paired t Test [Q1 (c)]	
Probability [Q2 (a)]	**Analysis of Covariance [Q6 (a)(b)]**
Sensitivity	
Specificity	**Spearman Rank-Order Correlation Coefficient [Q6 (c)]**
Predictive Value Positive	
Predictive Value Negative	**Kruskal-Wallis ANOVA [Q7]**
Chi-square Test of Independence [Q2 (b)]	**ANOVA**
	One-way ANOVA [Q8 (a)(b)]
Time Series: Autoregressive Model [Q3 (a)(b)]	Two-way ANOVA [Q8 (c)(d)]
	Multiple Regression [Q9 (a)(b)]
The Mann Whitney U Test [Q4]	**Partial Correlation Coefficient [Q9 (c)]**

In this appendix, we use selected data values from the published articles of well-respected journals such as the Journal of Speech and Hearing Disorders, the Journal of Speech and Hearing Research, and the American Journal of Epidemiology to illustrate **step-by-step calculation procedures** of several statistical methods. By doing so, we hope that readers will become familiar with some statistical techniques commonly used in the field of communication disorders. The exercises are intended to demonstrate the application and relevance of statistics to "real" problems encountered in the clinic or laboratory. A step-by-step approach to calculation is taken in order to clarify the meaning of concepts, identify the information needed to solve a set of problems, and minimize a heavy mathematical infrastructure. In some cases, n has been reduced or actual data values from various studies have been rounded to the nearest integer value to facilitate calculation.

CORRELATION, LINEAR REGRESSION, AND T-TEST

Q1. Conversations with children who are language impaired: Asking Questions. *Journal of Speech and Hearing Research,* **Vol. 36, 973–978, October 1993, by Johnson, J. R. et al.**

Samples of conversational language were elicited with a standardized interview protocol from 24 children, half with specific language impairment (SLI) and half with normally developing language (LN). Twelve LN children were compared to the other 12 SLI children by the mean length of utterance (MLU), the CYCLE (Curtiss Yamada Comprehensive Language Evaluation, Curtiss and Yamada, 1988) score, and the total number of child utterances (TCU). The results are shown in Table 1.

(a) Find the correlation coefficient between the MLU and the CYCLE for both groups. Interpret the result.
(b) Would it be suitable to use a linear regression model to predict the TCU from the MLU for the SLI group? If so, find an equation of a regression line.
(c) Do the MLU and CYCLE differ significantly between the two groups?

Solutions

(a) You may use the raw score method to calculate the correlation coefficient r directly from raw scores (see Chapter 6).

Step (1). Look up the raw score formula and determine what information you need for the calculation.

Formula

Let X be MLU scores and Y be CYCLE scores.

$$r_{XY} = \frac{n(\Sigma XY) - (\Sigma X)(\Sigma Y)}{\sqrt{[n\Sigma X^2 - (\Sigma X)^2][n\Sigma Y^2 - (\Sigma Y)^2]}}$$

Table 1(a). Description of Individual Subjects for SLI Group

GROUP	ID	MLU	CYCLE	TCU
SLI	1	1.9	0	232
	2	3.2	64	220
	3	3.3	37	246
	4	3.5	54	234
	5	3.9	12	131
	6	4.0	30	185
	7	4.6	27	157
	8	4.9	62	236
	9	4.9	56	193
	10	5.0	65	148
	11	5.2	70	188
	12	5.6	36	222

Table 1(b). Description of Individual Subjects for LN Group

GROUP	ID	MLU	CYCLE	TCU
LN	1	2.9	12	106
	2	3.2	30	185
	3	3.3	63	189
	4	3.6	54	178
	5	3.6	18	134
	6	4.2	38	162
	7	4.5	51	197
	8	4.6	59	186
	9	4.7	49	269
	10	4.8	66	165
	11	5.1	49	162
	12	5.9	64	202

Step (2).   Set up a table with headings for all the information you need for the formula and enter the score on X and Y (see Table 2).

Step (3).   At the bottom of the table make a row and enter in the sum of each column.

You will get $\Sigma X = 50.4$
$\Sigma X^2 = 220.46$
$\Sigma Y = 553$
$\Sigma Y^2 = 29033$
$\Sigma XY = 2433$

Step (4).   Calculate the correlation coefficient by substituting information in the formula and solving for r_{XY}.

$$r_{XY} = \frac{12(2433) - (50.4)(553)}{\sqrt{[12(220.46) - (50.4)^2][12(29033) - (553)^2]}}$$

$$= \frac{1324.8}{\sqrt{(105.36)(42587)}}$$

$$= \frac{1324.5}{2118.25}$$

$$= .625$$

Among LN students, there exists a moderate positive correlation between MLU scores and CYCLE scores.

Using the same steps, we could derive the following information for the SLI group (verify).

$\Sigma X = 50$ $\Sigma Y = 513$ $\Sigma XY = 2275.7$
$\Sigma X^2 = 220.78$ $\Sigma Y^2 = 27555$ $r_{XY} = .5223$

Table 2. Calculation Table for Correlation Coefficient

ID	X	X²	Y	Y²	XY
1	2.9	8.41	12	144	34.8
2	3.2	10.24	30	900	96
3	3.3	10.89	63	3969	207.9
4	3.6	12.96	54	2916	194.4
5	3.6	12.96	18	324	64.8
6	4.2	17.64	38	1444	159.6
7	4.5	20.25	51	2601	229.5
8	4.6	21.16	59	3481	271.4
9	4.7	22.09	49	2401	230.3
10	4.8	23.04	66	4356	316.8
11	5.1	26.01	49	2401	249.9
12	5.9	34.81	64	4096	377.6

	+)	+)	+)	+)	+)
	$\Sigma X = 50.4$	$\Sigma X^2 = 220.46$	$\Sigma Y = 553$	$\Sigma Y^2 = 29033$	$\Sigma XY = 2433$

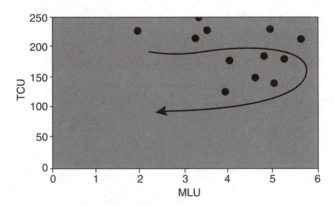

Figure 1. A scatter diagram describing TCU and MLU scores.

Again, there is a moderate positive correlation between MLU scores and CYCLE scores.

(b) First, we draw a scatter diagram to determine if there exists a linear relationship between MLU(X) and TCU(Y) (Figure 1).

The presence of an outlier score may change the nature of the relationship between two variables, especially if the sample size is very small. The researcher must decide whether or not to delete such a score from consideration. If the score is not deleted, we can use the following three methods to find the slope $b_{Y \cdot X}$ and the y intercept a.

Formula

(1) Given $\text{Cov}(X,Y)$ = covariance of X and Y

S^2x = variance of X.

Use the formula

$$b_{Y \cdot X} = \frac{Cov(X, Y)}{S^2_x}$$

(2) Given r_{XY} = correlation between X and Y
S_X = standard deviation of X
S_Y = standard deviation of Y

Use the formula

$$b_{Y \cdot X} = \frac{(r_{XY}) \cdot (S_Y)}{S_x}$$

(3) Given n = number of subjects
X = raw score on X
Y = raw score on Y

Use the formula

$$b_{Y \cdot X} = \frac{n(\Sigma XY) - (\Sigma X)(\Sigma Y)}{n(\Sigma X^2) - (\Sigma X)^2}$$

Use the formula (3) to find the slope $b_{Y \cdot X}$. Because we predict the TCU score (Y) from the MLU score (X), we make a table with headings for all information needed for the formula (see Table 3).

For SLI, we have:

Table 3. Calculation Table for the Slope and Y Intercept

ID	X	X²	Y	XY
1	1.9	3.61	232	440.8
2	3.2	10.24	220	704.0
3	3.3	10.89	246	811.8
4	3.5	12.25	234	819
5	3.9	15.21	131	510.9
6	4.0	16.00	185	740
7	4.6	21.16	157	722.2
8	4.9	24.01	236	1156.4
9	4.9	24.01	193	945.7
10	5.0	25.00	148	740
11	5.2	27.04	188	977.6
12	5.6	31.36	222	1243.2
	+)	+)	+)	+)
	$\Sigma X = 50$	$\Sigma X^2 = 220.78$	$\Sigma Y = 2392$	$\Sigma XY = 9811.6$

Calculate the slope by substituting all numerical values into the formula and solving for $b_{Y \cdot X}$.

$$b_{Y \cdot X} = \frac{12 \cdot (9811.6) - (50)(2392)}{12 \cdot (220.78) - (50)^2}$$

$$= \frac{-1860.8}{149.36}$$

$$= -12.458$$

The y intercept a can be given by:

$$a = \overline{Y} - b_{Y \cdot x} \cdot \overline{X}$$

$$= \left(\frac{2392}{12}\right) - (-12.458) \cdot \left(\frac{50}{12}\right)$$

$$= 199.333 - (-51.908)$$

$$= 251.241$$

The regression line (with an outlier score) is given by:

$$\hat{Y} = -12.458X + 251.241$$

By using the formula for correlation coefficient, it gives $r_{xy} = -.345$ (verify)
If we delete the outlier score such as ID 5 (3.9,131), then we would have

$$b_{Y \cdot X} = -14.144, \quad a = 264.821, \quad r_{xy} = -.472 \text{ (verify)}.$$

(c) To determine if there is a significant difference in MLU scores between the two groups, an independent t-test would be applied. As a prerequisite of an independent t-test, we must apply an F-test to determine the homogeneity of two variances. For the SLI group, the mean MLU score is calculated as

$$\overline{X}_{SLI} = \frac{\Sigma X}{n} = \frac{50}{12} = 4.17$$

Also, the variance of MLU score is given by:

$$S^2_{SLI} = \frac{n \cdot (\Sigma X^2) - (\Sigma X)^2}{n \cdot (n-1)} = \frac{12 \cdot (220.78) - (50)^2}{12 \cdot 11} = \frac{149.36}{132} = 1.13$$

For LN group, the mean MLU scores is:

$$\overline{X}_{LN} = \frac{\Sigma X}{n} = \frac{50.4}{12} = 4.2$$

the variance of MLU scores is also calculated as:

$$S^2_{LN} = \frac{n \cdot (\Sigma X^2) - (\Sigma X)^2}{n \cdot (n-1)} = \frac{12 \cdot (220.46) - (50.4)^2}{12 \cdot 11} = \frac{105.36}{132} = .80$$

Data values for SLI and LN are summarized as follows:

SLI	$\overline{X} = 4.17,$	$S^2 = 1.13,$	$n = 12.$
LN	$\overline{X} = 4.2,$	$S^2 = .80,$	$n = 12.$

Step (1). Apply an F-test to determine the homogeneity of two variances.

$$F \frac{S_2\text{larger}}{S_2\text{smaller}} = \frac{1.13}{.80} = 1.41 \text{ with d.f.} = (11,11).$$

F(.05) = 2.82 > 1.41, indicates that the p-value is greater than .05. Hence, distributions of the *two* groups' SLI and LN are homogeneous.

Step (2). Calculate an observed t-value and determine whether or not to reject H_0.

$H_0: \mu_{SLI} = \mu_{LN}$ or $\mu_{SLI} - \mu_{LN} = 0$
$H_1: \mu_{SLI} \neq \mu_{LN}$ or $\mu_{SLI} - \mu_{LN} \neq 0$

Formula for a homogeneous t value

$$t = \frac{(\overline{X}_1 - \overline{X}_2) - (\mu_1 - \mu_2)}{\sqrt{\dfrac{1}{n_1} + \dfrac{1}{n_2}} \cdot \sqrt{\dfrac{(n_1 - 1) \cdot S_1^2 + (n_2 - 1) \cdot S_2^2}{n_1 + n_2 - 2}}}$$

with d.f. = $n_1 + n_2 - 2$

where $(\mu_1 - \mu_2)$ represents a difference between two true population means, i.e., the value on the right side of H_o and $H_1(o)$.

$$t = \frac{(4.17 - 4.2) - 0}{\sqrt{\dfrac{1}{12} + \dfrac{1}{12}} \cdot \sqrt{\dfrac{(12 - 1) \cdot (1.13) + (12 - 1) \cdot .80}{12 + 12 - 2}}}$$

$$= \frac{-.03}{(.408)(.982)}$$

$$= -.0749$$

t = −0.749 with d.f. = 22 (compared to t (.025) = 2.074) has a p-value exceeding .05; therefore, the MLU did not differ significantly between the two groups.

For CYCLE scores, readers should verify the following results:

SLI	$\overline{X}$ = 42.75,	S^2 = 511.29,	n = 12
LN	$\overline{X}$ = 46.08,	S^2 = 322.63,	n = 12

Calculated F(.05) = $\dfrac{511.29}{322.63}$ = 1.58 was less than table value of F, therefore, we fail to

reject $H_o: \sigma^2_{SLI} = \sigma^2_{LN}$. Hence, two groups are homogeneous. Next, we apply a homogeneous independent t-test to determine the following hypotheses:

$H_0: \mu_{SLI} = \mu_{LN}$ or $\mu_{SLI} - \mu_{LN} = 0$
$H_1: \mu_{SLI} \neq \mu_{LN}$ or $\mu_{SLI} - \mu_{LN} \neq 0$

$$t = \frac{(42.75) - 46.08) - 0}{\sqrt{\dfrac{1}{12} + \dfrac{1}{12}} \cdot \sqrt{\dfrac{(12 - 1) \cdot (511.29) + (12 - 1) \cdot 322.63}{12 + 12 - 2}}}$$

$$= \frac{-3.33}{(.408)\cdot(20.42)}$$

$$= -.39 \text{ with d.f.} = 22$$

Calculated t = −.39 has a p-value exceeding .05; therefore, the CYCLE scores did not differ significantly between the two groups.

PROBABILITY AND CHI-SQUARE TEST OF INDEPENDENCE

Q2.   Otitis Media and Language Development At One Year of Age.
Wallace, I. F. et al. *Journal of Speech and Hearing Disorders.* Vol. 53, 245–251, August 1988.

Part I

The effect of otitis media on emerging language was examined in a group of one-year-olds. Based on pneumatic otoscopy, two groups were selected from the larger cohort of 65 subjects. Using otoscopy records, 15 subjects (nine high-risk infants and six healthy full-term infants) who had normal ratings in both ears during 80% or more of their visits were designated as otitis free. Another 12 subjects (9 high-risk infants and 3 healthy full-term infants) who demonstrated bilaterally positive otoscopy results during 30% or more of their visits were designated as otitis positive. Some of the demographic and perinatal data for the study are given in Table 4 for the 27 studied infants.

Table 4. Perinatal and Demographic Characteristics of Studied Children

CHARACTERISTIC	OTITIS POSITIVE (n = 12)	OTITIS FREE (n = 15)
Birthweight		
M	1782.1	2292.7
SD	878.0	1049.0
Gestational age		
M	33.8	35.9
SD	4.1	4.6
Maternal age		
M	27.4	23.3
SD	5.3	5.5
Race		
Black	6	10
Hispanic	5	5
White	1	0

Table 5. Ratings of Middle Ear Status Using Otoscopy and Tympanogram

Otoscopy

TYMPANOGRAM	CLEAR	SUSPECT	POSITIVE
Normal	160	31	7
Suspect	18	13	8
Positive	6	6	8

Part II

Otoscopic and tympanometric evaluations were conducted on 65 subjects between 40 weeks and 6 months of age postterm. A three-point otoscopy rating scale (i.e., clear, suspicious, positive) was used to categorize the tympanometric findings from each ear (i.e., negative, suspect, positive). Table 5 summarizes the results of the analysis for ears in which tympanometric and otoscopic examinations were completed on the same day.

(a) Using tympanometric results as indicative of disease status, find sensitivity, specificity, predictive value positive, and predictive value negative.
(b) Does agreement between the two measures occur? (Is there any independent relationship between them?)

Solutions

(a) Two rates that are often useful in the evaluation of a diagnostic test are the **sensitivity** rate and the **specificity** rate.

Sensitivity = Prob. (test result is positive given that the person carries a disease)

$$= \frac{\text{number of true positives}}{\text{number of true positives} + \text{number of false negatives}}$$

Specificity = Prob. (test result is negative given that the person does not carry a disease)

$$= \frac{\text{number of true negatives}}{\text{number of true negatives} + \text{number of false positives}}$$

Table 5 may be revised as in Table 6:

$$\text{Sensitivity} = \frac{8}{8 + 6} = \frac{8}{14} \text{ or } 57.1\%$$

$$\text{Specificity} = \frac{160}{160 + 7} = \frac{160}{167} \text{ or } 95.8\%$$

Because no diagnostic or screening test is perfect, it is impossible to increase both rates of the sensitivity and specificity of a test simultaneously. Clinicians must decide which rate should be maximized depending on the relative cost of obtaining a false positive result versus the cost of a false negative result. As can be seen from the calculations above and Table 6, the specificity rate is considerably higher than the sensitivity rate.

Other useful rates (for determining the accuracy of a diagnostic test) are called **Predictive Value Positive** and **Predictive Value Negative.** These rates can be calculated as:

Table 6. Calculation Table for True and False Positives

Otoscopy (Test Result)

TYMPANOGRAM (DISEASE STATUS)	CLEAR (NEGATIVES)	SUSPECT	POSITIVE (POSITIVES)
Normal (Negatives)	160 (True negatives)	31	7 (False positives)
Suspect	18	13	8
Positive (Positives)	6 (False negatives)	6	8 (True positives)

Predictive Value Positive = Prob. (a person carries a disease given that the test result is

$$\text{Positive)} = \frac{\text{number of true positives}}{\text{number of true positives} + \text{number of false positives}}$$

Predictive Value Negative = Prob (a person does not carry a disease given that test result

$$\text{is Negative)} = \frac{\text{number of true negatives}}{\text{number of true negatives} + \text{number of false negatives}}$$

In our example, Predictive Value Positive $= \dfrac{8}{7+8} = \dfrac{8}{15}$ or 53.3%

$$\text{Predictive Value Negative} = \frac{160}{160+6} = \frac{160}{166} \text{ or } 96.4\%$$

(b) Prior to calculating a chi-square test of independence, we must specify the null and alternative hypotheses.

H_o: Tympanogram and otoscopy results are independent (no agreement exists between the two measures.)

H_1: Tympanogram and otoscopy results are dependent. (Some agreement exists between the two measures.)

Compute the chi-square statistic following these steps:

Step (1).   Set up a chi-square table as in Table 7.

Table 7. A Chi-Square Table for Rating Middle Ear Status

Otoscopy

TYMPANOGRAM	CLEAR	SUSPECT	POSITIVE	ROW TOTAL
Normal	160	31	7	198
Suspect	18	13	8	39
Positive	6	6	8	20
Column total	184	50	23	257

Step (2).   Compute the expected frequency (E) for each cell. The formula for E is given by

$$\frac{\text{(the frequency of the row that the cell is in)} \cdot \text{(the frequency of the column that the cell is in)}}{\text{grand total}}$$

The calculations for this example are shown below. (Note that N = Normal, S = Suspect, P = Positive, and C = Clear)

$$E_{NC} = \frac{(198) \cdot (184)}{257} = 141.76$$

$$E_{NS} = \frac{(198) \cdot (50)}{257} = 38.52$$

$$E_{NP} = \frac{(198) \cdot (23)}{257} = 17.72$$

$$E_{SC} = \frac{(39) \cdot (184)}{257} = 27.92$$

$$E_{SS} = \frac{(39) \cdot (50)}{257} = 7.59$$

$$E_{SP} = \frac{(39) \cdot (23)}{257} = 3.49$$

$$E_{PC} = \frac{(20) \cdot (184)}{257} = 14.32$$

$$E_{PS} = \frac{(20) \cdot (50)}{257} = 3.89$$

$$E_{PP} = \frac{(20) \cdot (23)}{257} = 1.79$$

Step (3).   Construct a contingency table (Table 8) and enter the frequencies into O, E, $(O - E)^2$, and $\dfrac{(O - E)^2}{E}$, where O = the observed frequency.

Step (4).   Examine the following and decide how to proceed.

(a) If d.f. = 1, Yates' correction for continuity is applied. The method is explained in detail in Chapter 8.

(b) If d.f.>1, proceed with the computations.

For our example, d.f. = (row − 1)·(column − 1) = (3 − 1)·(3 − 1) = 4, which is greater than 1; therefore, we will calculate our observed chi-square value, denoted by χ^2_{obs} through the following formula:

$$\chi^2_{obs} = \frac{\Sigma \, (O - E)^2}{E} = \text{a total sum of } \frac{(O - E)^2}{E}$$

Table 8. Calculation Table for a Chi-Square Test of Independence

	O	E	(O − E)	(O − E)²	$\frac{(O - E)^2}{E}$
NC	160	141.76	18.24	332.70	2.35
NS	31	38.52	−7.52	56.55	1.47
NP	7	17.72	−10.72	114.92	6.49
SC	18	27.92	−9.92	98.41	3.52
SS	13	7.59	5.41	29.27	3.86
SP	8	3.49	4.51	20.34	5.83
PC	6	14.32	−8.32	69.22	4.83
PS	6	3.89	2.11	4.45	1.14
PP	8	1.79	6.21	38.56	21.54

$$\chi^2_{obs} = 2.35 + 1.47 + 6.49 + 3.52 + 3.86 + 5.83 + 4.83 + 1.14 + 21.54 = 51.03$$
$$\text{with d.f.} = 4.$$

Step (5). Find the critical value of χ^2, denoted by χ^2crit(α, d.f.), and conclude it.

Setting up $\alpha = .05$ with d.f. $= 4$, we get χ^2crit(.05, 4) $= 9.488$
Under the decision rule,

If $\chi^2_{obs} \geq \chi^2$crit(α, d.f.), we reject H$_o$
If $\chi^2_{obs} < \chi^2$crit(α, d.f.), we do not reject H$_o$

For our example, because $\chi^2_{obs} = 51.03 > \chi^2$crit(.05, 4) $= 9.488$, we must reject H$_o$. Hence, tympanogram and otoscopy measures are dependent (or related to each other) at the 5% level of significance ($\alpha = .05$).

TIME-SERIES ANALYSIS

Q3. From Pronoun Reversals to Correct Pronoun Usage: A Case Study of a Normally Developing Child
Journal of Speech and Hearing Disorders, Vol. 48, 394–402, November 1983, by Schiff-Myers, N. B.

A total of 1386 intelligible utterances were transcribed from audiotapes. Approximately 27% of these contained first-person and second-person pronouns. An additional 480 utterances with such pronouns were collected using hand-written notes. There were substantial developmental changes during the three observed periods, namely Time 1 (21 months), Time 2 (23 months), and Time 3 (25 months). Proportions of pronoun confusion and imitated utterances at different ages and linguistic levels are summarized in Table 9 below.

(a) Which statistical method would be suitable if you wish to predict the total number of utterances (TUT) at a specified time period, such as Time 4 (27 months) and Time 5 (29 months)?

(b) Perform the method you chose to predict TUT scores at Time 4 and Time 5.

Table 9. Proportion of Pronoun Confusion and Imitated Utterances in a Normal Child's Speech at Different Ages and Linguistic Levels.

	(TUT) TOTAL NUMBER OF UTTERANCE TYPES	% OF IMITATED UTTERANCES	% OF PRONOUN CONFUSION	MLU (MEAN LENGTH OF UTTERANCE)
Time 1 (21 months)	246	21	59	2.69
Time 2 (23 months)	418	9	26	3.82
Time 3 (25 months)	307	3	3	4.7

Solution

(a) We frequently encounter situations in which data become available in a time-ordered sequence. Analysis of this kind of data set has two main purposes: to describe a useful mathematical model for forecasting outcomes and then to actually use that model to forecast future values at a specified time period. Statistical methods used to accomplish these objectives are referred to as "time-series analyses." Such analyses generally consist of the following three major components:

(1) selecting a tentative model
(2) estimating the model parameters
(3) testing for adequacy of fit.

The most complex stage is the last component because the validity of forecasting procedures heavily depends on the historical data (prior distribution), i.e., we often predict the future value based on the assumption that future trends will behave as they have in the past. However, in the behavioral sciences, this assumption is rarely warranted for an extended time horizon; therefore, the model we present here is based on the Bayesian distribution. Such a distribution updates forecasted values (posterior distribution) as new data emerge (data distribution).

Given our example, a time-series analysis for a single-subject design is the most suitable model to predict future TUT scores, because the data are continuous and are to be updated whenever new data emerge. The formula for the time-series model used here is given as:

$$\hat{Y}_{t+1} = \mu + \varnothing(Y_t - \mu)$$

where $\hat{Y}_{t+1}$ (read "Y hat sub t + 1") = the future value at time t + 1.
   Y_t = the actual observed score at time t.
   $\mu = \overline{Y}$ = Sample mean (from 1 to t)

$$= \frac{\sum\limits_{i=1}^{t} Y_i}{n}$$

$\varnothing$ (read "phi") = the autocorrelation coefficient

$$= \frac{\sum\limits_{i=1}^{t-1} (Y_t - \mu)(Y_{t+1} - \mu)}{\sum\limits_{i=1}^{t-1} (Y_t - \mu)^2}$$

The time-series model may be considered as a regression model for a continuous data; therefore, $\varnothing$ may be interpreted as the rate of change from one time to another, and Y as the y intercept. The table TUT data give:

$$Y_1 = 246, \quad Y_2 = 418, \quad Y_3 = 307.$$

$$t = 3, \quad \mu = \bar{Y} = \frac{246 + 418 + 307}{3} = 323.67$$

$$= \frac{(246 - 323.67)\cdot(418 - 323.67) + (418 - 323.67)\cdot(307 - 323.67)}{(246 - 323.67)^2 + (418 - 323.67)^2}$$

$$= \frac{(-77.67)\cdot(94.33) + (94.33)\cdot(-16.67)}{(-77.67)^2 + (94.33)^2}$$

$$= \frac{(-7326.61 + (1572.48)}{14930.78}$$

$$= \frac{-8899.09}{14930.78}$$

$$= -.596$$

The equation for a time-series model for this particular set of data is

$$\hat{Y}_{t+1} = 323.67 - .596(Y_t - 323.67)$$

(b) Using the equation $\hat{Y}_{t+1} = 323.67 - .596(Y_t - 323.67)$ we could predict TUT score at time 4. It gives:

$$\hat{Y}_4 = 323.67 - .596(307 - 323.67)$$
$$= 333.61$$

The predicted TUT score at time 4 (on the basis of three previous times) is 333.61. Time-series analysis also allows us to forecast values for two future time periods. The procedure is similar to that for forecasting values for one time period. Symbolically, we write $\hat{Y}_{t+2}$ to describe the predicted score at $(t + 2)^{\text{th}}$ time period; we then have

$$\hat{Y}_{t+2} = \mu + \varnothing(\hat{Y}_{t+1} - \mu)$$

Alternatively, it is possible to express $\hat{Y}_{t+2}$ entirely in terms of μ, $\varnothing$, and the available observed scores. Substituting the expression for $\hat{Y}_{t+1}$ into the above equation gives

$$\hat{Y}_{t+2} = \mu + \varnothing[\mu + \varnothing(Y_t - \mu) - \mu]$$
$$= \mu + \varnothing^2(Y_t - \mu)$$

Based on the formula above, the predicted score of TUT at time 5 given that $t = 3$ is expressed as

$$\hat{Y}_5 = \mu + \varnothing(Y_3 - \mu)$$
$$= 323.67 + (-.596)^2[307 - 323.67]$$
$$= 317.75$$

Therefore, the predicted TUT score at time 5 is 317.75.

THE MANN-WHITNEY U TEST

Q4. **F2 Transitions During Sound/Syllable Repetitions of Children who Stutter and Predictions of Stuttering Chronicity**
Journal of Speech and Hearing Research, **Vol. 36, 883–896, October 1993, by Yaruss, J. S. and Contour, E. G.**

Thirteen children who stuttered were divided into two groups based on their predicted risk of continuing to stutter as measured by the Stuttering Prediction Instrument (SPI). The high-risk group consisted of seven male subjects with a mean age of 50.57 months, with a standard deviation of 10.95 months. The low-risk group consisted of five male subjects and one female subject with a mean age of 48.50 months, with a standard deviation of 12.18 months. Table 10 summarizes the children's reported ages at the time of onset of stuttering, their ages at the time of a videotaping session, and their ages at diagnostic evaluation.

> Determine whether there was a significant difference between the high-risk and low-risk groups for reported ages at the onset of stuttering (the first column of Table 10).

Solution

(a) First, we may wish to determine if the t-test's assumptions, such as normality and equal variances, are violated. Because sample sizes of both groups are relatively small, it is possible that the assumption of normality has been violated. Hence, the non-parametric version of the independent t-test (or unpaired t-test), called the **Mann-Whitney U Test,** might be appropriately applied.

The purpose of this test is to determine if two independent groups were drawn from the same population. The calculation of this statistic for our example data is illustrated in the following steps.

Step (1). State the hypotheses:

$H_o: \mu_H = \mu_L$
$H_1: \mu_H \neq \mu_L$

where H = High-risk and L = Low-risk.

Step (2). Compute the U statistic.

(i) First, we arrange the data by rank order from lowest to highest (see Table 11), noting the group membership. If two or more scores are tied for the same rank, average the ranks and assign the average rank to two or more scores.

(ii) Next, calculate the sum of the ranks for each group. Designate the larger sum of ranks as T_L.

Group H (High-risk) = 1 + 2.5 + 2.5 + 6.5 + 9.5 + 9.5 + 11 = 42.5

(iii) Group L (Low-risk) = 4.5 + 4.5 + 6.5 + 8 + 12 + 13 = 48.5

$$T_L = 48.5, \text{ because } 48.5 > 42.5$$

(iv) Compute U_1 and U_2 using the following formulas. The value of the Mann-Whitney U statistic is whichever value is smaller.

Table 10. Subjects' Ages on the Stuttering Severity Instrument and SPI

SUBJECT GROUP AND NUMBER	REPORTED AGE AT ONSET OF STUTTERING (MONTHS)	AGE AT AUDIO/ VIDEO TAPING (MONTHS)	AGE AT DIAGNOSTIC EVALUATION (MONTHS)
High risk			
1	28	34	36
2	24	47	51
3	28	48	46
4	42	48	48
5	42	50	50
6	43	57	59
7	30	70	72
Mean	33.86	50.57	51.71
(SD)	8.13	10.95	11.27
Low-risk			
1	29	36	41
2	30	36	42
3	29	41	44
4	48	57	62
5	41	58	54
6	57	63	65
Mean	39.00	48.50	51.33
(SD)	11.74	12.18	10.54

Table 11. Rank Order for the Mann-Whitney U Statistic

Score	24	28	28	29	29	30	30	41	42	42	43	48	57
Group	H	H	H	L	L	H	L	L	H	H	H	L	L
Rank	1	2.5	2.5	4.5	4.5	6.5	6.5	8	9.5	9.5	11	12	13

Formula:

$$U_1 = (n_L) \cdot (n_S) + \frac{n_L \cdot (n_L + 1)}{2} - T_L$$

$$U_2 = (n_L) \cdot (n_S) - U_1$$

where n_L = number of subjects in group with larger sum of ranks.
         n_S = number of subjects in group with smaller sum of ranks.
         T_L = larger sum of ranks.

For our example, we have:

$$n_L = 6, \quad n_S = 7, \quad T_L = 48.5$$

$$U_1 = (6) \cdot (7) + \frac{6 \cdot (6 + 1)}{2} - 48.5$$

$$= 42 + 21 - 48.5 = 14.5$$
$$U_2 = (6) \cdot (7) - 14.5$$
$$= 42 - 14.5$$
$$= 27.5$$

Therefore, U_1 (14.5) is the value of the Mann-Whitney U statistic.

Step (3).   Determine whether or not to reject H_o. To find the critical U value, consult Appendix C.6, which lists critical values for interpreting the Mann-Whitney U statistic. The table shows a critical value of 6 at $\alpha = .05$ with d.f = (6,7). Because the observed U value of 14.5 is greater than the critical value, the null hypothesis will be retained. For further practice in calculating the Mann-Whitney U test, readers may also wish to determine significance of between-group differences for age at audio/videotaping session and age at diagnostic evaluation (the second and third columns in Appendix C.6).

LATIN SQUARE DESIGN AND RANDOMIZED BLOCKED ANOVA

Q5.   **Effects of Temporal Alternations on Speech Intelligibility in Parkinsonian Dysarthria**
         Journal of Speech and Hearing Research, Vol. 37, 244–253, April 1994, by Hammen, V. L. et al.

The effect of two types of temporal alterations, paced and synthetic, on the intelligibility of parkinsonian dysarthric speech was investigated. Six speakers with idiopathic Parkinson's disease served as subjects. Paced temporal alterations were created by slowing each speaker to 60% of his/her habitual speaking rate. The synthetic alterations were created by modifying the habitual rate speech samples using digital signal processing. Three types of synthetic alterations were examined: Paused Altered, Speech Duration Altered, and a combination of both.

A total of 150 sentence files were created during the signal processing phase of the project, (5 sentences X 5 conditions [2 unmodified and 3 synthetic temporal alterations] X 6 speakers). A 5 X 5 Latin Square (Listeners X Sentences) was made for each subject, with the five conditions counterbalanced under the rows and columns of the square. The Latin Square table is shown in Table 12.

(a) Explain the advantages of the Latin square design briefly.
(b) Using the Latin square design, test the hypothesis that there is no significant differences among the five treatment conditions.

Table 12. Mean Percentage Intelligibility under Five Judges

Judges

Subject*	1	2	3	4	5
1	83(A)	88(B)	84(C)	81(D)	91(E)
2	83(B)	80(C)	50(D)	70(E)	81(A)
3	48(C)	54(D)	57(E)	54(A)	67(B)
4	21(D)	14(E)	14(A)	26(B)	26(C)
5	5(E)	3(A)	16(B)	6(C)	4(D)

*One subject was dropped from the analysis.

Solution

(a) The advantage of this design is that a reduced number of listeners are required to obtain measures of intelligibility. Because each listener is presented a different sentence for each condition, the problem of listener familiarity confounding the intelligibility measure is avoided. This design eliminates determining the reliability of the listeners using correlation methods. Therefore, relative homogeneity of the variables assigned to the rows and columns is assumed.

(b) Table 12 presents mean percentage intelligibility under five treatment conditions. An F value for testing treatment effects in a Latin square design may be obtained by substituting degrees of freedom into the general formula for the F statistic.

Notice that each score is a function of three possible influences: subjects, judges, and treatment conditions (five levels: A = Habitual Rate, B = Paced Habitual Rates, C = Pausal Alteration, D = Speech Duration Alteration, and E = Combined Alteration). Therefore, a full statistical model for the data may be written as:

$$Y_{ijk} = \mu + \alpha_j + \beta_k + \Pi_i + E_{ijk}.$$

where Y_{ijk} represents the score on the dependent variable for the $_i$th subject at the $_j$th level of treatment and $_k$th level of judges, μ is the grand mean parameter, α_j is the treatment effect parameter, β_k is the judge effect parameter, Π_i is the subject effect parameter, and E_{ijk} is the error term.

Because the Latin square model is strictly a main-effects model, it has no interaction effects. Therefore, the null hypothesis is written as:

$$H_o: \alpha_A = \alpha_B = \alpha_C = \alpha_D = \alpha_E$$

That is to say, every α_j becomes zero when H_o is true. Consequently, it gives

$$Y_{ijk} = \mu + \beta_k + \Pi_i + E_{ijk}.$$

We can now construct the mixed-effects RBANOVA (Randomized Blocked ANOVA) table to calculate the sum of squares (SS), degrees of freedom (d.f.), the mean squares (MS), and an F statistic (see Table 13).

Table 13. RBANOVA Calculation Table

JUDGE LEVELS	1	2	3	4	5	ROW TOTALS
Subjects						
1	83	88	84	81	91	427
2	83	80	50	70	81	364
3	48	54	57	54	67	280
4	21	14	14	26	26	101
5	5	3	16	6	4	34
COLUMN TOTALS	240	239	221	237	269	1206

k = 5 levels,   n = 5 subjects

Step (1).   Square the Grand Total and divide by $(n) \cdot (k)$, denoted by {1}

$$\{1\} = \frac{(1206)^2}{5.5} = 58177.44$$

Step (2).   Sum the squared row totals and divide by the number of treatment levels (k), denoted by {2} .

$$\{2\} = \frac{(427)^2 + (364)^2 + (280)^2 + (101)^2 + (34)^2}{5}$$

$$= 80916.4$$

Step (3).   Sum the square column totals and divide by the number of subjects (n), denoted by {3}.

$$\{3\} = \frac{(240)^2 + (239)^2 + (221)^2 + (237)^2 + (269)^2}{5}$$

$$= 58418.4$$

Step (4).   Square each individual score and find the sum of the squared scores, denoted by {4}.

$$(83)^2 + (88)^2 + (84)^2 + (81)^2 + (91)^2 + (83)^2 + (80)^2 + (50)^2 + (70)^2 + (81)^2 +$$
$$(48)^2 + (54)^2 + (57)^2 + (54)^2 + (67)^2 + (21)^2 + (14)^2 + (14)^2 + (26)^2 + (26)^2 +$$
$$(5)^2 + (3)^2 + (16)^2 + (6)^2 + (4)^2 = 82182$$

Step (5). Compute the sum of squares total (SS total), the sum of squares for judges (SS judges), the sum of squares for subjects (SS subjects), and the sum of squares for residual (SS residual).

SS total = {4} − {1} = 82182 − 58177.44 = 24004.56
SS judges = {3} − {1} = 58418.4 − 58177.44 = 240.46
SS subjects = {2} − {1} = 80916.4 − 58177.44 = 22738.96
SS residual = SS total − SS judges − SS subjects

$$= 24004.56 - 240.46 - 22738.96$$
$$= 1025.14$$

Step (6).   Calculate the degrees of freedom for treatments, subjects, residuals, and total. The full statistical model has one μ parameter, $(j - 1)$ independent α parameters, $(k - 1)$ independent β parameters, and $(i - 1)$ independent Π parameters.

$$\text{d.f. full} = \text{Total d.f.} - (j - 1) - (k - 1) - (i - 1)$$
$$= \{(5)(5) - 1\} - (5 - 1) - (5 - 1) - (5 - 1) = 12,$$

which is equal to the degrees of freedom of the denominator.
The restricted model has one μ parameter, $(k - 1)$ independent β parameters, and $(i - 1)$ independent parameters.
Thus, d.f. restricted = $\{(5)(5) - 1\} - (5 - 1) - (5 - 1) = 16$.
The difference (d.f. full) and (d.f. restricted) gives the degrees of freedom of the numerator, which gives $16 - 12 = 4$.

Step (7).   Calculate the F score for testing treatment effects in a Latin square design.

$$F = \frac{\text{SS treatment}/4}{\text{SS residual}/12}$$
$$\text{where SS treatment} = (i) \cdot \sum_{j=1}^{5} (\overline{Y}.j. - \overline{Y}...)^2$$
$$i = 5 \text{ subjects}$$

$\overline{Y}.j.$ = the mean value of each level
$\overline{Y}...$ = grand total mean

$$= \frac{1206}{25} = 48.24$$

$\overline{Y}_{.1.} = 47,\quad \overline{Y}_{.2.} = 56,\quad \overline{Y}_{.3.} = 48.8,\quad \overline{Y}_{.4.} = 42, \text{ and } \overline{Y}_{.5.} = 47.4$

SS treatment = $5 \cdot [(47 - 48.24)^2 + (56 + 48.24)^2 + (48.8 - 48.24)^2 + (42 - 48.24)^2 + (47.4 - 48.24)^2] = 508.56$

$$F_{obs} = \frac{508.56/4}{1025.14/12} = \frac{127.14}{85.43}$$

$$= 1.49$$

Step (8).   Under the decision rule, decide whether or not we reject H_o.

F_{crit} for treatment
F_{crit} (.05,4,12) = 3,26 > F_{obs} = 1.49

Therefore, we do not reject H_o. At a 5% level of significance, the five treatments have equal effects on intelligibility scores.

ANALYSIS OF COVARIANCE AND SPEARMAN RANK-ORDER CORRELATION COEFFICIENT

Q6.   Duration of Sound Prolongation and Sound/Syllable Repetition in Children Who Stutter: Preliminary Observations
Journal of Speech and Hearing Research. **Vol. 37, 254–253. April 1994, by Zebrowski, P. M.**

The purpose of the study was to measure the rate of sound/syllable repetitions (stutterings) per second in the conversational speech of school-age children who stutter. Nine randomly selected subjects were assigned to one of three treatment groups to reduce the rate of repetitions: A, B, and C. Suppose each subject was given a pretest to determine his or her severity level of stuttering prior to assignment. After the treatments, a posttest was administered and the data in Table 14 were collected. Note that the pretest is labeled as X, and the posttest is labeled as Y.

(a) What type of statistical analysis is the most suitable to test the null hypothesis that there is no treatment effect on the rate of repetition of sound/syllable per second? Explain why.

(b) Using the statistical analysis, test the null hypothesis.

Solution

(a) Given this problem, the analysis of covariance (ANCOVA) is a better method than ANOVA to determine individual differences among subjects. One of its advantages over ANOVA is that we can remove the portion of variance from subjects' posttest data values that is accounted for by the systematic differences among their pretest data values (covariant). This results in decreasing the *residual term*, which is in the denominator of the F ratio. When it is decreased, the size of the F-statistic increases while all other sources of covariance remain equal. In general, the ANCOVA is designed for the research question: "Are the observed differences due to chance, or do they reflect true population differences?"

   The ANCOVA is more powerful than ANOVA if the following assumptions are met:

(1) Independence of each score for pre- and posttest.
(2) Normality of pre- and post distributions.
(3) Homogeneity of variances for pre- and post-test distributions.
(4) Linearity: For each treatment, the regression of the post-test variable (Y) on the covariant (X) is linear in each group. If this assumption is not met, the ANCOVA should not be used. You can "eyeball" the relationship between X and Y to determine if they are linear.
(5) Homogeneity of regression slopes: The slopes of all groups are equal. This can be verified by "eyeballing" the similarity of the slopes across groups. If this assumption is violated, then the ANCOVA should not be used.

Table 14. Summary of the Rate of Repetitions of Three Treatment Groups

TREATMENT	A		B		C	
	X	Y	X	Y	X	Y
	2	1	5	3	3	3
	3	2	4	6	7	5
	4	3	6	6	5	4
Mean	3	2	5	5	5	4
SD	1	1	1	1.73	2	1
Variance	1	1	1	3	4	1

(6) Independence of covariant and treatments: the values on the covariant must not be affected by treatments. If this assumption is violated, then the ANCOVA should not be used.

(b) The information pertinent to the ANCOVA may be summarized in an ANCOVA table, as shown in Table 15.

The following steps may be used to fill in cells of the ANCOVA table.

Step (1). Calculate the adjusted sums of squares (SS treat) adj., (SS within) adj., (SS total) adj., and the sum of squares for the covariant, denoted by SScov. In order to find these values, we must calculate (SS treat), (SS within), and (SS total). Calculating the various types of sums of squares is tedious and time-consuming work; therefore, we show three treatment tables to derive such outcomes (Table 16).

Step (2). Find the square of the sum of the squared covariants between the groups, denoted by $(SSX_{between})^2$.

$$(SSX_{between})^2 = (\Sigma X_A)^2 + (\Sigma X_B)^2 - (\Sigma X_C)^2$$
$$= (9)^2 + (15)^2 + (15)^2$$
$$= 531$$

Step (3). Square the sum of the squared post scores between the group, denoted by $(SSY_{between})^2$.

$$(SSY_{between})^2 = (\Sigma Y_A)^2 + (\Sigma Y_B)^2 + (\Sigma Y_C)^2$$
$$= (6)^2 + (15)^2 + (12)^2$$
$$= 405$$

Step (4). Find the cross product of the sum of X and the sum of Y, for each group, denoted by $(SSXY_{between})$.

$$(SSXY_{between}) = (\Sigma X_A) \cdot (\Sigma Y_A) + (\Sigma X_B) \cdot (\Sigma Y_B) + (\Sigma X_C) \cdot (\Sigma Y_C)$$
$$= (9 \cdot 6) + (15 \cdot 15) + (15 \cdot 12)$$
$$= 459$$

Step (5). Find the total sum of X, (SSX_{total}), and the total sum of Y, (SSY_{total}).

$$(SSX_{total}) = (\Sigma X_A) + (\Sigma X_B) + (\Sigma X_C)$$
$$= 9 + 15 + 15$$
$$= 39$$

Table 15. General ANCOVA Calculation Table

ANCOVA Table

SOURCE	SUM OF SQUARES (SS)	DEGREES OF FREEDOM (D.F.)	MEAN SQUARES (MS)	F_{OBS} (F)
(Treatment) adj.				
(Within) adj.				
(Covariant) adj.				
Total				

Table 16. Summary of Necessary Calculations for SS adj and SS

Treatment A

X_A	X^2_A	Y_A	Y^2_A	$(X_A \cdot Y_A)$
2	4	1	1	2
3	9	2	4	6
4	16	3	9	12
9	29	6	14	20
ΣX_A	ΣX^2_A	ΣY_A	ΣY^2_A	$\Sigma X_A Y_A$

Treatment B

X_B	X^2_B	Y_B	Y^2_B	$(X_B \cdot Y_B)$
5	25	3	9	15
4	16	6	36	24
6	36	6	36	36
15	77	15	81	75
ΣX_B	ΣX^2_B	ΣY_B	ΣY^2_B	$\Sigma X_B Y_B$

Treatment C

X_C	X^2_C	Y_C	Y^2_C	$(X_C \cdot Y_C)$
3	9	3	9	9
7	49	5	25	35
5	25	4	16	20
15	83	12	50	64
ΣX_C	ΣX^2_C	ΣY_C	ΣY^2_C	$\Sigma X_C Y_C$

$$(SSY_{total}) = (\Sigma Y_A) + (\Sigma Y_B) + (\Sigma Y_C)$$
$$= 6 + 15 + 12$$
$$= 33$$

Step (6). Find the total of the cross product of X and Y (denoted by $SSXY_{total}$), the total of the squared X's (denoted by SSX^2_{total}), and the total of the squared Y's (denoted by SSY^2_{total}).

$$(SSXY_{total}) = (\Sigma X_A Y_A) + (\Sigma X_B Y_B) + (\Sigma X_C Y_C)$$
$$= 20 + 75 + 64$$
$$= 159$$

$$(SSX^2_{total}) = (\Sigma X^2_A) + (\Sigma X^2_B) + (\Sigma X^2_C)$$
$$= 29 + 77 + 83$$
$$= 189$$

$$(SSY^2_{total}) = (\Sigma Y^2_A) + (\Sigma Y^2_B) + (\Sigma Y^2_C)$$
$$= 14 + 81 + 50$$
$$= 145$$

Step (7). Using the values we derived in Step (6), find $(SSSY_{total})$, $(SSSX_{total})$, $(SSSY_{within})$, and $(SSSX_{within})$.

$$(SSSY_{total}) = (SSY^2_{total}) - \frac{(SSY_{total})^2}{N}$$

$$= 145 - \frac{(33)^2}{n_A + n_B + n_C}$$

$$= 145 - \frac{1089}{9}$$

$$= 145 - 121$$
$$= 24$$

where $n_A = 3$, $n_B = 3$, $n_C = 3$, $N = 3 + 3 + 3 = 9$, and $J = 3$ treatments.

$$(SSSX_{total}) = (SSX^2_{total}) - \frac{(SSX_{total})^2}{N}$$

$$= 189 - \frac{(39)^2}{9}$$

$$= 189 - 169$$
$$= 20$$

$$(SSSY_{within}) = (SSY^2_{total}) - \frac{(SSY_{between})^2}{J}$$

$$= 145 - \frac{405}{3}$$

$$= 145 - 135$$
$$= 10$$

$$(SSSX_{within}) = (SSX^2_{total}) - \frac{(SSX_{between})^2}{J}$$

$$= 189 - \frac{531}{3}$$

$$= 189 - 177$$
$$= 12$$

Step (8). Find the two sums of cross products (SCP_{total}) and (SCP_{within}), which will be used to find the adjusted sums of squares.

$$(SCP_{total}) = (SSXY_{total}) - \frac{(SSX_{total}) \cdot (SSY_{total})}{N}$$

$$= 159 - \frac{(39) \cdot (33)}{9}$$

$$= 159 - 143$$
$$= 16$$

$$(SCP_{within}) = (SSXY_{total}) - \frac{(SSXY_{between})}{J}$$

$$= 159 - \frac{459}{3}$$

$$= 159 - 153$$
$$= 6$$

Step (9). Using the values from Step (8), find $[(SSS_{total})adj.]$, $[(SSS_{treatment})adj.]$, and $[(SSS_{within})adj.]$.

$$[(SSS_{total})adj.] = [(SSSY_{total})adj.] - \frac{(SCP_{total})^2}{SSSX_{total}}$$

$$= 24 - \frac{(16)^2}{20}$$

$$= 11.2$$

$$[(SSS_{within})adj.] = [(SSSY_{within})adj.] - \frac{(SCP_{within})^2}{SSSX_{within}}$$

$$= 10 - \frac{(6)^2}{12}$$

$$= 7$$

$$[(SSS_{treatment})adj.] = [(SSSY_{total})adj.] - [(SSSY_{within})adj.]$$
$$= 11.2 - 7$$
$$= 4.2$$

Step (10). Find the sum of squares for the covariant, denoted by (SS_{cov}).

$$(SS_{cov}) = (SSSY_{within}) - [(SSSY_{within})adj.]$$
$$= 10 - 7$$
$$= 3$$

Step (11). Find degrees of freedom for the treatment (d.f. $_{treatment}$), within groups (d.f. $_{within}$), and the covariant (d.f.$_{cov}$).

$$d.f._{treatment} = (\text{total number of groups}) - 1$$
$$= 3 - 1$$
$$= 2$$

d.f.$_{within}$ = [(total number of groups)·(one less than the number of subjects in each group)]
$$-1$$

$$= [(3)\cdot(3 - 1)] - 1$$
$$= 6 - 1$$
$$= 5$$
$$d.f._{total} = N - 1$$
$$= 9 - 1$$
$$= 8$$

$$d.f._{cov} = d.f._{total} - d.f._{treatment} - d.f._{within}$$
$$= 8 - 5 - 2$$
$$= 1$$

Step (12). Calculate the mean squares for the treatment (MStreatment), within groups (MSwithin), and the covariant (MScov).

$$MStreatment = \frac{(SSS_{treatment})adj}{d.f._{treatment}}$$

$$= \frac{4.2}{2}$$

$$= 2.1$$

$$MSwithin = \frac{(SSS_{within})adj}{d.f._{within}}$$

$$= \frac{7}{5}$$

$$= 1.4$$

$$MScov = \frac{(SS_{cov})adj}{d.f._{cov}}$$

$$= \frac{3}{1}$$

$$= 3$$

Step (13). Calculate F_{obs} for the treatment and for the covariant.

$$F_{obs}(treatment) = \frac{MS\ treatment}{MS\ within}$$

$$= \frac{2.1}{1.4}$$

$$= 1.5$$

$$F_{obs}(covariant) = \frac{MS\ cov}{MS\ within}$$

$$= \frac{3}{1.4}$$

$$= 2.14$$

Step (14). Enter all values into the ANCOVA table (see Table 17).

Step (15). Use the decision rule to decide whether or not we reject the null hypothesis.

F_{crit} (.05, 2, 5) = 5.79 > F_{obs} = 1.5
We do not reject H_o
F_{crit} (.05, 1, 5) = 6.61 > F_{obs} = 2.14
We do not reject H_o

Table 17. A Final Summary of the ANCOVA Table

SOURCE	(SUM OF SQUARES)	(D.F.)	(MS)	(FOBS)
Treatment	4.2	2	2.1	1.5
Within	7	5	1.4	
Covariant	3	1	3	2.14
Total	14.2	8		

Table 18. Mean Age and Interval Since Onset for 11 Children Who Stutter

ID		AGE (YR.: MOS)	INTERVAL (MOS)
Subject	1	5.5	42
	2	5.7	39
	3	6.5	54
	4	6.8	21
	5	7.8	28
	6	8.3	63
	7	10.6	103
	8	11.0	67
	9	11.2	98
	10	11.3	65
	11	11.5	78

Therefore, there is neither treatment effects nor covariant effects (severity level) on the rate of repetition of sound/syllable per second.

(c) Table 18 describes the mean age and interval since onset (the length of time the children had exhibited stuttering problems) for 11 subjects from the same study as discussed above. Using Spearman rank-order correlation, determine whether or not age was significantly correlated with interval since onset.

Solution

Spearman rank-order correlation coefficient (r_s) is the suitable statistical analysis to answer the question because this nonparametric analysis could possibly avoid violating assumptions of normality and homogeneity of variance. The following steps lead to a derivation of r_s.

Step (1).   Convert the scores on Ages (X) to ranks. Do the same for the scores on Interval Y (see Table 19).

A rank of "1" is given to the lowest score, "2" to the next lowest score, and so on. The highest rank assigned must be the same value as the number of subjects in the sample. If two scores are tied for the same rank, average the ranks and assign the average rank to both scores.

Table 19. The Ranks of Ages and Intervals

ID	AGE (YRS: MOS)	RANK OF X (X_R)	INTERVAL (MOS)	RANK OF Y (Y_R)
1	5.5	1(the lowest)	42	4
2	5.7	2	39	3
3	6.5	3	54	5
4	6.8	4	21	1
5	7.8	5	28	2
6	8.3	6	63	6
7	10.6	7	103	11
8	11.0	8	67	8
9	11.2	9	98	10
10	11.3	10	65	7
11	11.5	11(the highest)	78	9

Step (2). Derive deviation scores of the rank of X and Y (Table 20).

Step (3). Calculate the covariance (Cov_{xy}) and the standard deviations of X and Y (S_X and S_Y), which are needed in the formula of the Spearman rank correlation coefficient r_{XY}.

$$Cov\,(X, Y) = \frac{\Sigma XY}{N - 1} = \frac{79}{10} = 7.9$$

$$S_X = \sqrt{\frac{\Sigma X^2}{N - 1}} = \sqrt{\frac{110}{10}} = \sqrt{11} = 3.32$$

$$S_Y = \sqrt{\frac{\Sigma X^2}{N - 1}} = \sqrt{\frac{110}{10}} = \sqrt{11} = 3.32$$

$$r_{XY} = \frac{Cov(X,Y)}{(SX)\cdot(SY)} = \frac{7.9}{(3.32)\cdot(3.32)} = .717$$

As expected, age was significantly correlated with the length of time the children had exhibited stuttering problems.

Q7. **The Operant Manipulation of Vocal Pitch in Normal Speakers**
Journal of Speech and Hearing Research, Vol. 14, 283–290, 1971,
by Moore, J. C. and Holbrook, A.

A device consisting of variable electronic filters and voice-actuated relays was used to raise or lower the vocal pitch of four normal-speaking subjects by the differential reinforcement of selected frequencies emitted by them during oral reading. The sequence of investigation with each subject was to measure the habitual pitch level (HPL), adjust the filters to a higher or lower range called conditioning pitch level (CPL), and establish the baseline responding rate at CPL. A fixed interval (FI) reinforcement schedule was alternated with a fixed ratio (FR) reinforcement schedule. Extinction trials (EXT) separated the four ex-

Table 20. The Deviation Scores of the Rank of X and Y

ID	X_R	$\bar{X}_R$	X	X^2	Y_R	$\bar{Y}_R$	Y	Y^2	XY
1	1	6	−5	25	4	6	−2	4	10
2	2	6	−4	16	3	6	−3	9	12
3	3	6	−3	9	5	6	−1	1	3
4	4	6	−2	4	1	6	−5	25	10
5	5	6	−1	1	2	6	−4	16	4
6	6	6	0	0	6	6	0	0	0
7	7	6	1	1	11	6	5	25	5
8	8	6	2	4	8	6	2	4	4
9	9	6	3	9	10	6	4	16	12
10	10	6	4	16	7	6	1	1	4
11	11	6	5	25	9	6	3	9	15
	$\bar{X}_R = 6$			$\Sigma X^2 = 110$	$\bar{Y}_R = 6$	$\Sigma Y^2 = 110$			$\Sigma XY = 79$

where $X = X_R - \bar{X}_R$ and $Y = Y_R - \bar{Y}_R$.

Table 21. The Results of Changes in Modal Fundamental Frequency of Subjects During Experimental Conditions for Four Participants

SUBJECTS	1	2	3	4
HPL	250	182	222	125
CPL	180	260	160	180
CR	200	240	175	175
FR	175	235	160	150
FI	180	250	175	160
EXT	255	200	195	120

perimental conditions with reinstatement by continuous reinforcement (CR) preceding each new condition. The results of changes in modal fundamental frequency during experimental conditions for four participants are summarized in Table 21.

Compute a Kruskal-Wallis one-way ANOVA on the data in Table 21 to determine whether or not there was a significant difference among the four subjects. Use $\alpha = .05$.

Solution

Step (1).   State the null (H_o) and alternative (H_a) hypotheses.

H_o: the four subjects are identical.
H_1: at least one subject differs from the others with respect to median performance scores.

Step (2).   Verify the following assumptions.

1. **Independence:** the data values are randomly assigned to respective groups independently.
2. **Minimum number of subjects:** the individual sample sizes are each at least 5.
3. **Shape of Distribution:** the groups have identical or symmetrical shapes.

Step (3).   Calculate the test statistic K. First we construct a data summary table for each subject and, regardless of group membership, rank (R) the scores from lowest to highest (Table 22). If two or more scores are equal, average the ranks and assign the average to each member of the tie.

Next, we calculate the mean square of the sum of ranks for each group, denoted by MS.

$$MS = \sum_{i=1}^{J} \frac{R^2 i}{n_i}$$

$$= \frac{(93.5)^2}{6} + \frac{(115)^2}{6} + \frac{(60)^2}{6} + \frac{(31.5)^2}{6}$$

$$= 1457.04 + 2204.17 + 600 + 165.38$$

$$= 4426.59$$

Finally, we calculate the K statistic and conclude it under the decision rule such that
(i) reject H_o if $K > \chi^2(\alpha, J - 1)$, where J = total number of groups.
(ii) Do not reject H_o if $K \leq \chi^2(\alpha, J - 1)$.

$$K = \frac{12}{N(N + 1)} \cdot (MS) - 3 \cdot (N + 1)$$

where N = total sample size. We now would be able to derive the observed K statistic and critical χ^2 value.

Given: N = 6 + 6 + 6 + 6 = 24 scores
              J = 4 groups (or 4 participants)
              MS = 4426.59

$$K = \frac{12}{24 \cdot (24 + 1)} \cdot (4426.59) - 3 \cdot (24 + 1)$$

$$= 88.53 - 75$$

Table 22. Ranks of Scores for Each Subject

Subject	1		2		3		4	
	Score	Rank	Score	Rank	Score	Rank	Score	Rank
	250	21.5	182	14	222	18	125	2
	180	12	260	24	160	5	180	12
	200	16.5	240	20	175	8.5	175	8.5
	175	8.5	235	19	160	5	150	3
	180	12	250	21.5	175	8.5	160	5
	255	23	200	16.5	195	15	120	1
Sums		93.5		115		60		31.5

$$= 13.53$$
$$\text{Critical } \chi^2(.05, 3) = 7.815 < 13.53$$

Therefore, we reject H_o; i.e., the observed difference is significant and the distributions of scores in the four subjects are not identical.

ONE-WAY AND TWO-WAY ANALYSIS OF VARIANCE

Q8. **Predictive Values of Routine Blood Pressure Measurements in Screening for Hypertension**
American Journal of Epidemiology, **Vol. 117, No. 4, 1990, by Rosner, B. and Polk, B. F.**

An epidemiologist conducted a study to compare systolic blood pressure and diastolic blood pressure for the purpose of hypertension detection in a range of healthy males and females of different ages. Although it was not a part of this study, assume that we were able to subdivide the sample into a group of nonstutterers and a group of stutterers. The results are summarized in Table 23.

Table 23. The Results of Systolic Blood Pressure and Diastolic Blood Pressure Levels for Participants

Systolic Blood Pressure (mm Hg)

AGE	GENDER	NONSTUTTERERS			STUTTERERS		
		M	SD	n	M	SD	n
Young							
30–49	M	126.8	14.3	262	135.6	19.0	41
30–49	F	119.7	15.9	172	130.8	21.3	52
Old							
50–69	M	136.5	19.6	179	145.1	22.8	42
50–69	F	135.7	21.0	196	145.1	23.7	47

Diastolic Blood Pressure (mm Hg)

AGE	GENDER	NONSTUTTERERS			STUTTERERS		
		M	SD	n	M	SD	n
Young							
30–49	M	82.2	10.9	262	87.8	13.7	41
30–49	F	77.1	10.8	172	84.6	14.2	52
Old							
50–69	M	83.6	11.5	179	89.2	14.0	42
50–69	F	80.4	11.3	196	87.8	13.8	47

(a) What statistical test procedure can be used to test for significant differences in diastolic blood pressure levels among the four groups (young males, young females, old males, and old females) within the nonstutterers?
(b) Perform the test mentioned in (a) and conclude it.
(c) What statistical test procedure can be used to test for significant differences of systolic blood pressure among young groups of stutterers and nonstutterers according to gender?
(d) Perform the test mentioned in (c) and conclude it.

Solution

(a) Whenever the means of more than two groups are to be compared, we frequently use the Analysis of Variance (ANOVA). For our example, we may start out by summarizing the results of four groups as follows.

Group:

1. (Young male nonstutterers) $\overline{Y}_1 = 82.2$, $S_1 = 10.9$, $n_1 = 262$
2. (Young female nonstutterers) $\overline{Y}_2 = 77.1$, $S_2 = 10.8$, $n_2 = 172$
3. (Old male stutterers) $\overline{Y}_3 = 83.6$, $S_3 = 11.5$, $n_3 = 179$
4. (Old female stutterers) $\overline{Y}_4 = 80.4$, $S_4 = 11.3$, $n_4 = 196$

where $\overline{Y}_i$ = the sample mean and S_i = the sample standard deviation.
Prior to ANOVA, we must verify the following assumptions.

(i) **Normality:** the data values within each group are normally distributed. The ANOVA procedures are relatively insensitive to the violation of the normality assumption, especially as the sample sizes increase, because of the effect of the central limit theorem.
(ii) **Homogeneity of variance:** The variances of the data values in each group are equal. Again, the ANOVA is relatively insensitive to the violation of homogeneity of variance if (i) all samples have the same or similar sizes, (ii) the sample size is large, and/or (iii) the largest sample standard deviation is no more than twice as large as the smallest sample standard deviation. If any one of the three conditions fail to be met, then we must use Bartlett's test for homogeneity of variance (available on SPSS, BMDP, or SAS software) to determine whether to use a nonparametric version of the ANOVA such as the Kruskal-Wallis test.

In summary, the flowchart in Figure 2 can help readers understand the general procedures for comparing the means of several independent groups.

(b) Using Bartlett's test, we could verify that the assumption of homogeneity of variance, along with the assumption of normality, has been met for the ANOVA.

Step (1).   State the null and alternative hypotheses.

H_o: $\mu_1 = \mu_2 = \mu_3 = \mu_4$ (All means are equal)
H_1: Not all means are equal.

Step (2).   Calculate the Between-Sum of Squares (SS_B) and the Within-Sum of Squares (SS_W).

Case (1).   If the raw data are available, then:

$$SS_B = \sum_{j=1}^{J} n_j \cdot (\overline{Y}_j - \overline{Y})^2 \text{ with d.f.} = J-1$$

$$SS_B = \sum_{j=1}^{J} \sum_{i=1}^{n_j} (Y_{ij} - \overline{Y}_j)^2 \text{ with d.f.} = \sum_{j=1}^{J} (n_j - 1)$$

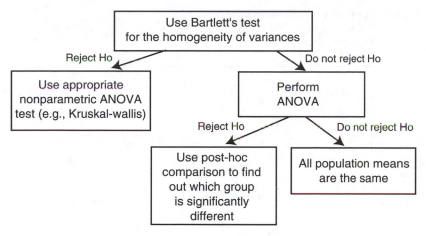

Figure 2. The general procedures for comparing the means of multiple groups.

where n_j = sample size of the jth group.
J = total number of groups
$\overline{Y}_j$ = the sample mean of the jth group
$\overline{Y}$ = the overall mean
Y_{ij} = the ith observed value of the jth group

Case (2). If the raw data are not available, then

$$SS_B = [\sum_{j=1}^{J} n_j \overline{Y}^2_j] - \left[\frac{(\sum_{j=1}^{J} n_j \overline{Y}_j)^2}{n} \right]$$

$$SSw = \sum_{j=1}^{J} (n_j - 1) \cdot S^2 j$$

$$\text{with d.f.} = \sum_{j=1}^{J} (n_j - 1)$$

For our example, we must use the formula in case (2) because the raw data are not available. One can now calculate SS_B and SS_W.

$$SS_B = [262 \cdot (182.2)^2 + 172 \cdot (77.1)^2 + 179 \cdot (83.6)^2 + 196 \cdot (80.4)^2]$$
$$- \left[\frac{\{(262 \cdot 82.2) + (172 \cdot 77.1) + (179 \cdot 83.6) + 196 \cdot (80.4)\}^2}{262 + 172 + 179 + 196} \right]$$

$$= [1770292.1 + 1022438.5 + 1251023.8 + 1266975.4] - \frac{(65520.4)^2}{809}$$

$$= 5310729.8 - 5306455.9$$
$$= 4273.9$$

$$SS_W = [(262 - 1) \cdot (10.9)^2 + (172 - 1) \cdot (10.8)^2$$
$$+ (179 - 1) \cdot (11.5)^2 + (196 - 1) \cdot (11.3)^2]$$
$$= 31009.41 + 19945.44 + 23540.5 + 24899.55$$
$$= 99394.9$$

Table 24. A Final Summary of One-Way ANOVA

SOURCES	SS	D.F.	$MS(=\dfrac{SS}{D.F.})$	$F(=\dfrac{MS_B}{MS_W})$
Between	4273.9	3	$\dfrac{4273.9}{3}=1424.63$	$F=\dfrac{1424.63}{123.47}$
Within	99394.9	805*	$\dfrac{99394.9}{85}=123.47$	$=11.54$

Step (3).　Construct the ANOVA table (Table 24) to calculate the F-ratio.
where J = 4 groups

$$MS_b = \frac{SS_b}{d.f._b} \quad \text{and} \quad MS_W = \frac{SS_w}{d.f._w}$$

$*d.f._W = (262 - 1) + (172 - 1) + (179 - 1) + (196 - 1) = 805$

Step (4).　Under the decision rule (at $\alpha = .05$), determine whether or not we reject H_o. $F_{crit}(.05, d.f. = 3, 805) = 2.60 < F_{obs} = 11.54$, therefore, we reject H_o. This tells us that the difference among the means of four groups are not equal.

(c)　The results according to gender are summarized in Table 25.

We are interested in the effects of both stuttering and gender on systolic blood pressure. These factors may be independent or they may be related to or interact with each other. One approach to the problem is to establish a two-way ANOVA model to detect the effects of stuttering, gender, and the combination of both factors on systolic blood pressure. There are two important assumptions for the two-way ANOVA that must be verified.

(i)　**Normality:** The data values within each cell are drawn from a population in which the data values are normally distributed. The two-way ANOVA is relatively insensitive to the violation of this assumption, particularly if n is large.

(ii)　**Homogeneity of Variances:** The variances of data values in the populations underlying all the cells of the design are equal. As in the case of the one-way ANOVA, we must use Bartlett's test for the homogeneity of variances to verify this assumption. Normally, the two-way ANOVA is relatively insensitive to the violation of this assumption if (i) the cell sizes are equal, (ii) sample size is large, and/or (iii) the largest sample standard deviation is no more than twice as large as the smallest sample standard deviation.

(d) Step (1).　Check all basic assumptions of a two-way ANOVA and determine whether or not it can be used.

Step (2).　If its assumptions are satisfied, we then construct the two-way ANOVA table (Table 26) to calculate all F values.

　　For the two-way ANOVA model, we can state the following three hypotheses.

1. H_o: There will be no gender effects on systolic blood pressure level after controlling for the effects of stuttering.

　　Use $F_{row} = \dfrac{MS\ row}{MS\ residual}$ to test it.

Table 25. Systolic Blood Pressure Among Young Groups of Nonstutterers and Stutterers According to Gender

STATUS (ROW EFFECT)	STUTTERING (COLUMN EFFECT)			
	NONSTUTTERERS		STUTTERERS	
Young males	M	126.8	M	135.6
	SD	14.3	SD	19.0
	n	262	n	41
Young females	M	119.7	M	130.8
	SD	15.9	SD	21.3
	n	172	n	52

Table 26. The General Two-Way ANOVA Table

SOURCE	SS	D.F.	MS	F
Row(Gender)	$\displaystyle\frac{\sum\limits_{i=1}^{r} Y_i^2\cdot}{C} - \frac{Y^2\cdot\cdot}{rc}$	$r - 1$	$\text{Row SS}/r - 1$	$F_{row} = \dfrac{\text{MS row}}{\text{MS residual}}$
Column (Stuttering)	$\displaystyle\frac{\sum\limits_{j=1}^{c} Y^2\cdot j}{r} - \frac{Y^2\cdot\cdot}{rc}$	$C - 1$	$\text{Column SS}/C - 1$	$F_{column} = \dfrac{\text{MS column}}{\text{MS residual}}$
Interaction (Gender + Stuttering)	$(\sum\limits_{i=1}^{r}\sum\limits_{j=1}^{c} \overline{Y}^2 ij - \frac{Y^2\cdot\cdot}{rc})$ $-$ Row SS $-$ Column SS	$(r - 1)\cdot$ $(C - 1)$	$\dfrac{\text{Interaction SS}}{(r - 1)(C - 1)}$	$F_{int.} = \dfrac{\text{MS interaction}}{\text{MS residual}}$
Residual (Error)		$n - rc$	$\sum\limits_{i=1}^{r}\sum\limits_{j=1}^{c} \dfrac{(n_{ij} - 1)\cdot(S^2_{ij})}{(n - rc)\cdot n_h}$	

2. H_o: There will be no stuttering effects on systolic blood pressure level after controlling for the effects of gender.

Use F column $= \dfrac{\text{MS column}}{\text{MS residual}}$ to test it.

3. H_o: There will be no interaction effects on systolic blood pressure level.

Use F interaction $= \dfrac{\text{MS interaction}}{\text{MS residual}}$ to test it.

An interaction effect between two variables is defined as one in which the effect of one variable depends on the level of the other variable. It may be asked "Is there a differential effect of stuttering on systolic blood pressure among different gender groups?" Such an interaction effect is important to understand in relation to the assumptions of the two-way ANOVA. If more than one treatment effect exists (namely, gender and stuttering), then we may expect to observe a treatment effect for both factors. To simplify the basic concept of an interaction effect, a graphic representation can be used. For our example, given the data below, systolic blood pressure levels can be plotted on the ordinate and the gender variable on the abscissa (see Figure 3).

STUTTERING		
GENDER	NONSTUTTERERS	STUTTERERS
MALE (M)	126.8	135.6
FEMALE (F)	119.7	130.8

To determine whether or not there is an interaction, the pattern for each pair of lines must be examined. If the lines intersect at a particular point, we could say that an interaction occurred. Otherwise, it can be concluded that there was no interaction between the two independent factors (variables). For our example, because there is no intersection point, it does not appear that systolic blood pressure was significantly affected by the interaction of gender and stuttering. Actual calculations would verify this fact.

4. Residual variances represent a measure of the amount of variability within the individual samples.

Before we calculate the sum of squares, we need to define some notations as follows:

(a) Calculate ROW SS (or SS $_{row}$)

$$SS_{row} = \frac{\sum\limits_{i=1}^{r} Y_i^{2.}}{C} - \frac{Y^2..}{rC}$$

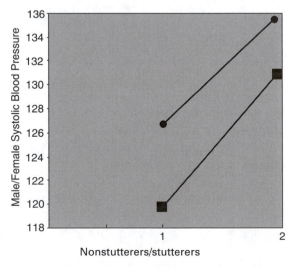

Figure 3. A graphical representation of an interaction effect by gender by stuttering.

where C = the total number of columns

r = the total number of rows

$$Yi\cdot = \sum_{j=1}^{C} \overline{Y}ij = \text{the total sum of the sample means of the jth column of the ith group.}$$

$$Y\cdot\cdot = \sum_{j=1}^{r} \sum_{j=1}^{C} \overline{Y}ij = \text{the total sum of the sample means of the ith row and jth column.}$$

(b) Calculate Column SS (or SS$_{\text{column}}$)

$$SS_{\text{column}} = \frac{\sum_{j=1}^{C} Y^2_j}{r} - \frac{Y^2\cdot\cdot}{rC}$$

where $Y\cdot j = \sum_{i=1}^{r} \overline{Y}ij = \text{the total sum of the sample means of the ith row of the jth group.}$

(c) Calculate the Interaction sum of squares (or SS interaction):

$$SS_{\text{interaction}} = \left(\sum_{i=1}^{r} \sum_{j=1}^{c} \overline{Y}^2ij - \frac{Y^2\cdot\cdot}{rC} \right) - SS_{\text{row}} - SS_{\text{column}}$$

Returning to our example, we first need c, r, (Yi·), (Y·j) and (Y··).

$C = 2$ (a total of two columns)

$r = 2$ (a total of two rows)

i = first row = $\overline{Y}_1\cdot = \overline{Y}_{11} + \overline{Y}_{12} = 126.8 + 135.6 = 262.4$

i = second row = $\overline{Y}_2\cdot = \overline{Y}_{21} + \overline{Y}_{22} = 119.7 + 130.8 = 250.5$

j = first column = $\overline{Y}\cdot_1 = \overline{Y}_{11} + \overline{Y}_{21} = 126.8 + 119.7 = 246.5$

j = second column = $\overline{Y}\cdot_2 = \overline{Y}_{12} + \overline{Y}_{22} = 135.6 + 130.8 = 266.4$

$\overline{Y}\cdot\cdot = \overline{Y}_{11} + \overline{Y}_{12} + \overline{Y}_{21} + \overline{Y}_{22} = 512.9$

We now have:

$$SS_{\text{row}} = \frac{(262.4)^2 + (250.5)^2}{2} - \frac{(512.9)^2}{2\cdot2}$$

$$= 35.402$$

$$\text{d.f.}_{\text{row}} = 2 - 1 = 1$$

$$MS_{\text{row}} = \frac{35.402}{1} = 35.402$$

$$SS_{\text{column}} = \frac{(246.5)^2 + (266.4)^2}{2} - \frac{(512.9)^2}{2\cdot2}$$

$$= 99.002$$

$$\text{d.f.}_{\text{column}} = 2 - 1 = 1$$

$$M.S._{\text{column}} = \frac{99.002}{1} = 99.002$$

$$SS_{\text{interaction}} = [(126.8)^2 + (135.6)^2 + (119.7)^2 + (130.8)^2] - \frac{(512.9)^2}{2\cdot2}$$

$$- 35.402 \, (SS_{\text{row}}) - 99.002 \, (SS_{\text{column}})$$

$$= 1.323$$

d.f. $_{\text{interaction}}$ = $(2 - 1) \cdot (2 - 1) = 1$

$$\text{M.S.}_{\text{interaction}} = \frac{1.323}{1} = 1.323$$

Next, we would calculate the mean square of residuals, denoted by MS_{residual}. To do so, we need the value of n_h.

$$\frac{1}{n_h} = \left[\left(\frac{1}{262} + \frac{1}{41} + \frac{1}{172} + \frac{1}{52} \right) \Big/ 4 \right]$$

$$= .0133$$

$$n_h = \frac{1}{.0133} = 75.188$$

Thus,

$$MS_{\text{residual}} = \frac{[(261 \cdot (14.3)^2 + 40 \cdot (19.0)^2 + 171 \cdot (15.9)^2 + 51 \cdot (21.3)^2]}{[(262 + 41 + 172 + 52) - 4] \cdot (75.188)}$$

$$= 3.41$$

$$\text{d.f. }_{\text{residual}} = (262 + 41 + 172 + 52) - 4 = 523$$

Finally, we must answer the following three questions:

Question 1. Is there a gender effect on systolic blood pressure level after controlling for the effect of stuttering?

   H_o: Not Significant
   H_1: Significant

Calculate an F_{row} ratio.

$$F_{\text{row}} = \frac{MS \text{ row}}{MS \text{ residual}} = \frac{35.402}{3.41} = 10.38 > F_{\text{crit}} (.05, 1.523) = 3.84$$

Hence, we reject H_o, i.e., the effects of gender is significant at α = 5%.

Question 2. Is there a stuttering effect on systolic blood pressure level after controlling for the effect of gender?

   H_o: Not Significant
   H_1: Significant

Calculate an F_{column} ratio.

$$F_{\text{column}} = \frac{MS \text{ column}}{MS \text{ residual}} = \frac{99.002}{3.41} = 29.033 > F_{\text{crit}} (.05, 1,523) = 3.84$$

Hence, we reject H_o; i.e., the effect of stuttering is significant.

Question 3. Is there an interaction effect on systolic blood pressure level?

   H_o: Not Significant
   H_1: Significant

Calculate an $F_{\text{interaction}}$ ratio.

$$F_{interaction} = \frac{MS\ interaction}{MS\ residual} = \frac{1.323}{3.41} = 0.388 < F_{crit}\ (.05,\ 1,523) = 3.84$$

Hence we do not reject H_o, i.e. the interaction effect is not significant.
These results above are displayed in Table 27.

When we interpret the results of a two-way ANOVA, we start with the interaction effect. If it is not significant, we must go back to find out which main effect (or possibly both) caused the significant effect. If the result is statistically significant, we examine the data for an interaction effect.

Given our example, the results imply that systolic blood pressure levels were affected by the factors of gender and stuttering independently of one another.

MULTIPLE REGRESSION

Q9. Duration of Sound Prolongation and Sound/Syllable Repetition in Children who Stutter: Preliminary Observations
Journal of Speech and Hearing Research, **Vol. 37, 254–263, April 1994.**
by Zebrowski, P. M.

The purpose of this study was to measure the duration of sound prolongations and sound/syllable repetitions in the conversational speech of school-age children who stutter. The correlation coefficients (r) between age, the duration of sound prolongations (SP), and the duration of sound/syllable repetitions (SSR) are summarized in Table 28.

(a) With this information, predict the SSR score of an incoming child whose age is 9.5 years old with an SP score of 720.
(b) Find the multiple correlation coefficient (r), and test its significance at $\alpha = 5\%$.
(c) Find the standardized partial regression coefficients (β), and determine which of the independent variables is the best predictor of SSR.

Solution

(a) There are three primary reasons why many researchers might want to use multiple regression analysis. They are as follows:

   (i) By establishing the functional relationship between one dependent variable (Y) and a group of two or more independent variables ($X_1, X_2, \ldots, X_K$), the analysis will indicate how each of two or more independent variables (Xs) predicts the dependent variable (Y).

   (ii) If one has no prior knowledge or empirical evidence for choosing a group of predictor variables, the multiple regression analysis will help to find which variables are associated most with a particular dependent variable.

Table 27. Two-way ANOVA for Systolic Blood Pressure

SOURCES	SS	D.F.	MS	F-STATISTICS	DECISION
Gender	35.402	1	35.402	10.89	Significant
Stuttering	99.002	1	99.002	30.46	Significant
Interaction	1.323	1	1.323	0.407	Not Significant
Residuals		523	3.41		

Table 28. The Correlation Coefficients Between Age, Sound Prolongations, and Sound/Syllable Repetitions

Correlations (N = 14)	AGE (A)	SOUND PROLONGATIONS (SP)	SOUND/SYLLABLE REPETITIONS (SSR)
A	1.00		
SP	.36	1.00	
SSR	−.14	.05	1.00
Means	8.2	706	724
Standard deviations	2.4	296	145

(iii) A researcher might wish to test a theory to see if the sample data support the theory. Suppose the theory suggests that the SSR score is influenced not only by age, but also by the SP score. A multiple regression analysis can be used to determine whether or not the SP score will add anything to the prediction of the SSR score beyond what can be predicted from age.

The idea behind multiple regression analysis is very similar to that of simple linear regression. In simple linear regression, we predict one variable (Y) from another variable (X). In multiple regression analysis, we have two or more variables $(X_1, X_2, \ldots, X_K)$ to predict one variable. Symbolically, a general equation for multiple regression analysis is given by

$$\hat{Y} = b_0 + b_1 X_1 + b_2 X_2 + \ldots + b_K X_K$$

where

$$\hat{Y} = \text{predictive value of Y}$$
$$b_0 = \text{y intercept}$$
$$(b_1, \ldots b_K) = \text{partial regression coefficients.}$$
$$(X_1, \ldots X_K) = \text{independent variables.}$$

The set of the partial regression coefficients tells us how strong each X (the predictor) is associated with Y (the predicted score).

In simple linear regression, r^2 gives a measure of the proportion of variance in Y that is predictable from X. The multiple correlation coefficient (r) can be squared (r^2) to measure the proportion of variance in Y that is predictable from several X's.

The reader should be aware of the complexities of calculating partial regression coefficients of multiple regression analysis that have more than two independent variables. When there are three or more independent variables, the mathematical deviation of a set of partial regression coefficients becomes increasingly abstract and difficult; therefore, the calculation of b's (slopes) will be limited to a multiple regression with two independent variables. (Most statistical software packages will calculate partial regression coefficients).

Imagine that we have one dependent variable (Y) and two predictor variables (X_1, X_2), and we wish to graph them in three-dimensional space. The graph that looks like the lines where the adjoining walls come together, extending from the floor to the ceiling, is the Y axis (Figure 4).

To plot sample data points, we simply take a set of values (Y, X_1, X_2) for each individual value in a data set, locate them on their respective axis, and then find the point in space where those values meet. By repeating this process until all subjects are plotted, the result is a collection of points suspended in space representing the data.

The multiple regression equation is the best-fit plane, not a line, through our swarm of points. The best-fit plane represents the predicted values at Y for a linear combination of X_1 and X_2. So, whenever you wish to predict the value of Y, you can locate the point on the plane where X_1 and X_2 meet and then find the corresponding value of Y. This Y is the predictive value of Y, denoted by $\hat{Y}$.

The y intercept of the multiple regression, denoted by b_0, is the point on the Y axis where the regression plane intersects that axis. At this point, X_1 and X_2 are both equal to 0; therefore,

$$b_0 = \overline{Y} - b_1\overline{X}_1 - b_2\overline{X}_2$$

The partial regression coefficients give the relationship between Y and (X_1, X_2) for our example. The partial correlation coefficient b_1 represents the association between Y and X_1 while X_2 is constant; b_2 represents the association between Y and X_2 while X_1 is constant. The formulas for b_1 and b_2 are given by:

$$b_1 = \left[\frac{r yx_1 - (r yx_2)\cdot(r x_1 x_2)}{1 - r^2 x_1 x_2} \right] \cdot \left(\frac{Sy}{Sx_1} \right)$$

$$b_2 = \left[\frac{r yx_2 - (r yx_1)\cdot(r x_1 x_2)}{1 - r^2 x_1 x_2} \right] \cdot \left(\frac{Sy}{Sx_2} \right)$$

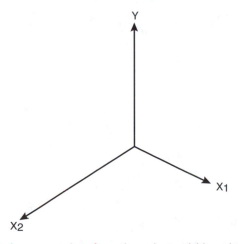

Figure 4. A graphical representation of one dependent variable and two predictor variables.

where:

r_{YX_1} = correlation between Y and X_1
r_{YX_2} = correlation between Y and X_2
$r_{X_1X_2}$ = correlation between X_1 and X_2
S_{X_1} = standard deviation of X_1
S_{X_2} = standard deviation of X_2
S_Y = standard deviation of Y
b_1 = partial regression coefficient of X_1
b_2 = partial regression coefficient of X_2

For our example, we can find the multiple regression equation describing Y (SSR) for a linear combination of X_1 (Age) and X_2 (SP).

$$\hat{Y} = b_0 + b_1X_1 + b_2X_2$$

Step (1).   Find b_1 and b_2.
b_1 = partial regression coefficient of Age

$$= \left[\frac{r_{SSR, Age} - (r_{SSR, SP}) \cdot (r_{Age, SP})}{1 - r^2_{Age, SP}} \right] \cdot \left(\frac{S_{SSr}}{S_{Age}} \right)$$

$$= \left[\frac{(-.14) - (.05) \cdot (.36)}{1 - (.36)^2} \right] \cdot \left(\frac{145}{2.4} \right)$$

$$= \left(\frac{-.158)}{.8704} \right) \cdot (60.417)$$

$$= -10.967$$

b_2 = partial regression coefficient of SP

$$= \left[\frac{r_{SSR, SP} - (r_{SSR, Age}) \cdot (r_{SP, Age})}{1 - r^2_{SP, AGE}} \right] \cdot \left(\frac{S_{SSR}}{S_{SP}} \right)$$

$$= \left[\frac{(.05) - (-.14) \cdot (.36)}{1 - (.36)^2} \right] \cdot \left(\frac{145}{296} \right)$$

$$= \left(\frac{.1004}{.8704} \right) \cdot (.490)$$

$$= 0.0565$$

Step (2).   Find the y intercept b.

$$b_o = \overline{Y}_{SSR} - (b_{Age} \cdot \overline{X}_{Age}) - (b_{sp} \cdot \overline{X}_{sp})$$

Given:

$\overline{Y}_{SSR}$ = the sample mean of SSR = 724
b_{Age} = −10.967
$\overline{X}_{Age}$ = the sample mean of Age = 8.2
b_{sp} = .0565
$\overline{X}_{sp}$ = the sample mean of Sp = 706

Hence, b_o = 724 − (−10.967)·(8.2) − (.0565)·(706)
= 774.040

Step (3). Compute the value of $\hat{Y}$ using the multiple regression formula.
Recall that our hypothetical child is 9.5 years old and has a score of 720 on SP.
$\hat{Y}$ = the best predictive SSR score given that he/she is 9.5 years old and has 720 on SP.
$\hat{Y} = 774.04 + (-10.967) \cdot (9.5) + (.0565) \cdot (720)$
  $= 710.534$

(b) R^2 is a measure of the proportion of variance in Y (SSR) accounted for by X_1 (Age) and X_2 (SP). The value of R^2 can be calculated through the formula below.

$$R^2 = \frac{r^2_{YX_1} + r^2_{YX_2} - 2(r_{YX_1})(r_{YX_2})(r_{X_1X_2})}{1 - r^2_{X_1X_2}}$$

or, for our example,

$$R^2 = \frac{r^2_{SSR, Age} + r^2_{SSR, SP} - 2(r_{SSR, Age})(r_{SSR, SP})(r_{Age, SP})}{1 - r^2_{Age, SP}}$$

$$= \frac{(-.14)^2 + (.05)^2 - 2(-.14) \cdot (.05)(.36)}{1 - (.36)^2}$$

$$= \frac{.02714}{.8704}$$

$$= .0312 \text{ or } 3.12\%$$

This result tells us that approximately 3.12% of the variance in SSR scores can be accounted for by the linear combination of Age and SP scores.
Next, we will test the significance of R^2.

Step (1). State the null and alternative hypotheses.

  $H_0: R^2 = 0$ (Not significant)
  $H_1: R^2 \neq 0$ (Significant)

Step (2). Calculate the observed F (F_{obs})

$$F_{obs} = \frac{R^2/K}{(1 - R^2)/(N - K - 1)}$$

with d.f. = Numerator K, Denominator N − K − 1
Where R^2 = square of multiple correlation coefficient
    K = number of independent variables
    N = number of subjects

Our example gives:

$$F_{obs} = \frac{(.0312)/2}{(1 - .0312)/(14 - 2 - 1)}$$

with d.f. = Numerator 2, Denominator 11

$$= \frac{.0156}{.9688/11}$$

$$= .177$$

Step (3).   Find the critical value of F (F_{crit}) and conclude it under the decision rule.

Because $F_{obs} = .177 < F_{crit} (.05, 2, 11) = 3.98$, we do not reject H_0 and conclude that there is no significant association between SSR scores and the combination of Age and SP scores.

(c) If the researcher wishes to determine which of the independent variables are the best predictors of Y, he or she will have to examine the partial regression coefficients in relation to each other, i.e., the researcher must calculate the standardized regression coefficients, denoted by the β (beta), to determine the strength of associations between Y and each X. This calculation is shown below.

Step (1).   Calculate $\hat{\beta}$ age and $\hat{\beta}$ sp

$$\hat{\beta}\ age = b_{age} \cdot \frac{S_{age}}{S_{SSR}}$$

$$= (-10.967) \cdot \frac{2.4}{145}$$

$$= -.182$$

$$\hat{\beta}\ sp = b_{sp} \cdot \frac{S_{sp}}{S_{SSR}}$$

$$= (.0565) \cdot \frac{296}{145}$$

$$= .115$$

Step (2).   Take the absolute values of $\hat{\beta}$ age and $\hat{\beta}$ sp.

$$|\hat{\beta}\ age| = |-.182| = .182$$
$$|\hat{\beta}\ sp| \ \ = |.115| = .115$$

This indicates that age is a slightly better predictor of SSR than SP is.

APPENDIX B.
Calculation of the Power
of a Statistical Test

Ideally, one wants to avoid (or at least minimize) making both Type I and Type II errors at the same time. Unfortunately, the two errors always work against one another. That is to say, if one tries to decrease α (type I error), one is likely to increase b (type II error), and vice versa. In most cases, researchers pay more attention to a Type II error, because it is β that determines the **power** of a statistical test, denoted by $(1 - \beta)$.

The power represents the probability of rejecting a false null hypothesis correctly, i.e., it is the ability of a statistical test to detect a difference between the mean under H_o and the mean under H_1 when it exists. For example, researchers might suspect that the mean IQ score of a certain group of children is 105. Knowing the population mean score (μ) under the null hypothesis is 100, and the standard deviation (σ) is 15, the alternative mean is 105 for n = 36.

How do we calculate power of this test? The following steps are necessary for calculating power.

Step 1.   State H_o and H_1

H_o: $\mu_o = 100$
H_1: $\mu_1 = 105$

Step 2.   Draw a diagram of two sampling distributions.

Figure A

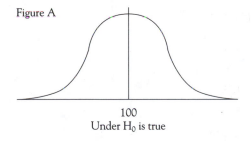

100
Under H_0 is true

vs

Figure B

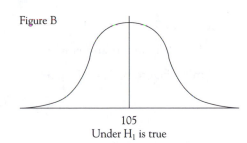

105
Under H_1 is true

273

Step 3. Set up α (say, .05) and drop a line down through Zcritical to meet Figure B. The point at which this line meets the abscissa in Figure B is referred to as μ_M. Shade in the "rejection areas" for both diagrams.

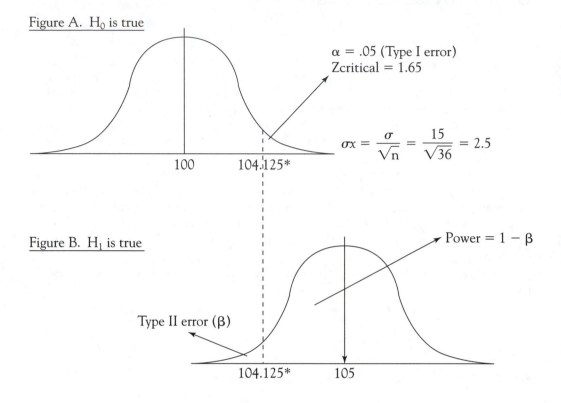

Figure A. H_0 is true

$\alpha = .05$ (Type I error)
Zcritical = 1.65

$\sigma x = \dfrac{\sigma}{\sqrt{n}} = \dfrac{15}{\sqrt{36}} = 2.5$

100   104.125*

Figure B. H_1 is true

Power = $1 - \beta$

Type II error (β)

104.125*   105

* $100 + (1.65)2.5 = 104.125$, therefore $\mu_M = 104.125$

Step 4.   Calculate β and power

Under Figure B, Z is calculated as

$$Z = \frac{104.125 - 105}{2.5} = -.35$$

Therefore, the probability of β is calculated as $50\% - 13.68\% = 36.32\%$.

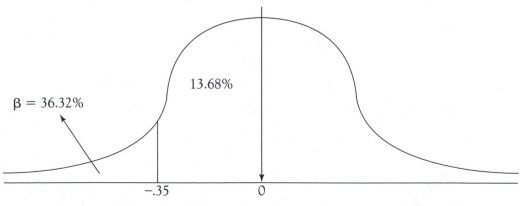

13.68%

$\beta = 36.32\%$

−.35   0

Hence, the power of the test is given by:

$$100\% - 36.32\% = 63.68\%$$

This means that given a specific alternative hypothesis, researchers will correctly reject a false null hypothesis about 63.68% of the time.

It is extremely important to do what you can to increase the power of a test. The following are some factors that influence power.

(i) Sample size (n): The power of a statistical test increases as the sample size increases, because increasing the sample size decreases the variability in the sampling distribution, which eventually increases the power.

(ii) Significance level (α): As α increases, the power of a statistical test also increases, because the ability to detect a difference when it exists becomes better if you use a less credible level of significance.

(iii) Standard deviation (s or σ): The power of a statistical test increases if the standard deviation (s or σ) decreases.

In summary, the following decision table may be useful for understanding types of errors and power.

	H_o is True	H_o is False
Do not reject H_o	Correct Decision $(1 - \alpha)$	Type II Error (β)
Reject H_o	Type I Error (α)	Correct Decision Power $(1 - \beta)$

APPENDIX C.
The Tables

The Standard Normal Distribution
Areas under the standard normal curve from 0 to z for various values of z.

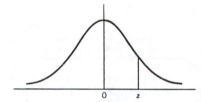

z	.00	.01	.02	.03	.04	.05	.06	.07	.08	.09
0.0	.0000	.0040	.0080	.0120	.0160	.0199	.0239	.0279	.0319	.0359
0.1	.0398	.0438	.0478	.0517	.0557	.0596	.0636	.0675	.0714	.0754
0.2	.0793	.0832	.0871	.0910	.0948	.0987	.1026	.1064	.1103	.1141
0.3	.1179	.1217	.1255	.1293	.1331	.1368	.1406	.1443	.1480	.1517
0.4	.1554	.1591	.1628	.1664	.1700	.1736	.1772	.1808	.1844	.1879
0.5	.1915	.1950	.198 5	.2019.	.2054	.2088	.2123	.2157	.2190	.2224
0.6	.2258	.2291	.2324	.2357	.2389.	.2422	.2454	.2486	.2518	.2549
0.7	.2580	.2612	.2642	.2673	.2704	.2734	.2764	.2794	.2823	.2852
0.8	.2881	.2910	.2939	.2967	.2996	.3023	.3051	.3078	.3106	.3133
0.9	.3159	.3186	.3212	.3238	.3264	.3289	.3315	.3340	.3365	.3389
1.0	.3413	.3438	.3461	.3485	.3508	.3531	.3554	.3577	.3599	.3621
1.1	.3643	.3665	.3686	.3708	.3729	.3749	.3770	.3790	.3810	.3830
1.2	.3849	.3869	.3888	.3907	.3925	.3944	.3962	.3980	.3997	.4015
1.3	.4032	.4049	.4066	.4082	.4099	.4115	.4131	.4147	.4162	.4177
1.4	.4192	.4207	.4222	.4236	.4251	.4265	.4279	.4292	.4306	.4319

The Standard Normal Distribution
Areas under the standard normal curve from 0 to z for various values of z.

z	.00	.01	.02	.03	.04	.05	.06	.07	.08	.09
1.5	.4332	.4345	.4357	.4370	.4382	.4394	.4406	.4418	.4429	.4441
1.6	.4452	.4463	.4474	.4484	.4495	.4505	.4515	.4525	.4535	.4545
1.7	.4554	.4564	.4573	.4582	.4591	.4599	.4608	.4616	.4625	.4633
1.8	.4641	.4649	.4656	.4664	.4671	.4678	.4686	.4693	.4699	.4706
1.9	.4713	.4719	.4726	.4732	.4738	.4744	.4750	.4756	.4761	.4767
2.0	.4772	.4778	.4783	.4788	.4793	.4798	.4803	.4808	.4812	.4817
2.1	.4821	.4826	.4830	.4834	.4838	.4842	.4846	.4850	.4854	.4857
2.2	.4861	.4864	.4868	.4871	.4875	.4878	.4881	.4884	.4887	.4890
2.3	.4893	.4896	.4898	.4901	.4904	.4906	.4909	.4911	.4913	.4916
2.4	.4918	.4920	.4922	.4925	.4927	.4929	.4931	.4932	.4934	.4936
2.5	.4938	.4940	.4941	.4943	.4945	.4946	.4948	.4949	.4951	.4952
2.6	.4953	.4955	.4956	.4957	.4959	.4960	.4961	.4962	.4963	.4964
2.7	.4965	.4966	.4967	.4968	.4969	.4970	.4971	.4972	.4973	.4974
2.8	.4974	.4975	.4976	.4977	.4977	.4978	.4979	.4979	.4980	.4981
2.9	.4981	.4982	.4982	.4983	.4984	.4984	.4985	.4985	.4986	.4986
3.0	.4987	.4987	.4987	.4988	.4988	.4989	.4989	.4989	.4990	.4990
3.1	.4990	.4991	.4991	.4991	.4992	.4992	.4992	.4992	.4993	.4993
3.2	.4993	.4993	.4994	.4994	.4994	.4994	.4994	.4995	.4995	.4995
3.3	.4995	.4995	.4995	.4996	.4996	.4996	.4996	.4996	.4996	4997
3.4	.4997	.4997	.4997	.4997	.4997	.4997	.4997	.4997	.4997	.4998
3.5	.4998	.4998	.4998	.4998	.4998	.4998	.4998	.4998	.4998	.4998
3.6	.4998	.4998	.4999	.4999	.4999	.4999	.4999	.4999	.4999	.4999
3.7	.4999	.4999	.4999	.4999	.4999	.4999	.4999	.4999	.4999	.4999
3.8	.4999	.4999	.4999	.4999	.4999	.4999	.4999	.4999	.4999	.4999
3.9	.49995	.49995	.49996	.49996	.49996	.49996	.49996	.49996	.49997	.49997
4.0	.49997									
4.5	.499997									
5.0	.4999997									

Student's *t* Distribution

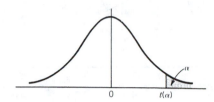

df	t(.005)	t(.01)	t(.025)	t(.05)	t(.10)	t(.25)
1	63.657	31.821	12.706	6.314	3.078	1.000
2	9.925	6.965	4.303	2.920	1.886	0.816
3	5.841	4.541	3.182	2.353	1.638	.765
4	4.604	3.747	2.776	2.132	1.533	.741
5	4.032	3.365	2.571	2.015	1.476	0.727
6	3.707	3.143	2.447	1.943	1.440	.718
7	3.499	2.998	2.365	1.895	1.415	.711
8	3.355	2.896	2.306	1.860	1.397	.706
9	3.250	2.821	2.262	1.833	1.383	.703
10	3.169	2.764	2.228	1.812	1.372	0.700
11	3.106	2.718	2.201	1.796	1.363	.697
12	3.055	2.681	2.179	1.782	1.356	.695
13	3.012	2.650	2.160	1.771	1.350	.694
14	2.977	2.624	2.145	1.761	1.345	.692
15	2.947	2.602	2.131	1.753	1.341	0.691
16	2.921	2.583	2.120	1.746	1.337	.690
17	2.898	2.567	2.110	1.740	1.333	.689
18	2.878	2.552	2.101	1.734	1.330	.688
19	2.861	2.539	2.093	1.729	1.328	.688
20	2.845	2.528	2.086	1.725	1.325	0.687
21	2.831	2.518	2.080	1.721	1.323	.686
22	2.819	2.508	2.074	1.717	1.321	.686
23	2.807	2.500	2.069	1.714	1.319	.685
24	2.797	2.492	2.064	1.711	1.318	.685
25	2.787	2.485	2.060	1.708	1.316	0.684
26	2.779	2.479	2.056	1.706	1.315	.684
27	2.771	2.473	2.052	1.703	1.314	.684
28	2.763	2.467	2.048	1.701	1.313	.683
29	2.756	2.462	2.045	1.699	1.311	.683
Large	2.576	2.326	1.960	1.645	1.282	.674

The Chi-Square Distribution

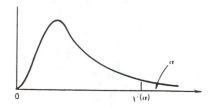

df	$\chi^2(.995)$	$\chi^2(.99)$	$\chi^2(.975)$	$\chi^2(.95)$	$\chi^2(.90)$	$\chi^2(.10)$	$\chi^2(.05)$	$\chi^2(.025)$	$\chi^2(.01)$	$\chi^2(.005)$
1	—	—	0.001	0.004	0.016	2.706	3.841	5.024	6.635	7.879
2	0.010	0.020	0.051	0.103	0.211	4.605	5.991	7.378	9.210	10.597
3	0.072	0.115	0.216	0.352	0.584	6.251	7.815	9.348	11.345	12.838
4	0.207	0.297	0.484	0.711	1.064	7.779	9.488	11.143	13.277	14.860
5	0.412	0.554	0.831	1.145	1.610	9.236	11.071	12.833	15.086	16.750
6	0.676	0.872	1.237	1.635	2.204	10.645	12.592	14.449	16.812	18.548
7	0.989	1.239	1.690	2.167	2.833	12.017	14.067	16.013	18.475	20.278
8	1.344	1.646	2.180	2.733	3.490	13.362	15.507	17.535	20.090	21.955
9	1.735	2.088	2.700	3.325	4.168	14.684	16.919	19.023	21.666	23.589
10	2.156	2.558	3.247	3.940	4.865	15.987	18.307	20.483	23.209	25.188
11	2.603	3.053	3.816	4.575	5.578	17.275	19.675	21.920	24.725	26.757
12	3.074	3.571	4.404	5.226	6.304	18.549	21.026	23.337	26.217	28.299
13	3.565	4.107	5.009	5.892	7.042	19.812	22.362	24.736	27.688	29.819
14	4.075	4.660	5.629	6.571	7.790	21.064	23.685	26.119	29.141	31.319
15	4.601	5.229	6.262	7.261	8.547	22.307	24.996	27.488	30.578	32.801
16	5.142	5.812	6.908	7.962	9.312	23.542	26.296	28.845	32.000	34.267
17	5.697	6.408	7.564	8.672	10.085	24.769	27.587	30.191	33.409	35.718
18	6.265	7.015	8.231	9.390	10.865	25.989	28.869	31.526	34.805	37.156
19	6.844	7.633	8.907	10.117	11.651	27.204	30.144	32.852	36.191	38.582
20	7.434	8.260	9.591	10.851	12.443	28.412	31.410	34.170	37.566	39.997
21	8.034	8.897	10.283	11.591	13.240	29.615	32.671	35.479	38.932	41.401
22	8.643	9.542	10.982	12.338	14.042	30.813	33.924	36.781	40.289	42.796
23	9.260	10.196	11.689	13.091	14.848	32.007	35.172	38.076	41.638	44.181
24	9.886	10.856	12.401	13.848	15.659	33.196	36.415	39.364	42.980	45.559
25	10.520	11.524	13.120	14.611	16.473	34.382	37.652	40.646	44.314	46.928
26	11.160	12.198	13.844	15.379	17.292	35.563	38.885	41.923	45.642	48.290
27	11.808	12.879	14.573	16.151	18.114	36.741	40.113	43.194	46.963	49.645
28	12.461	13.565	15.308	16.928	18.939	37.916	41.337	44.461	48.278	50.993
29	13.121	14.257	16.047	17.708	19.768	39.087	42.557	45.722	49.588	52.336
30	13.787	14.954	16.791	18.493	20.599	40.256	43.773	46.979	50.892	53.672
40	20.707	22.164	24.433	26.509	29.051	51.805	55.758	59.342	63.691	66.766
50	27.991	29.707	32.357	34.764	37.689	63.167	67.505	71.420	76.154	79.490
60	35.534	37.485	40.482	43.188	46.459	74.397	79.082	83.298	88.379	91.952
70	43.275	45.442	48.758	51.739	55.329	85.527	90.531	95.023	100.425	104.215
80	51.172	53.540	57.153	60.391	64.278	96.578	101.879	106.629	112.329	116.321
90	59.196	61.754	65.647	69.126	73.291	107.565	113.145	118.136	124.116	128.299
100	67.328	70.065	74.222	77.929	82.358	118.498	124.342	129.561	135.807	140.169

The F Distribution: Values of F (.05)

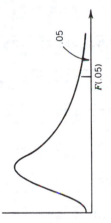

$F(.05)$

Degrees of freedom of the numerator

$df_2 \backslash df_1$	1	2	3	4	5	6	7	8	9	10	12	15	20	24	30	40	60	120	∞
1	161·4	199·5	215·7	224·6	230·2	234·0	236·8	238·9	240·5	241·9	243·9	245·9	248·0	249·1	250·1	251·1	252·2	253·3	254·3
2	18·51	19·00	19·16	19·25	19·30	19·33	19·35	19·37	19·38	19·40	19·41	19·43	19·45	19·45	19·46	19·47	19·48	19·49	19·50
3	10·13	9·55	9·28	9·12	9·01	8·94	8·89	8·85	8·81	8·79	8·74	8·70	8·66	8·64	8·62	8·59	8·57	8·55	8·53
4	7·71	6·94	6·59	6·39	6·26	6·16	6·09	6·04	6·00	5·96	5·91	5·86	5·80	5·77	5·75	5·72	5·69	5·66	5·63
5	6·61	5·79	5·41	5·19	5·05	4·95	4·88	4·82	4·77	4·74	4·68	4·62	4·56	4·53	4·50	4·46	4·43	4·40	4·36
6	5·99	5·14	4·76	4·53	4·39	4·28	4·21	4·15	4·10	4·06	4·00	3·94	3·87	3·84	3·81	3·77	3·74	3·70	3·67
7	5·59	4·74	4·35	4·12	3·97	3·87	3·79	3·73	3·68	3·64	3·57	3·51	3·44	3·41	3·38	3·34	3·30	3·27	3·23
8	5·32	4·46	4·07	3·84	3·69	3·58	3·50	3·44	3·39	3·35	3·28	3·22	3·15	3·12	3·08	3·04	3·01	2·97	2·93
9	5·12	4·26	3·86	3·63	3·48	3·37	3·29	3·23	3·18	3·14	3·07	3·01	2·94	2·90	2·86	2·83	2·79	2·75	2·71
10	4·96	4·10	3·71	3·48	3·33	3·22	3·14	3·07	3·02	2·98	2·91	2·85	2·77	2·74	2·70	2·66	2·62	2·58	2·54
11	4·84	3·98	3·59	3·36	3·20	3·09	3·01	2·95	2·90	2·85	2·79	2·72	2·65	2·61	2·57	2·53	2·49	2·45	2·40
12	4·75	3·89	3·49	3·26	3·11	3·00	2·91	2·85	2·80	2·75	2·69	2·62	2·54	2·51	2·47	2·43	2·38	2·34	2·30
13	4·67	3·81	3·41	3·18	3·03	2·92	2·83	2·77	2·71	2·67	2·60	2·53	2·46	2·42	2·38	2·34	2·30	2·25	2·21
14	4·60	3·74	3·34	3·11	2·96	2·85	2·76	2·70	2·65	2·60	2·53	2·46	2·39	2·35	2·31	2·27	2·22	2·18	2·13
15	4·54	3·68	3·29	3·06	2·90	2·79	2·71	2·64	2·59	2·54	2·48	2·40	2·33	2·29	2·25	2·20	2·16	2·11	2·07
16	4·49	3·63	3·24	3·01	2·85	2·74	2·66	2·59	2·54	2·49	2·42	2·35	2·28	2·24	2·19	2·15	2·11	2·06	2·01
17	4·45	3·59	3·20	2·96	2·81	2·70	2·61	2·55	2·49	2·45	2·38	2·31	2·23	2·19	2·15	2·10	2·06	2·01	1·96
18	4·41	3·55	3·16	2·93	2·77	2·66	2·58	2·51	2·46	2·41	2·34	2·27	2·19	2·15	2·11	2·06	2·02	1·97	1·92
19	4·38	3·52	3·13	2·90	2·74	2·63	2·54	2·48	2·42	2·38	2·31	2·23	2·16	2·11	2·07	2·03	1·98	1·93	1·88
20	4·35	3·49	3·10	2·87	2·71	2·60	2·51	2·45	2·39	2·35	2·28	2·20	2·12	2·08	2·04	1·99	1·95	1·90	1·84
21	4·32	3·47	3·07	2·84	2·68	2·57	2·49	2·42	2·37	2·32	2·25	2·18	2·10	2·05	2·01	1·96	1·92	1·87	1·81
22	4·30	3·44	3·05	2·82	2·66	2·55	2·46	2·40	2·34	2·30	2·23	2·15	2·07	2·03	1·98	1·94	1·89	1·84	1·78
23	4·28	3·42	3·03	2·80	2·64	2·53	2·44	2·37	2·32	2·27	2·20	2·13	2·05	2·01	1·96	1·91	1·86	1·81	1·76
24	4·26	3·40	3·01	2·78	2·62	2·51	2·42	2·36	2·30	2·25	2·18	2·11	2·03	1·98	1·94	1·89	1·84	1·79	1·73
25	4·24	3·39	2·99	2·76	2·60	2·49	2·40	2·34	2·28	2·24	2·16	2·09	2·01	1·96	1·92	1·87	1·82	1·77	1·71
26	4·23	3·37	2·98	2·74	2·59	2·47	2·39	2·32	2·27	2·22	2·15	2·07	1·99	1·95	1·90	1·85	1·80	1·75	1·69
27	4·21	3·35	2·96	2·73	2·57	2·46	2·37	2·31	2·25	2·20	2·13	2·06	1·97	1·93	1·88	1·84	1·79	1·73	1·67
28	4·20	3·34	2·95	2·71	2·56	2·45	2·36	2·29	2·24	2·19	2·12	2·04	1·96	1·91	1·87	1·82	1·77	1·71	1·65
29	4·18	3·33	2·93	2·70	2·55	2·43	2·35	2·28	2·22	2·18	2·10	2·03	1·94	1·90	1·85	1·81	1·75	1·70	1·64
30	4·17	3·32	2·92	2·69	2·53	2·42	2·33	2·27	2·21	2·16	2·09	2·01	1·93	1·89	1·84	1·79	1·74	1·68	1·62
40	4·08	3·23	2·84	2·61	2·45	2·34	2·25	2·18	2·12	2·08	2·00	1·92	1·84	1·79	1·74	1·69	1·64	1·58	1·51
60	4·00	3·15	2·76	2·53	2·37	2·25	2·17	2·10	2·04	1·99	1·92	1·84	1·75	1·70	1·65	1·59	1·53	1·47	1·39
120	3·92	3·07	2·68	2·45	2·29	2·17	2·09	2·02	1·96	1·91	1·83	1·75	1·66	1·61	1·55	1·50	1·43	1·35	1·25
∞	3·84	3·00	2·60	2·37	2·21	2·10	2·01	1·94	1·88	1·83	1·75	1·67	1·57	1·52	1·46	1·39	1·32	1·22	1·00

Degrees of freedom of the denominator

The F Distribution: Values of F (.025)

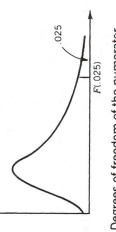

Degrees of freedom of the numerator

df_2 \ df_1	1	2	3	4	5	6	7	8	9	10	12	15	20	24	30	40	60	120	∞
1	647.8	799.5	864.2	899.6	921.8	937.1	948.2	956.7	963.3	968.6	976.7	984.9	993.1	997.2	1001	1006	1010	1014	1018
2	38.51	39.00	39.17	39.25	39.30	39.33	39.36	39.37	39.39	39.40	39.41	39.43	39.45	39.46	39.46	39.47	39.48	39.49	39.50
3	17.44	16.04	15.44	15.10	14.88	14.73	14.62	14.54	14.47	14.42	14.34	14.25	14.17	14.12	14.08	14.04	13.99	13.95	13.90
4	12.22	10.65	9.98	9.60	9.36	9.20	9.07	8.98	8.90	8.84	8.75	8.66	8.56	8.51	8.46	8.41	8.36	8.31	8.26
5	10.01	8.43	7.76	7.39	7.15	6.98	6.85	6.76	6.68	6.62	6.52	6.43	6.33	6.28	6.23	6.18	6.12	6.07	6.02
6	8.81	7.26	6.60	6.23	5.99	5.82	5.70	5.60	5.52	5.46	5.37	5.27	5.17	5.12	5.07	5.01	4.96	4.90	4.85
7	8.07	6.54	5.89	5.52	5.29	5.12	4.99	4.90	4.82	4.76	4.67	4.57	4.47	4.42	4.36	4.31	4.25	4.20	4.14
8	7.57	6.06	5.42	5.05	4.82	4.65	4.53	4.43	4.36	4.30	4.20	4.10	4.00	3.95	3.89	3.84	3.78	3.73	3.67
9	7.21	5.71	5.08	4.72	4.48	4.32	4.20	4.10	4.03	3.96	3.87	3.77	3.67	3.61	3.56	3.51	3.45	3.39	3.33
10	6.94	5.46	4.83	4.47	4.24	4.07	3.95	3.85	3.78	3.72	3.62	3.52	3.42	3.37	3.31	3.26	3.20	3.14	3.08
11	6.72	5.26	4.63	4.28	4.04	3.88	3.76	3.66	3.59	3.53	3.43	3.33	3.23	3.17	3.12	3.06	3.00	2.94	2.88
12	6.55	5.10	4.47	4.12	3.89	3.73	3.61	3.51	3.44	3.37	3.28	3.18	3.07	3.02	2.96	2.91	2.85	2.79	2.72
13	6.41	4.97	4.35	4.00	3.77	3.60	3.48	3.39	3.31	3.25	3.15	3.05	2.95	2.89	2.84	2.78	2.72	2.66	2.60
14	6.30	4.86	4.24	3.89	3.66	3.50	3.38	3.29	3.21	3.15	3.05	2.95	2.84	2.79	2.73	2.67	2.61	2.55	2.49
15	6.20	4.77	4.15	3.80	3.58	3.41	3.29	3.20	3.12	3.06	2.96	2.86	2.76	2.70	2.64	2.59	2.52	2.46	2.40
16	6.12	4.69	4.08	3.73	3.50	3.34	3.22	3.12	3.05	2.99	2.89	2.79	2.68	2.63	2.57	2.51	2.45	2.38	2.32
17	6.04	4.62	4.01	3.66	3.44	3.28	3.16	3.06	2.98	2.92	2.82	2.72	2.62	2.56	2.50	2.44	2.38	2.32	2.25
18	5.98	4.56	3.95	3.61	3.38	3.22	3.10	3.01	2.93	2.87	2.77	2.67	2.56	2.50	2.44	2.38	2.32	2.26	2.19
19	5.92	4.51	3.90	3.56	3.33	3.17	3.05	2.96	2.88	2.82	2.72	2.62	2.51	2.45	2.39	2.33	2.27	2.20	2.13
20	5.87	4.46	3.86	3.51	3.29	3.13	3.01	2.91	2.84	2.77	2.68	2.57	2.46	2.41	2.35	2.29	2.22	2.16	2.09
21	5.83	4.42	3.82	3.48	3.25	3.09	2.97	2.87	2.80	2.73	2.64	2.53	2.42	2.37	2.31	2.25	2.18	2.11	2.04
22	5.79	4.38	3.78	3.44	3.22	3.05	2.93	2.84	2.76	2.70	2.60	2.50	2.39	2.33	2.27	2.21	2.14	2.08	2.00
23	5.75	4.35	3.75	3.41	3.18	3.02	2.90	2.81	2.73	2.67	2.57	2.47	2.36	2.30	2.24	2.18	2.11	2.04	1.97
24	5.72	4.32	3.72	3.38	3.15	2.99	2.87	2.78	2.70	2.64	2.54	2.44	2.33	2.27	2.21	2.15	2.08	2.01	1.94
25	5.69	4.29	3.69	3.35	3.13	2.97	2.85	2.75	2.68	2.61	2.51	2.41	2.30	2.24	2.18	2.12	2.05	1.98	1.91
26	5.66	4.27	3.67	3.33	3.10	2.94	2.82	2.73	2.65	2.59	2.49	2.39	2.28	2.22	2.16	2.09	2.03	1.95	1.88
27	5.63	4.24	3.65	3.31	3.08	2.92	2.80	2.71	2.63	2.57	2.47	2.36	2.25	2.19	2.13	2.07	2.00	1.93	1.85
28	5.61	4.22	3.63	3.29	3.06	2.90	2.78	2.69	2.61	2.55	2.45	2.34	2.23	2.17	2.11	2.05	1.98	1.91	1.83
29	5.59	4.20	3.61	3.27	3.04	2.88	2.76	2.67	2.59	2.53	2.43	2.32	2.21	2.15	2.09	2.03	1.96	1.89	1.81
30	5.57	4.18	3.59	3.25	3.03	2.87	2.75	2.65	2.57	2.51	2.41	2.31	2.20	2.14	2.07	2.01	1.94	1.87	1.79
40	5.42	4.05	3.46	3.13	2.90	2.74	2.62	2.53	2.45	2.39	2.29	2.18	2.07	2.01	1.94	1.88	1.80	1.72	1.64
60	5.29	3.93	3.34	3.01	2.79	2.63	2.51	2.41	2.33	2.27	2.17	2.06	1.94	1.88	1.82	1.74	1.67	1.58	1.48
120	5.15	3.80	3.23	2.89	2.67	2.52	2.39	2.30	2.22	2.16	2.05	1.94	1.82	1.76	1.69	1.61	1.53	1.43	1.31
∞	5.02	3.69	3.12	2.79	2.57	2.41	2.29	2.19	2.11	2.05	1.94	1.83	1.71	1.64	1.57	1.48	1.39	1.27	1.00

Degrees of freedom of the denominator

The F distribution: Values of F (.01)

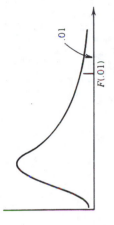

$F(.01)$

Degrees of freedom of the numerator

$df_2 \backslash df_1$	1	2	3	4	5	6	7	8	9	10	12	15	20	24	30	40	60	120	∞
1	4052	4999·5	5403	5625	5764	5859	5928	5981	6022	6056	6106	6157	6209	6235	6261	6287	6313	6339	6366
2	98·50	99·00	99·17	99·25	99·30	99·33	99·36	99·37	99·39	99·40	99·42	99·43	99·45	99·46	99·47	99·47	99·48	99·49	99·50
3	34·12	30·82	29·46	28·71	28·24	27·91	27·67	27·49	27·35	27·23	27·05	26·87	26·69	26·60	26·50	26·41	26·32	26·22	26·13
4	21·20	18·00	16·69	15·98	15·52	15·21	14·98	14·80	14·66	14·55	14·37	14·20	14·02	13·93	13·84	13·75	13·65	13·56	13·46
5	16·26	13·27	12·06	11·39	10·97	10·67	10·46	10·29	10·16	10·05	9·89	9·72	9·55	9·47	9·38	9·29	9·20	9·11	9·02
6	13·75	10·92	9·78	9·15	8·75	8·47	8·26	8·10	7·98	7·87	7·72	7·56	7·40	7·31	7·23	7·14	7·06	6·97	6·88
7	12·25	9·55	8·45	7·85	7·46	7·19	6·99	6·84	6·72	6·62	6·47	6·31	6·16	6·07	5·99	5·91	5·82	5·74	5·65
8	11·26	8·65	7·59	7·01	6·63	6·37	6·18	6·03	5·91	5·81	5·67	5·52	5·36	5·28	5·20	5·12	5·03	4·95	4·86
9	10·56	8·02	6·99	6·42	6·06	5·80	5·61	5·47	5·35	5·26	5·11	4·96	4·81	4·73	4·65	4·57	4·48	4·40	4·31
10	10·04	7·56	6·55	5·99	5·64	5·39	5·20	5·06	4·94	4·85	4·71	4·56	4·41	4·33	4·25	4·17	4·08	4·00	3·91
11	9·65	7·21	6·22	5·67	5·32	5·07	4·89	4·74	4·63	4·54	4·40	4·25	4·10	4·02	3·94	3·86	3·78	3·69	3·60
12	9·33	6·93	5·95	5·41	5·06	4·82	4·64	4·50	4·39	4·30	4·16	4·01	3·86	3·78	3·70	3·62	3·54	3·45	3·36
13	9·07	6·70	5·74	5·21	4·86	4·62	4·44	4·30	4·19	4·10	3·96	3·82	3·66	3·59	3·51	3·43	3·34	3·25	3·17
14	8·86	6·51	5·56	5·04	4·69	4·46	4·28	4·14	4·03	3·94	3·80	3·66	3·51	3·43	3·35	3·27	3·18	3·09	3·00
15	8·68	6·36	5·42	4·89	4·56	4·32	4·14	4·00	3·89	3·80	3·67	3·52	3·37	3·29	3·21	3·13	3·05	2·96	2·87
16	8·53	6·23	5·29	4·77	4·44	4·20	4·03	3·89	3·78	3·69	3·55	3·41	3·26	3·18	3·10	3·02	2·93	2·84	2·75
17	8·40	6·11	5·18	4·67	4·34	4·10	3·93	3·79	3·68	3·59	3·46	3·31	3·16	3·08	3·00	2·92	2·83	2·75	2·65
18	8·29	6·01	5·09	4·58	4·25	4·01	3·84	3·71	3·60	3·51	3·37	3·23	3·08	3·00	2·92	2·84	2·75	2·66	2·57
19	8·18	5·93	5·01	4·50	4·17	3·94	3·77	3·63	3·52	3·43	3·30	3·15	3·00	2·92	2·84	2·76	2·67	2·58	2·49
20	8·10	5·85	4·94	4·43	4·10	3·87	3·70	3·56	3·46	3·37	3·23	3·09	2·94	2·86	2·78	2·69	2·61	2·52	2·42
21	8·02	5·78	4·87	4·37	4·04	3·81	3·64	3·51	3·40	3·31	3·17	3·03	2·88	2·80	2·72	2·64	2·55	2·46	2·36
22	7·95	5·72	4·82	4·31	3·99	3·76	3·59	3·45	3·35	3·26	3·12	2·98	2·83	2·75	2·67	2·58	2·50	2·40	2·31
23	7·88	5·66	4·76	4·26	3·94	3·71	3·54	3·41	3·30	3·21	3·07	2·93	2·78	2·70	2·62	2·54	2·45	2·35	2·26
24	7·82	5·61	4·72	4·22	3·90	3·67	3·50	3·36	3·26	3·17	3·03	2·89	2·74	2·66	2·58	2·49	2·40	2·31	2·21
25	7·77	5·57	4·68	4·18	3·85	3·63	3·46	3·32	3·22	3·13	2·99	2·85	2·70	2·62	2·54	2·45	2·36	2·27	2·17
26	7·72	5·53	4·64	4·14	3·82	3·59	3·42	3·29	3·18	3·09	2·96	2·81	2·66	2·58	2·50	2·42	2·33	2·23	2·13
27	7·68	5·49	4·60	4·11	3·78	3·56	3·39	3·26	3·15	3·06	2·93	2·78	2·63	2·55	2·47	2·38	2·29	2·20	2·10
28	7·64	5·45	4·57	4·07	3·75	3·53	3·36	3·23	3·12	3·03	2·90	2·75	2·60	2·52	2·44	2·35	2·26	2·17	2·06
29	7·60	5·42	4·54	4·04	3·73	3·50	3·33	3·20	3·09	3·00	2·87	2·73	2·57	2·49	2·41	2·33	2·23	2·14	2·03
30	7·56	5·39	4·51	4·02	3·70	3·47	3·30	3·17	3·07	2·98	2·84	2·70	2·55	2·47	2·39	2·30	2·21	2·11	2·01
40	7·31	5·18	4·31	3·83	3·51	3·29	3·12	2·99	2·89	2·80	2·66	2·52	2·37	2·29	2·20	2·11	2·02	1·92	1·80
60	7·08	4·98	4·13	3·65	3·34	3·12	2·95	2·82	2·72	2·63	2·50	2·35	2·20	2·12	2·03	1·94	1·84	1·73	1·60
120	6·85	4·79	3·95	3·48	3·17	2·96	2·79	2·66	2·56	2·47	2·34	2·19	2·03	1·95	1·86	1·76	1·66	1·53	1·38
∞	6·63	4·61	3·78	3·32	3·02	2·80	2·64	2·51	2·41	2·32	2·18	2·04	1·88	1·79	1·70	1·59	1·47	1·32	1·00

Degrees of freedom of the denominator

Critical Values for the Wilcoxon Signed-Rank Test for n = 5 to 50

One-Sided	Two-Sided	n = 5	n = 6	n = 7	n = 8	n = 9	n = 10	n = 11	n = 12	n = 13	n = 14	n = 15	n = 16
α = .05	α = .10	1	2	4	6	8	11	14	17	21	26	30	36
α = .025	α = .05		1	2	4	6	8	11	14	17	21	25	30
α = .01	α = .02			0	2	3	5	7	10	13	16	20	24
α = .005	α = .01				0	2	3	5	7	10	13	16	19

One-Sided	Two-Sided	n = 17	n = 18	n = 19	n = 20	n = 21	n = 22	n = 23	n = 24	n = 25	n = 26	n = 27	n = 28
α = .05	α = .10	41	47	54	60	68	75	83	92	101	110	120	130
α = .025	α = .05	35	40	46	52	59	66	73	81	90	98	107	117
α = .01	α = .02	28	33	38	43	49	56	62	69	77	85	93	102
α = .005	α = .01	23	28	32	37	43	49	55	61	68	76	84	92

One-Sided	Two-Sided	n = 29	n = 30	n = 31	n = 32	n = 33	n = 34	n = 35	n = 36	n = 37	n = 38	n = 39
α = .05	α = .10	141	152	163	175	188	201	214	228	242	256	271
α = .025	α = .05	127	137	148	159	171	183	195	208	222	235	250
α = .01	α = .02	111	120	130	141	151	162	174	186	198	211	224
α = .005	α = .01	100	109	118	128	138	149	160	171	183	195	208

One-Sided	Two-Sided	n = 40	n = 41	n = 42	n = 43	n = 44	n = 45	n = 46	n = 47	n = 48	n = 49	n = 50
α = .05	α = .10	287	303	319	336	353	371	389	408	427	446	466
α = .025	α = .05	264	279	295	311	327	344	361	379	397	415	434
α = .01	α = .02	238	252	267	281	297	313	329	345	362	380	398
α = .005	α = .01	221	234	248	262	277	292	307	323	339	356	373

Critical Values for a Mann-Whitney Test.

Critical values for a one-tailed test at $\alpha = 0.01$ (roman type) and $\alpha = 0.005$ (boldface type) and for a two-tailed test at $\alpha = 0.02$ (roman type) and $\alpha = 0.01$ (boldface type).

n_2 \ n_1	1	2	3	4	5	6	7	8	9	10	11	12	13	14	15	16	17	18	19	20
1	—[b]	—	—	—	—	—	—	—	—	—	—	—	—	—	—	—	—	—	—	—
2	—	—	—	—	—	—	—	—	—	—	—	—	0	0	0	0	0	0	1	1
	—	—	—	—	—	—	—	—	—	—	—	—	—	—	—	—	—	—	0	0
3	—	—	—	—	—	—	0	0	1	1	1	2	2	2	3	3	4	4	4	5
	—	—	—	—	—	—	—	—	0	0	0	1	1	1	2	2	2	2	3	3
4	—	—	—	—	0	1	1	2	3	3	4	5	5	6	7	7	8	9	9	10
	—	—	—	—	—	0	0	1	1	2	2	3	3	4	5	5	6	6	7	8
5	—	—	—	0	1	2	3	4	5	6	7	8	9	10	11	12	13	14	15	16
	—	—	—	—	0	1	1	2	3	4	5	6	7	7	8	9	10	11	12	13
6	—	—	—	1	2	3	4	6	7	8	9	11	12	13	15	16	18	19	20	22
	—	—	—	0	1	2	3	4	5	6	7	9	10	11	12	13	15	16	17	18
7	—	—	0	1	3	4	6	7	9	11	12	14	16	17	19	21	23	24	26	28
	—	—	—	0	1	3	4	6	7	9	10	12	13	15	16	18	19	21	22	24
8	—	—	0	2	4	6	7	9	11	13	15	17	20	22	24	26	28	30	32	34
	—	—	—	1	2	4	6	7	9	11	13	15	17	18	20	22	24	26	28	30
9	—	—	1	3	5	7	9	11	14	16	18	21	23	26	28	31	33	36	38	40
	—	—	0	1	3	5	7	9	11	13	16	18	20	22	24	27	29	31	33	36
10	—	—	1	3	6	8	11	13	16	19	22	24	27	30	33	36	38	41	44	47
	—	—	0	2	4	6	9	11	13	16	18	21	24	26	29	31	34	37	39	42
11	—	—	1	4	7	9	12	15	18	22	25	28	31	34	37	41	44	47	50	53
	—	—	0	2	5	7	10	13	16	18	21	24	27	30	33	36	39	42	45	48
12	—	—	2	5	8	11	14	17	21	24	28	31	35	38	42	46	49	53	56	60
	—	—	1	3	6	9	12	15	18	21	24	27	31	34	37	41	44	47	51	54
13	—	0	2	5	9	12	16	20	23	27	31	35	39	43	47	51	55	59	63	67
	—	—	1	3	7	10	13	17	20	24	27	31	34	38	42	45	49	53	56	60
14	—	0	2	6	10	13	17	22	26	30	34	38	43	47	51	56	60	65	69	73
	—	—	1	4	7	11	15	18	22	26	30	34	38	42	46	50	54	58	63	67
15	—	0	3	7	11	15	19	24	28	33	37	42	47	51	56	61	66	70	75	80
	—	—	2	5	8	12	16	20	24	29	33	37	42	46	51	55	60	64	69	73
16	—	0	3	7	12	16	21	26	31	36	41	46	51	56	61	66	71	76	82	87
	—	—	2	5	9	13	18	22	27	31	36	41	45	50	55	60	65	70	74	79
17	—	0	4	8	13	18	23	28	33	38	44	49	55	60	66	71	77	82	88	93
	—	—	2	6	10	15	19	24	29	34	39	44	49	54	60	65	70	75	81	86
18	—	0	4	9	14	19	24	30	36	41	47	53	59	65	70	76	82	88	94	100
	—	—	2	6	11	16	21	26	31	37	42	47	53	58	64	70	75	81	87	92
19	—	1	4	9	15	20	26	32	38	44	50	56	63	69	75	82	88	94	101	107
	—	0	3	7	12	17	22	28	33	39	45	51	56	63	69	74	81	87	93	99
20	—	1	5	10	16	22	28	34	40	47	53	60	67	73	80	87	93	100	107	114
	—	0	3	8	13	18	24	30	36	42	48	54	60	67	73	79	86	92	99	105

Critical Values for a Mann-Whitney Test

Critical values for a one-tailed test at $\alpha = 0.05$ (roman type) and $\alpha = 0.025$ (boldface type) and for a two-tailed test at $\alpha = 0.10$ (roman type) and $\alpha = 0.05$ (boldface type).

n_2 \ n_1	1	2	3	4	5	6	7	8	9	10	11	12	13	14	15	16	17	18	19	20
1	—	—	—	—	—	—	—	—	—	—	—	—	—	—	—	—	—	—	0	0
	—	—	—	—	—	—	—	—	—	—	—	—	—	—	—	—	—	—	—	—
2	—	—	—	—	0	0	0	1	1	1	1	2	2	2	3	3	3	4	4	4
	—	—	—	—	—	—	—	0	0	0	0	1	1	1	1	1	2	2	2	2
3	—	—	0	0	1	2	2	3	3	4	5	5	6	7	7	8	9	9	10	11
	—	—	—	0	1	1	2	2	3	3	4	4	5	5	6	6	7	7	8	8
4	—	—	0	1	2	3	4	5	6	7	8	9	10	11	12	14	15	16	17	18
	—	—	—	0	1	2	3	4	4	5	6	7	8	9	10	11	11	12	13	13
5	—	0	1	2	4	5	6	8	9	11	12	13	15	16	18	19	20	22	23	25
	—	—	0	1	2	3	5	6	7	8	9	11	12	13	14	15	17	18	19	20
6	—	0	2	3	5	7	8	10	12	14	16	17	19	21	23	25	26	28	30	32
	—	—	1	2	3	5	6	8	10	11	13	14	16	17	19	21	22	24	25	27
7	—	0	2	4	6	8	11	13	15	17	19	21	24	26	28	30	33	35	37	39
	—	—	1	3	5	6	8	10	12	14	16	18	20	22	24	26	28	30	32	34
8	—	1	3	5	8	10	13	15	18	20	23	26	28	31	33	36	39	41	44	47
	—	0	2	4	6	8	10	13	15	17	19	22	24	26	29	31	34	36	38	41
9	—	1	3	6	9	12	15	18	21	24	27	30	33	36	39	42	45	48	51	54
	—	0	2	4	7	10	12	15	17	20	23	26	28	31	34	37	39	42	45	48
10	—	1	4	7	11	14	17	20	24	27	31	34	37	41	44	48	51	55	58	62
	—	0	3	5	8	11	14	17	20	23	26	29	33	36	39	42	45	48	52	55
11	—	1	5	8	12	16	19	23	27	31	34	38	42	46	50	54	57	61	65	69
	—	0	3	6	9	13	16	19	23	26	30	33	37	40	44	47	51	55	58	62
12	—	2	5	9	13	17	21	26	30	34	38	42	47	51	55	60	64	68	72	77
	—	1	4	7	11	14	18	22	26	29	33	37	41	45	49	53	57	61	65	69
13	—	2	6	10	15	19	24	28	33	37	42	47	51	56	61	65	70	75	80	84
	—	1	4	8	12	16	20	24	28	33	37	41	45	50	54	59	63	67	72	76
14	—	2	7	11	16	21	26	31	36	41	46	51	56	61	66	71	77	82	87	92
	—	1	5	9	13	17	22	26	31	36	40	45	50	55	59	64	67	74	78	83
15	—	3	7	12	18	23	28	33	39	44	50	55	61	66	72	77	83	88	94	100
	—	1	5	10	14	19	24	29	34	39	44	49	54	59	64	70	75	80	85	90
16	—	3	8	14	19	25	30	36	42	48	54	60	65	71	77	83	89	95	101	107
	—	1	6	11	15	21	26	31	37	42	47	53	59	64	70	75	81	86	92	98
17	—	3	9	15	20	26	33	39	45	51	57	64	70	77	83	89	96	102	109	115
	—	2	6	11	17	22	28	34	39	45	51	57	63	67	75	81	87	93	99	105
18	—	4	9	16	22	28	35	41	48	55	61	68	75	82	88	95	102	109	116	123
	—	2	7	12	18	24	30	36	42	48	55	61	67	74	80	86	93	99	106	112
19	0	4	10	17	23	30	37	44	51	58	65	72	80	87	94	101	109	116	123	130
	—	2	7	13	19	25	32	38	45	52	58	65	72	78	85	92	99	106	113	119
20	0	4	11	18	25	32	39	47	54	62	69	77	84	92	100	107	115	123	130	138
	—	2	8	13	20	27	34	41	48	55	62	69	76	83	90	98	105	112	119	127

Partial Listing of Scholastic and Professional Journals Relevant to the Field of Communication Disorders

A.A.C., Augmentative and Alternative Communication
A.S.H.A., Journal of the American Speech-Language-Hearing Association
Academic Therapy
Acta Oto-Laryngologica
Acta Sympolica
Alzheimer's Disease and Associated Disorders
American Annals of the Deaf
American Journal of Audiology
American Journal of Mental Deficiency
American Journal of Otolaryngology
American Journal of Otology
American Journal of Speech-Language Pathology
American Journal on Mental Retardation
Annals of Dyslexia
Annals of Neurology
Annals of Otology, Rhinology, and Laryngology
Aphasiology
Applied Linguistics
Applied Psycholinguistics
Archives of Otolaryngology
Archives of Otolaryngology—Head and Neck Surgery
Audecibel
Audiology; A journal of auditory communication
Auris, Nasus, Larynx
Australian Journal of Human Communication Disorders

Behavior Research and Therapy
Brain and Cognition
Brain and Language
Brain Injury
British Journal of Audiology
British Journal of Disorders of Communication

Child Language Teaching and Therapy
Cleft Palate Bulletin
Cleft Palate Journal
Cleft Palate—Craniofacial Journal
Clinical Linguistics & Phonetics

Clinics in Communication Disorders
Cognitive Neuropsychology
Cognitive Rehabilitation

D.S.H. Abstracts
Developmental Medicine & Child Neurology
Dysphagia

Ear and Hearing
European Journal of Disorders of Communication
Exceptional Children

Folia Phoniatrica
Folia Phoniatrica et Logopaedica

Health Communication
Hearing Journal
Hearing Rehabilitation Quarterly
Human Communication
Human Communication Canada

Index to Speech, Language, & Hearing Journal Titles, 1954–78
Intervention in School and Clinic

Journal of Computer Users in Speech and Hearing
Journal of Auditory Research
Journal of Autism and Developmental Disorders
Journal of Child Language
Journal of Childhood Communication Disorders
Journal of Cognitive Neuroscience
Journal of Cognitive Rehabilitation
Journal of Communication Disorders
Journal of Fluency Disorders
Journal of Head Trauma Rehabilitation
Journal of Learning Disabilities
Journal of Motor Behavior
Journal of Rehabilitation of the Deaf
Journal of Special Education
Journal of Speech and Hearing Research
Journal of the Academy of Rehabilitative Audiology
Journal of the Acoustical Society of America
Journal of the American Academy of Audiology
Journal of the American Audiology Society
Journal of the American Auditory Society
Journal of the American Deafness and Rehabilitation Association
Journal of Voice
Journal of Speech-Language Pathology and Audiology/Revue . . .

Language and Cognitive Processes
Language and Language Behavior Abstracts

Language Testing
Language, Speech and Hearing Services in Schools
Laryngoscope
Learning Disability Quarterly
Linguistics and Language Behavior Abstracts

Memory & Cognition
Mind & Language

Newsounds

Otolaryngology—Head and Neck Surgery

Perspectives in Education and Deafness
Perspectives on Dyslexia
Phonetica

R.A.S.E. Remedial and Special Education
Reading and Writing
Rehabilitation Literature
Remedial and Special Education

Seminars in Hearing
Seminars in Speech and Language
Sign Language Studies
Specific Learning Disabilities Gazette

Topics in Early Childhood Special Education
Topics in Language Disorders

Volta Review
Volta Voices

APPENDIX E.
ASHA Handbook of Presenter Information[1]

....

DEAR ASHA PRESENTER,

This manual has been prepared to help you develop and deliver a successful presentation at the ASHA Annual Convention and other educational programs. We hope the following information helps you to provide a positive, practical educational experience for program participants. We understand that some of the following information will seem elementary to the accomplished presenter. We have compiled this handbook with speakers of all levels of experience in mind. If you have any questions about the information listed in this handbook, please call us anytime.

Convention and Meetings Division
American Speech-Language-Hearing Association
10801 Rockville Pike
Rockville, MD 20852
301-897-5700

---

[1]Reproduced with permission. American Speech-Language-Hearing Association, Rockville, Maryland.

GENERAL PRESENTER INFORMATION

1. **Schedule**

   It is very important that all sessions keep to the schedule, so be sure to begin and end your sessions on time. Take the first few minutes to outline your objectives for the session. Don't forget to allow time for audience participation and questions and answers.

2. **Room Set-up and Audiovisual Equipment**

   At the beginning of each day, ASHA staff will be checking each meeting room to ensure proper set-up and audiovisual equipment. Rooms are set for the entire day, so there may be equipment there that you did not request. Feel free to use any equipment that is already set up. AV technicians are available if you are unsure how to use a piece of equipment. If a piece of equipment you requested is not there, please let the AV technicians or ASHA staff know. A speaker-ready room will be available in every building where program sessions are being held. Each ready room will have a slide previewer available and additional equipment to help you prepare for your session. Locations will be announced. There will also be an AV office in each building for any questions you may have.

   All rooms will be equipped with an overhead, 35mm slide projector, and one microphone. Any additional equipment was to have been requested on the original program submission. Additional equipment cannot be requested on site.

3. **Session Evaluations**

   Session evaluations will be placed in every room before each session to allow attendees to provide feedback. Please remind attendees to complete an evaluation and turn it in directly to you at the end of the session. These are for your information and do not need to be turned in to ASHA.

4. **Handouts**

   ASHA encourages the use of handout materials for your session. If you wish to provide handouts, please bring 200 copies with you. A business center will be available on site if you need more copies. Short Course and Institute presenters will receive additional information regarding handouts prior to the Convention.

5. **CEU Information**

   On the podium in each room, there will be a card which lists continuing education verification codes (attendance codes). **Please announce the code which corresponds to your session AT THE END OF THE SESSION.** Attendees may not get credit for the course if the attendance code is not read.

   If you are teaching an **Institute or Short Course,** please remind participants that there is a separate CEU form for these courses, and they must turn their continuing education participant form in AT THE END OF THE SESSION.

   If you are teaching a **Seminar** of any length, remind participants to record their attendance on their Seminar CEU form and turn that form in before they leave the Convention.

6. **Audiotaping**

   ASHA plans to audiotape most of the presentations at the Convention. Please let us know as soon as possible if you do not wish to have your session audiotaped.

   If your session is taped, you are entitled to one free copy. Please pick it up at the on-site cassette sales booth.

7. **Presenter Recognition**

   ASHA appreciates your contribution to the success of the Convention. We will gladly send a letter to your employer advising them of your contribution. Please complete the speaker recognition form in the back of this pamphlet. Letters will be mailed following the Convention.

PLANNING AND PREPARATION

The following guidelines should help you plan a solid, well-structured presentation:

- Find out how much time you have to speak and plan your presentation accordingly.
- Be sure your presentation covers what your abstract or the brochure describes so that attendees' expectations are met.
- Find out who the audience is and determine what you want them to know. Remember that the average attendee has 5–10 years of experience.
- State your objectives in the beginning of your presentation and prepare concluding points for the end, before questions and discussion.
- Put yourself in the participant's place. Project enthusiasm and interest in your topic.
- Try to relax. Most people are nervous presenting before a group. Focusing on a responsive person in the audience helps you connect with the audience. Remember, the audience wants to hear what you have to say.
- Effective learning is a partnership. Reinforce this by interacting with your audience. Ask questions and invite comments.

INVOLVING THE AUDIENCE

One of the most frequent criticisms of educational programs is that they are conducted in a passive format; the speaker imparts knowledge while the audience listens impassively. Here are some ways to keep the audience involved and interested:

- **Ask for their questions.** All session types include time for questions and answers. Be prepared! Before your presentation, think about what questions could be asked; formulate brief, clear answers to each and rehearse those answers. Develop some questions of your own to ask the audience if the question and answer period begins slowly. Throughout your presentation, ask questions of the group, if only for them to answer in their mind.

  During your presentation, answer questions to clarify ambiguities immediately. Postpone questions related to resolving a specific problem to the end of the session. If someone asks a question that you can't answer, don't panic! You have several options:

  - Say that you will locate the answer and get back to him or her.
  - Suggest appropriate resources that will provide the answer.
  - Ask for suggestions from other members of the audience.

- **Have attendees work** with a partner or a small group to discuss scenarios, problems, or to share experiences, and use case studies, group discussions, role playing, etc. to keep your presentation moving.
- **Ask the attendees** how they plan to apply your information.
- **Use samples** (if applicable), quizzes, strategic plans or other hands-on documentation for the audience to work with during the session.

SPEAKING SKILLS

Here are some tips to help you feel more relaxed, organized, and confident:

Organize your materials in the way that is most comfortable to you: script, outline, 3″ x 5″ cards, pictures, etc.

Rehearse! This helps to work the bugs out of your presentation and add polish and smoothness. Note: a rehearsal usually runs about 20% shorter than the final presentation. Plan ahead!

Concentrate on deep breathing and relaxing.

Make your opening simple and exciting. Be able to explain your topic or theme in one or two sentences that are free of professional jargon.

Try to maintain a natural pace. Use natural gestures and voice inflection to add interest to your presentation. Much of communication is nonverbal, so how you look, sound, and come across is very important. Project enthusiasm for your subject without preaching.

Talk to your audience, not at them. Use eye contact often, ideally 90% of the time. Do not read your speech or presentation! Speak clearly, and speak directly into the microphone.

Speak in short and simple sentences. Choose your major points carefully and reinforce each point with examples or stories from your experience.

Never apologize for yourself or your credentials. Do not criticize anything about the session, city, or the setting. Never indicate that you don't have enough time to cover a point you've made, even if you don't. The audience is immediately disappointed.

Your conclusion must be memorable.

Don't run over your time limit.

Incorporate the traits that attract and hold your attention when you see a favorite speaker or presenter.

Arrive early. Get comfortable, find the lights, check the AV and the room setup. Preparation and open communication are the keys to a successful presentation.

ABOUT YOUR AUDIENCE: ADULT LEARNERS

"What's in it for me?"

Adult learners are different from other types of audiences. They bring a wealth of experience to the session and have highly tangible reasons for attending a certain presentation:

- Hot topic
- Continuing Education credits
- Networking opportunity
- Upgrade their skills
- Need information
- Reputation of sponsor/speaker

Adult learners are goal-oriented and less flexible than other learners. They want a speaker to "provide activities, guidance, and materials that facilitate learning." They are more interested in a performance-based model of education, where the emphasis is on:

- Learning
- Processing information
- Applying new knowledge

The delivery/instructional method is as/more important than the quality of the information. Audiences want to get involved in the learning process. Adults want:

- Active involvement in the learning process
- To practice what they are learning
- A physical and emotional atmosphere conducive to learning
- To use their experience to reinforce and give meaning to learning
- To focus on problems and how to solve them; this puts learning in context

Chinese Proverb—
  Tell me, *I'll forget*
  Show me, *I may remember*
  But involve me, *and I'll understand*

PROGRAM DEVELOPMENT

6 Steps to Develop a Quality Presentation:

- **Assess Need**
  What's the problem/issue I want to address?
- **Analyze Audience**
  Who will come? What needs do they have to be filled? How can I best fulfill their needs in regard to this issue?
- **Learning Outcomes**
  What are the three things I want listeners to go away with? i.e., "Participants will learn . . . 1, 2, 3."
- **Content and Methods**
  What type of information is most needed by the audience? Research data? Hands-on experience? Case Studies?
  What method should I use to impart this information to the audience? Small group interaction? Problem-solving sessions?
- **Program Delivery**
  Am I prepared?
- **Evaluate Program**
  How did I do?

PUTTING TOGETHER A SUCCESSFUL PRESENTATION

Because the learning needs of participants vary, it is very importnt to provide a variety of instructional methods throughout the session. The outline of teaching approaches below gives an introduction to strategies you might use in presenting.

Presentation Methods

- Lecture
- Panel
- Case study
- Films/videotape/slides

Audience Participation/Discussion Methods

- Question/answer periods
- Guided large group discussions
- Small group activity
- Simulation methods
- Role playing/interview
- Simulation exercises

Audiovisual Materials

Carefully selected and prepared AV materials can be an integral part of any presentation. They offer variation for different learning styles and keep the audience stimulated. Be sure to preview the tapes, set up the AV equipment, move the film or tape to the starting point, and be ready to troubleshoot or move into another form of presenting the material if the machines malfunction.

People generally remember 20% of what they hear, 30% of what they see, and 50% of what they both see and hear. Use audiovisual materials to reinforce the major themes of your presentation.

SPECIAL INSTRUCTIONS FOR POSTER SESSION PRESENTERS

Poster sessions present a special challenge to the presenter and a more personal educational experience for the attendee. Some tips to work with:

Make your poster simple but visually stimulating. Stick to a limited number of main points on the poster. You can elaborate on these points on an individual basis. Make any pictures, charts or graphs large enough to be seen from a distance of 5–10 feet.

Handouts are an excellent complement to a poster session. Summarize your main points or conclusions on a brief handout. You may also wish to add additional references and information on how to reach you for more information. We suggest you bring 250 handouts, but you may need more depending on the popularity of your subject.

Be prepared with a general outline of your findings or objectives; anticipate questions and prepare answers; and involve your audience by asking them questions (Have you experienced this? What did you do?).

Poster sessions offer a unique opportunity to get to know the people you are presenting to. Be ready with a greeting to each person who approaches the board. Handle each attendee on an individual basis. Get to know them and have fun.

SPEAKER RECOGNITION FORM

Yes, I would like a letter written to my supervisor regarding my participation in the ASHA Annual Convention

_____

Presenter Name

_____

Presentation Title

_____

Type of Session

If you are presenting multiple sessions, additional presentation titles can be attached on a separate sheet.

Person to whom letter should be mailed:

_____

Name

_____

Affiliation

_____

Address

_____

City   State   Zip

Glossary

....

A-B design: The most basic of the Small-N (time series) designs in which observations are made over a period of time to establish a "baseline" (A) for the subsequent comparison of retest data. Next, a treatment (B) is introduced (independent variable), and changes in the dependent variable are noted.

A-B-A design: A type of Small-N design in which a baseline condition is first established, followed by a treatment condition, and, finally, by the withdrawal of the treatment condition (a return to baseline).

A-B-A-B (reversal): The most commonly used of the Small-N designs. First, a baseline phase is established. Second, treatment is introduced. Third, treatment is withdrawn. Fourth, treatment is introduced once again to assess its reliability. A variation of this design involves substituting an independent variable in the final B condition that is different from the first B condition.

Anabolic thinking: A critical thinking process that involves building up or assembling complex structures from more elementary components(i.e., crafting a research plan or proposal based on the separate elements of previous research).

Abscissa: The horizontal axis of a graph.

Abstract: A concise summary of the research problem investigated, the methods used, the highlights of the results, and their statistical significance.

Alternating treatment design: Two treatments, A and B, are alternated randomly as they are applied to a single subject. The results are examined to determine whether one of the treatments is more effective than the other treatment.

Analysis of covariance (ANCOVA): One of the parametric ANOVA designs that allows for the statistical adjustment of data values of a dependent variable in accord with known quantities of one or more unwanted variables that the investigator might wish to control.

Analysis of variance (ANOVA): A method for analyzing population variances of two or more groups in order to make inferences about the population.

ANOVAR designs: Designs that entail the comparison of two or more groups and the use of ANOVA statistical techniques.

Applied behavior analysis: An approach that emphasizes manipulating and measuring aspects of the observable behavior of individual subjects as opposed to groups of subjects.

A posteriori conclusion: A conclusion drawn from inductive reasoning based on actual facts or research outcomes.

A priori conclusion: A conclusion drawn from deductive reasoning based on prior beliefs or expectations.

Bartlett test: Frequently used to determine whether the assumption of *homogeneity of variance among groups* is met, thereby allowing for the use of any parametric ANOVA.

Baseline: The measured rate of responding prior to introducing an intervention or treatment.

Bayes' method (rule): A mathematical basis for determining the degree to which a prior belief corresponds with the actual facts of subsequent observations. Statistically, a formula for computing the conditional probability of one event $P(A|B)$ from the conditional probability of another event, $P(B|A)$.

Bernouli theorem: A theorem that states that the relative frequency of an observed event will approximate its probable frequency of future occurrence if observed over an indefinitely long series of trials.

Between-groups variance: The amount of variation between means owing to a systematic treatment effect. Also known as "systematic experimental variance."

Bimodal: A distribution that has two modes.

Biomedical computer programs P-series (BMDP): An advanced statistical software package that is especially suitable for many medical and biological applications.

Bivariate relationship: The relationship between two variables.

Bonferroni t procedure: A method for making a priori pairwise comparisons of group means; used in cases in which the researcher wishes to increase the power of the test. Also called the Dunn multiple comparison procedure.

Catabolic thinking: A type of critical thinking process in which the various parts of a complex problems or structure, such as a research article, are broken down for the evaluation of each component.

Causal explanation: Explanation for the observed relations among events based on the presumption that one is the cause (antecedent event) and the other is the effect (consequent event).

Central limit theorem: In general, this theorem states that sample means tend to be normally distributed, provided that the size of the sample is sufficiently large.

Central tendency: Measures that reflect the average size of a frequency distribution such as the mean, median, or mode.

Changing-criterion design: A variation of the Small-N designs. First, a series of behavioral criteria are established. A treatment is then introduced and its effectiveness is judged based on the extent to which the response level of a target behavior matches the preset criteria.

Chebyshev's theorem: States that, for any data set, at least $100 \cdot (1-(1/k)^2)\%$ of all data values are lying within k standard deviations of the mean, where $k > 1$.

Chi-square test (χ^2 test): Used for evaluating hypotheses about the relationship between nominal variables having two or more independent categories.

Cluster sampling: A multistage sampling procedure in which smaller samples are selected from larger units or clusters. Often used to assure balanced geographical representation.

Coefficient of variation: The ratio of the mean to the standard deviation.

Conditional probability: The probability of one event occurring given that another event has already occurred.

Confidence interval testing: The statistical means of estimating (with confidence) the interval that contains the population parameter.

Confounding effect: The consequence of an extraneous variable that produces an unwanted influence on the dependent variable.

Constructs: Concepts refined to a degree as to serve as premises for theories.

Construct validity: The degree to which a particular test or measuring instrument actually measures the theoretical construct under investigation.

Content validity: The extent to which a particular test or measurement is judged to be representative of the behavior or skills it is designed to assess.

Contingency table: A two-dimensional table used to illustrate the frequencies of responses for two or more nominal or quantitative variables in various combinations.

Continuous variables: Observations that can potentially take on any value including fractional units of measurement along some line segment or interval.

Control group: The group of subjects to whom the independent variable is not assigned or applied.

Controlled experimental studies: Designs that entail the active and systematic manipulation of one or more independent variables.

Correlation: The statistical method that describes the relationship between two or more variables.

Correlation coefficient (r): A measure used to denote a range of relations among variables in which $+1$ expresses a perfect positive correlation and -1 expresses a perfect negative correlation.

Correlated variable: When the measure of one variable changes with or predicts the measure of a second variable, the variables are said to be *correlated*.

Counterbalancing: A method that controls for the effects of one condition preceding another by "balancing" the order in which they are administered to subjects so that each subject is exposed to each condition an equal number of times.

Covariance: The degree to which two or more variables vary together.

Criterion variable: The performance variable (Y) that is estimated from another *predictor variable* (X). Also called the outcome or dependent variable.

Crossover design: An experimental design in which each group of subjects receives both a control and an experimental treatment. This is accomplished by alternating the sequence of treatments administered.

Cross tabulation: A means of examining the relationships among two or more variables by organizing their frequency distributions into two or more categories, as portrayed in a contingency table.

Cross-validation: A technique commonly used in conjunction with regression analysis to determine how well a data set obtained from one sample of subjects can be generalized to another set of subjects.

Data probability: An intermediate mathematical probability of new sample data prior to deriving a posterior probability.

Data set: A well-defined aggregate of characteristics that serve to categorize or classify experience.

Deductive reasoning: A logical thought process that begins with a general premise or law presumed to be true that is then used to explain a specific observation.

Degrees of freedom: The number of scores in a distribution that are allowed to vary (remain free). In a single sample, this index number is expressed as the number of scores minus one; denoted by $n-1$.

Dependent events: Those events whose probability is influenced by the occurrence of other events.

Dependent variable: The consequence or effect caused by assigning or manipulating the independent variable.

Descriptive question: A question that asks about the objective or empirical features of objects or events without regard to their interrelationship.

Descriptive statistics: Measures, such as percentages, averages, and standard deviations, used to summarize, condense, and organize data into a more convenient and interpretable form.

Descriptive studies: Studies designed to observe, illustrate, record, classify, or by other means make clear the distinctive features of research variables.

Deviation: The difference between each data value in a distribution and the mean.

Dichotomous variables: Variables that only have two outcomes, i.e., male/female, yes/no, normal/abnormal etc.

Difference question: A question that entails comparison of between-group differences in a search for causal explanations.

Discrete variables: Values of observations that can potentially assume or constitute a sequence of isolated or separated points along a number line represented by integers.

Discriminant analysis: A statistical method for determining which dependent variables among a set of such variables are most responsible for discriminating among groups.

Distribution-free statistics: Distributions that are free of assumptions about the shape of the underlying population distribution and that employ nonparametric tests.

Effect size: An index of the magnitude of the effect of the independent variable; the degree to which the phenomenon of interest exists in the population.

Empirical doctrine: A doctrine that nothing can be said to exist until it is actually observed to exist to some degree.

Event: A collection of several possible outcomes from a sample space, i.e., an event is a subset of the sample space.

Expected frequency: The probability estimate (or theoretical frequency) for a cell of a contingency table.

Experimental analysis of behavior: See *applied behavioral analysis*.

Experimental group: The group of subjects to whom the independent variable is applied.

Experimenter effects: Also known as the Rosenthal effect. Conscious or unconscious bias held by an experimenter that can influence the outcome of a study.

Ex post facto studies: Studies that lack purposeful experimental manipulation of an independent variable and that search for past causes of an observed phenomenon.

External validity: The degree to which the results of a study can be generalized to a population from which a sample was drawn.

F distribution: A distribution that can be used to test the equality of two or more population variances.

Factor analysis: A statistical method for organizing data so that existing relationships among numerous variables can be more readily identified and comprehended. This is accomplished by reducing a large number of observations into a small number of key indicators of underlying constructs.

Factor loadings: The final step of factor analysis used to determine the degree to which the measure correlates with a certain factor.

Factors: Measures that are found to be correlated.

False negative: A negative test result when the person actually has the disorder or disease in question.

False positive: A positive test result when the person actually does not have the disorder or disease in question.

Freidman two-way analysis of variance by ranks: A nonparametric test especially useful for randomized block designs in which a block consists of three or more repeated measures obtained from the same subject.

"Frequentist" definition of probability: The expected frequency of an event in a long run(i.e., in a very long series of repeated trials under highly similar conditions).

Goodness-of-fit: A type of chi-square test that evaluates the extent to which a set of observations follows a theoretical distribution of some kind.

Hawthorne effect: Changes in performance in subjects' performance when they believe that they have attracted the attention of significant others or have been "singled out" for observation.

Homogeneity (homoscedasticity): A statistical assumption that the standard deviation of the dependent variable within two or more groups is the same regardless of the level of the independent variable administered, i.e., the two populations are assumed to have equal variances. The validity of this assumption is important in the use of ANOVA and multiple regression techniques.

Hypothesis testing: The scientific means of investigating problems under controlled, empirical conditions. Statistically, this entails determining whether a probability estimate of a population parameter is justifiable based on the research findings.

Independent events: The occurrence of one event has no effect on the probability of the occurrence of the other event.

Independent variable: A variable that is manipulated or assigned to determine its influence on the dependent variable. Also known as the antecedent condition or cause.

Inductive gap: The gap between current knowledge based on previous studies and the predicted outcomes of future experiments.

Inductive reasoning: A logical thought process wherein a general theory or set of laws are derived from specific observations or individual cases.

Inferential statistics: A type of statistics that allow an investigator to generalize results from a particular sample to the population from which the sample was drawn.

Institutional review board (IRB): A group of diverse individuals charged with reviewing research proposals of investigators and their compliance with regulations for protecting the rights of human and animal subjects.

Interaction effect: The joint effect of two independent variables(e.g., how the two treatments combine or interact to influence certain outcomes).

Intercorrelations: A list that shows the results of correlating each test item with all other test items.

Interobserver reliability: The consistency of judgments between two or more observers based on measurements or ratings made at the same point in time.

Interval probability estimate: A range of values within which the true probability for a particular event is likely to fall.

Interval scale: A scale that possesses the properties of a nominal and an ordinal scale. In addition, data values are distributed at equal intervals along a continuous number line, but the line contains no meaningful zero.

Internal validity: The degree to which the results of a research study are directly attributable to the influence of an independent variable as opposed to some unwanted or extraneous influence.

Intraobserver reliability: The consistency of judgments within the same observer, based on measurements or ratings made at different points in time.

Joint distribution: A distribution that describes how two variables are related to one another.

Joint probability: The probability that two or more events will occur simultaneously or in succession.

kappa (κ) formula: A statistical method for determining the interobserver or intraobserver agreement for nominal measures.

Kruskal-Wallis one-way analysis of variance by ranks (KWANOVA): A nonparametric version of the one-way ANOVA and an extension of the Mann-Whitney U test; it is useful for deciding whether the distribution of scores in the populations underlying each group are identical. Like other nonparametric tests, ranks are substituted in order to represent the dependent variable.

Latin square: A repeated measures design in which the presentation of conditions is counterbalanced so that each occurs in each sequential position of a block.

e.g., ABCD
BDAC
CADB
DCBA

The number of sequences should equal the number of conditions, and each condition should both precede and follow each of the other conditions.

Linear regression: A statistical method that predicts the best estimated value of a dependent variable from an independent variable when a linear relationship between two variables exists.

Linear relationship: A relationship between two variables that can be depicted by a straight line drawn through a number of given points when a scatterplot of the two variables is constructed.

Mann-Whitney U test: A highly useful nonparametric test analog of the unpaired t-test for two independent samples concerned with the equality of medians rather than means.

Matched random assignment: A sampling technique that combines matching and random assignment of subjects to groups.

Matched samples: Samples achieved by restricting the degree to which subjects in different groups are allowed to differ by pairing them according to particular qualitative or quantitative characteristics.

Meta-analysis: Statistical methods that allow for the analysis and summary of the results of two or more independent experiments.

Metamorphism: The notion that complex mental structures or symbolic representations, existing a priori in the mind of an artist or scientist, can lead to subsequent creations or new discoveries.

Method of association: The method that merely describes the relationship (correlation) among two or more events without reference to causation.

Method of constant stimuli: The method that requires that several comparison stimuli be randomly paired with a fixed standard.

Method of difference: Two effects are typically examined: one of these effects is examined when preceded by the presumed cause, and the other is examined when the presumed cause is absent.

MINITAB: A statistical software package appropriate for an introduction to computerized statistical analysis techniques. Data values can be stored and displayed in columns and rows like a spreadsheet.

Multigroup designs: Three or more groups are used to examine different treatment effects resulting from alternative independent variables or from different levels of the same independent variable.

Multiple baseline designs: Small-N designs that involve the application of a treatment to different baselines at different times. Appropriate for the analysis of a treatment influence across different subjects, behaviors, or settings.

Multiple regression: Regression techniques for determining the relationship between one dependent variable and two or more independent variables (i.e., Y is predicted from X_1, $X_2 \ldots$, etc).

Multiplication rule: A formula for calculating the probability of the joint or successive occurrence of two or more events based on more than one observation.

Multivariate analysis of variance (MANOVA): A statistical technique designed for problems in which there is more than one dependent variable under investigation.

Multivariate relationship: The relationship between more than two variables.

Mutually exclusive events: Events that cannot occur together in the context of the same experiment.

Negatively skewed: A distribution in which the tail points to the left (negative) side of the curve, signifying that the proportion of high scores in the distribution is greater than for low scores.

Nominal scale: A scale of measurement in which data can only be named or counted and in which numbers are used solely for purposes of classification or labeling.

Nonequivalent comparison group design: Entails the use of at least two nonrandom comparison groups, both of whom are pretested prior to treatment. Subsequently, the groups are posttested to examine between-group differences.

Nonexperimental research: Research in which no attempt is made to achieve randomization in subject assignment to conditions, nor is there an effort to manipulate the variables under study.

Nonparametric statistics: Statistical methods that do not depend on a knowledge of the population distribution or its parameters. Such techniques are well suited for situations in which the population distributions are skewed or unknown, especially when the sample size is small.

Nonrandom sampling: Sampling techniques in which the probability for subject selection is unknown.

Nonsignificant difference: A statistical finding that should be interpreted to mean "not yet proved" or "inconclusive."

Null hypothesis (H_0): A statement of statistical equality (no significant relationship between two or more variables).

Objective language: Communicates an observation according to the empirical attributes of the phenomenon observed.

Observed frequency: The actual counts recorded in one cell of a contingency table.

One-group pretest posttest design: This pre-experimental design allows for the comparison of pretest and posttest data subsequent to treatment. However, because no control group is used, there is inadequate control for internal and external validity.

One-shot case study: The weakest of the pre-experimental designs. The presumed effect of some treatment is evaluated ex post facto. No pretest is given, nor is a control group used to control for sources of internal invalidity. Also called the one-group posttest design.

One-way ANOVA: The simplest of the ANOVA designs, involving the analysis of a single factor.

Operant: A class of behavior whose acquisition and rate of emission is dependent on its consequences (reinforcing stimuli).

Operant level: See *baseline*.

Operationism: A doctrine that emphasizes the importance of defining the quantitative meaning of theoretical terms in accordance with specified measurements or observations.

Ordinal scale: Possesses the properties of a nominal scale. In addition, data can be arranged in order or ranked, but quantitative differences between data values (i.e., how much larger or smaller one value is than another) cannot be determined.

Ordinate: The vertical axis of a graph.

Organismic variable: Relatively stable physical or psychological characteristics that are not subject to active experimental manipulation (e.g., age, sex, gender, height, weight, intelligence, etc.).

P-value: The actual probability that a test statistic in a hypothesis test is at least as extreme as the value obtained.

Pairing design: A study that involves dependent, correlated, or related samples.

Paradigm shift: A notable change in a mode of thinking or model for doing things.

Parameter: A number or quantity used to describe characteristics of a population.

Parametric statistic: Statistical methods that depend on a knowledge of the population distribution.

Pearson product-moment correlation (r): Computes a parametric correlation coefficient, reflecting the association between two variables measured on a continuous scale.

Phenomena: The observable characteristics of objects and events.

Pie chart: A graphical method for representing the proportion of a data set following into certain categories in the form of a circle containing wedges.

Pilot investigation: A preliminary study useful in planning and rehearsing the steps involved in a more extensive research project.

Planned (a priori) comparisons: Methods that allow for the analysis of a limited number of pairwise comparisons of means prior to performing ANOVA.

Population: All of the subjects within a well-defined group to whom the research findings are applied. An all-inclusive data set about which a conclusion or causal inference is drawn.

Positively skewed: A distribution in which the tail points to the right (positive) side of the curve, signifying that the proportion of low scores in the distribution is greater than for high scores.

Posterior probability: The conditional probability calculated by using Bayes' rule. It represents the predictive value of a positive test or a negative test.

Post hoc comparisons: Statistical methods for comparing means after performing ANOVA. See Scheffé's method and Tukey's method.

Posttest-only control group design: The most basic version of the true experimental designs. Given the assumption that randomization has effectively balanced extraneous between-group differences, only a posttest is given following treatment to avoid the potential sensitizing influence of a pretest on performance.

Power of the test: The probability of rejecting a false null hypothesis, i.e., the probability of reaching a correct decision. It is calculated as "1-(type II error)" or symbolically, $1-\beta$.

Practice effect: The facilitative influence of previous testing on performance measures, resulting from familiarity, experience, or learning.

Predictive studies: Studies that seek to describe the degree to which one variable is predictive of another variable.

Predictive validity: The degree to which a particular measure or procedure is able to accurately predict some other variable or performance outcome.

Predictive value negative (PV⁻): The probability that a person does not carry a disorder or disease, given that the test result is negative.

Predictive value positive (PV⁺): The probability that a person carries a disorder or disease, given that the test result is positive.

Predictor variable: The variable (X) that is used to predict performance on another *criterion variable* (Y). Also called the independent variable.

Pre-experimental design: Studies that fail to meet at least two of the three criteria necessary for a true experiment.

Pretest-posttest control group design: The most commonly used of the true experimental designs. Two groups of subjects are randomly assigned to either an experimental condition, in which treatment (X) is administered, or to a control condition in which no treatment is given.

Prior probability: The unconditional probability used in the numerator of Bayes' rule. It represents the prevalence of a disease prior to performing an actual diagnostic test.

Probability estimate: The relative degree of certainty versus uncertainty about a particular research outcome. Statistically, a ratio reflecting long-run percentages for the generality of observed results.

Probability studies: Studies that attempt to forecast statistical outcomes based on a priori assumptions and/or empirical evidence.

Problem making: Deductive reasoning processes emanating from a general theory or explanatory model that leads to a research hypothesis.

Problem solving: Inductive reasoning processes in which the data derived from an experiment are used to support or refute a research hypothesis.

Prognosis: A prediction of the outcome of a proposed course of treatment for a given case.

Qualitative research: Strategies that emphasize nonnumerical data collection methods such as observations, interviews, etc. When numbers are used, typically they are intended to code, classify, or simply represent the presence or absence of the quality under study.

Quantitative research: The collection of numerical measures of behavior under controlled conditions that can be subjected to statistical analysis.

Quasi-experiments: Studies that satisfy all of the requirements of a true experiment with the exception of random assignment.

Random assignment: An effort to establish equivalent groups by randomly assigning subjects from the available subject pool to various treatments or conditions.

Random errors: Errors that are due to unknown causes of variation.

Random selection: A method in which a sample of subjects or observations is drawn from a population in such a way that each subject or observation has an equal chance of being represented.

Randomized-blocks analysis of variance (RBANOVA): Used for determining whether the differences between two or more groups may be due to chance or to systematic differences among the groups. It is especially appropriate for within-subject designs in which repeated measures of the same subject are made.

Range: The difference between the lowest and highest values in a distribution.

Ratio Scale: The most powerful of the numerical measurements scales. Possesses the properties of all others.

Regression analysis: A statistical means of determining the nature of the relationship between two variables based on estimating or predicting the value of one from the other.

Regression line: The best-fitted straight line through a joint distribution that represents predicted values of the dependent variable for each value of the independent variable.

Relationship question: A question that asks about the degree to which an observed phenomenon may change in association with other variables (e.g., age, gender, cognitive ability, etc.).

Reliability: The consistency of a test or measurement procedure. Statistically, the extent to which departures from a true score reflect random errors of measurement.

Research hypothesis (H_1): A problem statement derived from theoretical reasoning, prior data, or both; used for predicting associative or causal relations among variables. Also termed the *alternative hypothesis*.

Response amplitude: The amount or magnitude of a response as it is measured, perceived, or judged to exist.

Response duration: The time during which a response is observed to continue.

Response frequency: The total number of response units observed to occur or measured per unit of time (rate).

Response latency: The time it takes for a response to occur following some specified event.

Sample: A collection of some of the elements drawn from a population.

Sampling error: The expected amount of variance in a distribution of scores that is due to chance alone.

Sampling frame: A full listing of all subjects in a targeted population that one wishes to sample.

Sample space: The collection of all possible distinct outcomes that can occur when an experiment is performed.

Scheffé's method: One of the post hoc multiple comparison methods used to determine which specific group means among the various comparisons are significantly different from other means. It is highly useful when the sample sizes among the comparison groups are unequal.

Scientific method: Certain systematic thinking and action processes involving the control and measurement of variables that lead to valid and reliable answers to a question.

Selection bias: Factors that preclude or interfere with the establishment of equivalent groups.

Serendipity: The process of accidentally discovering valuable information while exploring an unrelated problem.

Significance level: The probability value selected or predetermined for rejecting the null hypothesis. Conventionally, the cutoff value between results attributed to chance and results attributed to a systematic influence is set at either $p < .05$ or $p < .01$. *p values* are also called *alpha levels*.

Simple random sampling: A technique in which each member of a population has a chance equal to that of every other member of the population of being selected for a sample.

Slope (b): The general magnitude or rate of change that describes how two variables go together.

Solomon four-group design: A design that attempts to control for certain interaction effects between a pretest and an independent variable and their combined influence on a dependent variable.

Spearman rank-correlation (rho): A nonparametric analog of the Pearson product-moment correlation computed on two variables with ranked scores.

Speculative language: Descriptions or definitions that are largely based on the unobservable or intuitive perceptions of an individual.

Standard deviation (σ, SD): The square root of variance.

Standard error of the mean ($\sigma_{\bar{x}}$, SEM): An estimate of the expected deviation of sample means from the true population mean as a result of chance or measurement errors.

Standard score (Z): A score based on the number of standard deviation units away from the mean on which its raw score equivalent lies.

Static-group comparison design: A type of pre-experimental design in which the performance of two groups is compared, one group receiving treatment and the other not receiving treatment. No effort is made to pretest subjects nor to randomly assign subjects to groups.

Statistic: A number derived by counting or measuring sample observations drawn from a population that is used in estimating a population parameter.

Statistical conclusion validity: The relative truth upon which the statistical conclusions of a study are based.

Statistical Package for the Social Sciences (SPSS): One of the most widely used packages for statistical analysis, designed for educational, social, and behavioral science research.

Statistical regression: The tendency for extreme scores in a data set, on repeated testing, to move toward the average score of a distribution.

Stratified random sampling: A technique in which random samples are drawn from defined subgroups (strata) of a population to assure adequate representation of members within each subgroup.

Subjective view: An estimate of probability that reflects a person's opinion or "best guess" based on prior experience.

Syllogism: A deductive form of reasoning introduced by Aristotle in which a conclusion is drawn from two previous statements.

Symmetric distribution: A distribution curve shaped in such a way that, if a vertical line is drawn through its center, the portion on one side of the curve is a mirror image of the other side.

Systematic errors: Uncontrolled systematic influences that can bias the outcome of an experiment by causing the scores in a distribution to consistently lean in one direction or another.

Systematic random sampling: A parsimonious way of drawing a sample from a large population when a membership list is available. A sampling interval size such as every tenth name on a list may be used to define the sampling frame.

Systematic variance: Systematic differences between the scores of two or more groups resulting from the assignment or active manipulation of the independent variable.

t-distribution: A bell-shaped distribution, usually associated with small sample size ($n \leq 30$). The basis for the so-called Student t-test used in null hypothesis testing.

Test-retest reliability: The extent to which a certain test or measuring procedure yields consistent findings when repeatedly administered to the same subjects.

Test sensitivity: The probability that the test result is positive given that the person has the disorder or disease.

Test specificity: The probability that the test result is negative given that the person does not have the disorder or disease.

Theory: A systematic structure of thought for guiding scientific inquiry and for organizing new facts as they emerge.

Time-series design: Repeated measures of a dependent variable are made before and after administering an independent variable.

True experiment: Distinguished from other designs on the basis of one or more of the following factors: random assignment of subjects to at least two groups, use of a control group, and active manipulation of an independent variable.

True score: One that should result as the consequence of repeated sampling over a very long series of trials under ideal conditions, using a perfect test instrument.

Tukey's method: One of the post hoc multiple comparison methods used to determine which specific group means among the various comparisons are significantly different from others. It is highly useful when the sample sizes among comparison groups are equal.

Two-way ANOVA: The ANOVA design involving two independent variables.

Type I error (alpha α): The rejection of a null hypothesis when it is true. Results in a false-positive conclusion.

Type II error (beta β): The retention of a null hypothesis when it is false. Results in a false-negative conclusion.

Unconditional probability: The probability of one event occurring independent of another event.

Variables: The factors described by constructs that are capable of assuming different values.

Variability: The degree of fluctuation in a population of scores when sampled.

Variance (σ^2, s^2): A measure of the dispersion in a distribution of observations in a population or sample, i.e., the average of the squared deviations from the mean.

Vicious circularity: Results when an answer is based on the question and the question is based on the answer.

Wilcoxon matched-pairs signed-ranks test: A commonly used nonparametric analog of the paired t-test that utilizes information about both the magnitude and direction of differences for pairs of scores.

Within-group variance: The degree of error variance that may involve both sampling errors and measurement errors.

Y intercept (a): The value of a dependent variable when not influenced by an independent variable.

Yates' correction for continuity: The chi-square formula exclusively designed for degrees of freedom $=1$. The correction deals with the inconsistency between the theoretical chi-square distribution and the actual distribution having 1 degree of freedom by subtracting 0.5 from the numerator of each term in the chi-square test prior to squaring the term.

Z distribution: A bell-shaped distribution, usually associated with a large sample size ($n > 30$). Also termed the standard normal distribution where the mean$=0$ and the standard deviation$=1$.

Z score: The amount of deviation of a score (X) from the mean of the distribution divided by the standard deviation.

Z test: The test for examining the significance of differences between means based on the Z distribution.

References

Adams, M. R., Freeman, F. J.,& Conture, E. G. (1984). Laryngeal dynamics of stutterers. In R. F. Curlee & W. H. Perkins (Eds.), *Nature and treatment of stuttering: New directions*. San Diego: College-Hill Press.

Alley, M. (1987). *The craft of scientific writing*. Englewood Cliffs, NJ: Prentice-Hall.

American Speech-Language-Hearing Association, (1989, April). Final report of the task force on research. Research Bulletin, Rockville, MD.

Anastasi, A. (1988). *Psychological testing* (6th ed.). New York: McGraw Hill.

Andrews, B., Guitar, B., & Howie, P. (1980). Meta-analysis of the effects of stuttering treatment. *Journal of Speech and Hearing Disorders*, 45, 387–307.

Aram, D., Scott, D., Shaywitz, S. E., Fletcher, J. M., & Francis, D. J. (1994). *Project II. Emergence of reading disability in children with early language impairments*. NIH-NICHD Program Project: 5P0l HD21888–07. Project Leader: D. Aram, Emerson College, Boston, MA.

Armstrong, J. S. (1980). Unintelligible management research and academic prestige. *Interfaces*, 10, 80.

Attanasio, J.S. (1994). Inferential statistics and treatment efficacy studies in communication disorders. *Journal of Speech and Hearing Research*, 37, 755–759.

Baer, D. M. (1975). In the beginning there was a response. In E. Ramp & G. Semb (Eds.), *Behavior analysis: Areas of research and application*. Englewood Cliffs, NJ: Prentice-Hall.

Bakan, D. (1966). The test of significance in psychological research. *Psychological Bulletin*, 66, 423–437.

Bales, R. (1950). *Interaction process analysis*. Cambridge, MA: Addison Wesley.

Baumgartner, J. M., & Brutten, G. J. (1983). Expectancy and heart rate as predictors of the speech performance of stutterers. *Journal of Speech and Hearing Research*, 26, 383–388.

Barresi, B. (1996). *Proper name recall in older and younger adults: The contributions of word uniqueness and strategies*. Unpublished doctoral dissertation, Emerson College, Boston, Massachusetts.

Bayes, T. (1763). Essay toward solving a problem in the doctrine of chances. *Philosophical transactions*. Royal Society, London, 53, 370–418. (Reprinted in Biometrika, 1958, 45, 293–315).

Bloodstein, O. (1974). The rules of early stuttering. *Journal of Speech and Hearing Disorders*, 39, 379–394.

Bloodstein, O. (1987). *A handbook on stuttering*. Chicago: National Easter Seal Society.

Boulding, K. E. (1978). *Ecodynamics: A new theory of societal evolution*. Beverly Hills, CA: Sage.

Brady, J.V. (1958). Ulcers in executive monkeys. Scientific American, 199, 95–100.

Browner, W. S., Newman, T. B., Cummings, S. R, & Hulley, S. B. (1988). Getting ready to estimate sample size: Hypotheses and underlying principles. In S. B. Hulley & S. R. Cummings (Eds.), *Designing clinical research*. Baltimore: Williams & Wilkins.

Brutten, G. J. (1975). Typography, assessment and behavior change strategies. In J. Eisenson, Jr. (Ed.), *Stuttering: A second symposium*. New York: Harper & Row.

Brutten, G. J., & Janssen, P. (1981). *A normative and factor analysis study of the responses of Dutch and American stutterers to the speech situation checklist*. Proceedings, 18th Congress International Association of Logopedics & Phoniatrics, Washington, DC: American Speech-Language-Hearing Association.

Bursztajn, H. J., Feinbloom, R. I., Hamm, R. M., & Brodsky, A. (1990). *Medical choices-medical chances*. New York: Routledge.

Campbell, D. T. (1969). Reforms as experiments. *American Psychologist*, 24,409–429.

Campbell, D. T., & Stanley, J. C. (1966). *Experimental and quasi-experimental designs for research*. Chicago: Rand McNally.

Cannon, W. B. (1945). *The way of an investigation*. New York: W.W. Norton.

Carver, R. P. (1983). The case against statistical significance testing. In P. Hauser-Cram & F. C. Martin (Eds.), *Essays on educational research: Methodology, testing and application*. Cambridge, MA: Harvard Education Review, Reprint No. 16.

Cohen, J. (1960). A coefficient of agreement for nominal scales. *Educational and Psychological Measurement*, 20, 37–46.

Cohen, J. (1977). *Statistical power analysis for the behavioral sciences* (Rev. ed.). New York: Academic Press.

Colton, T. (1974). *Statistics in medicine*. Boston: Little, Brown.

Cook, T. D., & Campbell, D. T. (1979). *Quasi-experimentation*. Chicago: Rand McNally.

Cook, T. D., Cox, F. L., & Mark, M. M. (1977). Randomized and quasi-experimental designs in evaluation research: An introduction. In L. Rutman (Ed.), *Evaluation research methods: A basic guide*. Beverly Hills: Sage.

Cooper, H. M., & Lemke, K. M. (1991). On the role of meta-analysis in personality and social psychology. *Personality and Social Psychology Bulletin, 17*, 245–251.

Cornett, R. O. (1967). Cued speech. *American Annals of the Deaf, 112*, 3–13.

Crichton, M. (1975). Medical obfuscation: Structure and function. *New England Journal of Medicine, 293*, 1257.

Curtiss, S., & Yamada, J. (1988). *Curtiss Yamada comprehensive language evaluation*. Unpublished test. University of California, Los Angeles.

Dallenbach, K. M. (1951). A puzzle picture with a new principle of concealment. *American Journal of Psychology, 64*, 431.

Dember, W. N., & Jenkins, J. J. (1970). *General psychology: Modeling behavior and experience*. Englewood Cliffs, NJ: Prentice-Hall.

Dewey, J. (1922). *Human nature and conduct*. New York: Holt, Rinehart and Winston.

Dunn, L. M., & Dunn, L. M. (1981). *Peabody Picture Vocabulary Test-Revised*. Circle Pines, MN: American Guidance Service.

Emerick, L. L., & Hatten, J. T. (1979). *Diagnosis and evaluation in speech pathology* (2nd ed.). Englewood Cliffs, NJ: Prentice-Hall.

Eysenck, H. L. (1983). Special review [review of M. L. Smith, G. V. Glass, & T. I. Miller, The benefits of psychotherapy]. *Behavior Research and Therapy, 21*, 315–320.

Filstead, W. J. (Ed.), (1970). *Qualitative methodology: Firsthand involvement with the social world*. Chicago: Markam.

Franke, R. H., & Kaul, J. D. (1978). The Hawthorne experiments: First statistical interpretation. *American Sociological Review, 43*, 623–253.

Fry, D. B. (1979). *The physics of speech*. Cambridge: Cambridge University Press.

Gartland, J. J. (1993). *Medical writing and communicating*. Frederick, MD: University Publishing Group.

Gelfand, D. M., & Hartmann, D. P. (1984). *Child behavior analysis and therapy*. New York: Pergamon Press.

Glass, G. V. (1977). Integrating findings: The meta-analysis of research. *Review of Research in Education, 5*, 351–379.

Glass, G. V., Willson, V. L., & Gottman, J. M. (1975). *Design and analysis of time-series experiments*. Boulder: Colorado Associated University Press.

Good, I. J. (1950). *Probability and weighing of evidence*. London: Griffin.

Gorsuch, R. L. (1983). *Factor analysis*. Hillsdale, NJ: Lawrence Erlbaum Associates.

Gregory, R. L. (1968). Visual illusions. *Scientific American, 219* (5), 66.

Guilford, J. P. (1950). *Fundamental statistics in psychology and education* (2nd ed.). New York: McGraw-Hill.

Guilford, J. P. (1956). *Fundamental statistics in psychology and education* (3rd ed.). New York: McGraw-Hill.

Hammen, V. L., Yorkston, K. M., & Minifie, F. D. (1974). Effects of temporal alterations on speech intelligibility in Parkinson's dysarthria. *Journal of Speech and Hearing Research, 37*, 244–253.

Hayes, W. L. (1973). *Statistics for the social sciences* (2nd ed.). New York: Holt, Rinehart & Winston.

Herson, M., & Barlow, D. H. (1976). *Single case experimental designs: Strategies for studying behavior change in the individual*. New York: Pergamon Press.

Hoover, K. R. (1976). *The elements of social scientific thinking*. New York: St. Martin's Press.

Iverson, G. R. (1984). *Bayesian statistical inference*. Newbury Park, CA: Sage.

James, W. (1890). *The principles of psychology*. 2 vols. New York: Henry Holt.

Jerger, J. (1963). Viewpoint. *Journal of Speech and Hearing Research, 6*, 301.

Jerger, J., Burney, P., Maulden, L., & Crump, B. (1993). Predicting hearing loss from the acoustic reflex. In B. Alford & S. Jerger (Eds.), *Clinical audiology: The Jerger perspective*. San Diego: Singular Publishing Group.

Johnson, J. R., Miller, J. F., Curtis, S., & Tallal, P. (1993). Conversations with children who are language impaired: Asking questions. *Journal of Speech and Hearing Research, 36*, 973–978.

Kaplan, E., Goodglass, H., & Weintraub, S. (1983). *Boston Naming Test*. Philadelphia: Lea & Febiger.

Kazdin, A. E. (1978). *History of behavior modification*. Baltimore: University Park Press.

Kazdin, A. E. (1982). *Single-case research designs: Methods for clinical and applied settings*. New York: Oxford University Press.

Kent, R. D., & Reed, C. (1992). *The acoustic analysis of speech*. San Diego: Singular.

Kerlinger, F. N. (1964). *Foundations of behavioral research*. New York: Holt, Rinehart & Winston.

Kerlinger, F. N. (1973). *Foundations of behavioral research* (2nd ed.). New York: Holt, Rinehart & Winston.

Kerlinger, F. N. (1986). *Foundations of behavioral research* (3rd ed.). New York: Holt, Rinehart & Winston.

Krasner, L. (1971). Behavior therapy. *Annual Review of Psychology, 22*, 483–532.

Kuhn, T. S. (1970). *The structure of scientific revolutions* (2nd ed.). Chicago: University of Chicago Press.

Lass, N. J., Ruscello, D. M., Pannbacker, M. D., Middleton, G. F., Schmitt, J. F., & Scheuerle, J. F. (1995). Career selection and satisfaction in the professions. *Asha, 37*, 48–51.

Liebert, R. M., & Liebert, L.L. (1995). *Science and behavior: An introduction to methods of psychological research*. Englewood Cliffs, NJ: Prentice-Hall.

Liebow, E. (1967). *Tally's corner: A study of street corner negro men*. Boston: Little, Brown.

Lundberg, G. A., Schragg, C. C.; Larson, O. N.; & Catton, Jr. W. R. (1968). *Sociology* (4th ed.). New York: Harper & Row.

Maxwell, A. E. (1970). *Basic statistics in behavioral research*. Baltimore: Penguin.

Maxwell, D. L., & Satake, E. (1993). *Applications of Bayesian statistics to the diagnosis of stuttering*. American Speech-Language-Hearing Association, Anaheim, California.

McGuigan, F. J. (1994). *Biological psychology: A cybernetic science*. Englewood Cliffs, NJ: Prentice-Hall.

McGuigan, F. J. (1993) *Experimental psychology. Methods of research*. Englewood Cliffs, NJ: Prentice-Hall.

Melton, A. W. (1962) Editorial. *Journal of Experimental Psychology, 64*, 553–557.

Menyuk, P., & Looney, P. (1972). Relationships among components of the grammar in language disorder. *Journal of Speech and Hearing Research, 15*, 395–406.

Merton, R. K. (1959). Notes on problem-finding in sociology. In R. K. Merton, L. Broom, & L. Conttrell, Jr. (Eds.), *Sociology today: Problems and prospects*. New York: Basic Books.

Milgram, S. (1977). *Subject reaction. The neglected factor in the ethics of experimentation*. Hastings Center Report, October.

Mishler, E. G. (1983). Meaning in context: Is there any other kind? In P. Hauser-Cram & F. C. Martin (Eds.), *Essays on educational research: Methodology, testing and application*. Cambridge, MA: Harvard Educational Review, Reprint No. 16.

Moore, J. C., & Holbrook, A. (1971). The operant manipulation of vocal pitch in normal speakers. *Journal of Speech and Hearing Research, 14*, 283–290.

Morrison, D. E., & Henkel, R. E. (1970). Significance tests in behavioral research: Skeptical conclusions and beyond. In D. E. Morrison & R. E. Henkel (Eds.), *The significance test controversy: A reader*. Chicago: Aldine.

Nicholls, G. H. & Ling, D. (1982). Cued speech and the reception of spoken language. *Journal of Speech and Hearing Research, 25*, 262–269.

Noldus, L. P. (1991). The observer: A software system for collection and analysis of observational data. *Behavior Research Methods, Instruments, and Computers, 23*, 415–429.

Norman, G. R., & Streiner, D. L. (1986). *PDQ Statistics*. Philadelphia: B. C. Decker.

Nunnally, J. C. (1978). *Psychometric theory* (2nd ed.). New York: McGraw-Hill.

Nye, C., Turner, I. Summarizing articulation disorder treatment effects: A meta-analysis. (1990). In L. B. Olswang, C. K. Thompson, S. F. Warren, & N. J. Minghetti (Eds.), *Treatment efficacy research in communication disorders*. Rockville, MD: American Speech-Language-Hearing Foundation.

Olmstead, D. (1971). *Out of the mouth of babes*. The Hague: Mouton.

Panagos, J. M., & Prelock, P. A. (1982). Phonological constrains on the sentence productions of language-disordered children. *Journal of Speech and Hearing Research, 25*, 171–177.

Peters, W. S. (1987). *Counting for something: Statistical principles and personalities*. New York: Springer-Verlag.

Piaget, J. (l932). *The language and thought of the child*. New York: Harcourt, Brace.

Pillimer, D. B., & Light, R. J. (1983). Synthesizing outcomes: How to use research evidence from many studies. *Harvard Education Review, 50*, 176–195 (b).

Pirsig, R. M. (1974). *Zen and the art of motorcycle maintenance*. New York: Bantam.

Poincaré, H. (1913). *The foundations of science*. New York: Science Press.

Pratt, S. R., Heintzelman, A. T. & Deming, S. E. (1993). The efficacy of using the IBM speech viewer vowel accuracy module to treat young children with hearing Impairment. *Journal of Speech and Hearing Research, 36*, 1063–1974.

Prizant, B. M. (1992). Childhood autism rating scale (review). In J. Conoley & J. Kramer (Eds.), Mental measurements yearbook. Lincoln: Buros Institute, University of Nebraska-Lincoln.

Pruzansky, S. (1973). Clinical investigation of the experiments of nature. In *Orofacial anomalies: Clinical and research implications*. ASHA Reports, number 8, 63.

Records, N. L., & Tomblin, J. B. (1994). Clinical decision making: Describing the decision rules of practicing speech-language pathologists. *Journal of Speech and Hearing Research, 37*, 144–156.

Riley, G. D. (1972). A stuttering severity instrument for children and adults. *Journal of Speech and Hearing Disorders, 37*, 314–320.

Riley, G. D. (1986). *A stuttering severity instrument for children and adults* (revised). Austen, TX: Proed.

Rosenthal, R., & Jacobson, L. (1966). *Experimenter effects in behavioral research*. New York: Appleton-Century-Crofts.

Rosenthal, R., & Jacobson, L. (1968). *Pygmalion in the classroom: Teacher expectation and pupils' intellectual development*. New York: Holt, Rhinehart & Winston.

Rossi, P. H., Freeman, H. W., & Wright, S. R. (1979). *Evaluation: A systematic approach*. Beverly Hills, CA: Sage.

Rosner, B., & Polk, B. F. (1983). Predictive valves of routine blood pressure measurements in screening for hypertension. *American Journal of Epidemiology, 117*, 429–444.

Rutter, M. Attention deficit disorder/hyperkinetic syndrome: Conceptual and research issues regarding diagnosis and classification (1989). In T. Sagvolden & T. Archer (Eds.), *Attention deficit disorder: Clinical and basic research*. Hillsdale, NJ: Lawrence Erlbaum.

Rvachew, S. (1994). Speech perception training can facilitate sound production learning. *Journal of Speech and Hearing Research, 37*, 347–357.

Sachs, H. S., Berrier, J., Reitman, D., Ancora-Berk, V. A., & Chalmers, T. C. (1987). Meta-analysis of randomized controlled trials. *New England Journal of Medicine, 316*, 450–455.

Satake, E., & Maxwell, D. L. (1995). *Application of Bayesian statistics: Determining accuracy of diagnosis of stuttering*. American Statistical Association, Pittsburgh, Pennsylvania.

Schiff-Myers, N. B. (1983). Pronoun reversals to correct pronoun usage: A case study of a normally developing child. *Journal of Speech and Hearing Disorders, 48*, 394–402.

Schopler, E., Reichler, R., & Renner, B. (1988). *The childhood autism rating scale*. Los Angeles: Western Psychological Services.

Shaffir, W. B., & Stebbins, R. A. (Eds.) (1991). *Experiencing fieldwork: An inside view of qualitative research*. Newbury Park, CA: Sage.

Shaughnessy, J. J., & Zechmeister, E. B. (1994). *Research methods in psychology*. New York: McGraw-Hill.

Shavelson, R. J. (1988). Statistical reasoning for the behavioral sciences (2nd ed.). Boston: Allyn and Bacon.

Shipley, K. G. (Ed.) (1982). *A style guide for writers in communicative disorders*. Tucson, AZ: Communication Skill Builders.

Shriberg, L. D., Kwiatkowski, J., & Gruber, F. A. (1994). Developmental phonological disorders II: Short-term speech-sound normalization. *Journal of Speech and Hearing Research, 37*, 1127–1150.

Sidman, M. (1960). *Tactics of scientific research*. New York: Basic Books.

Siegel, S. (1956). *Nonparametric statistics for the behavioral sciences*. New York: McGraw-Hill.

Singer, C. (1959). *A history of scientific ideas*. New York: Dorset Press.

Siu, R. H. (1957). *The tao of science*. Cambridge, MA: M.I.T. Press.

Skinner, B. F. (1956). A case study in scientific method. *American Psychologist, 11*, 221–233.

Skinner, B. F. (1938). *The behavior of organisms*. New York: Appleton-Century-Crofts.

SPSS Reference Guide (1990). Chicago: SPSS, Inc.

Stevens, S. S. (1960). *Handbook of experimental psychology* (3rd ed.). New York: John Wiley & Sons.

Strunk, W., Jr., & White, E. B. (1979). *The elements of style*. (3rd ed.). New York: MacMillan.

Thayer, N., & Dodd, B. (1996). Auditory processing and phonologic disorders. *Audiology, 35*, 37–44.

Thomas, D. S.(1929). Statistics in social research. *The American Journal of Sociology, 35*, 1–9.

Thorndike, E. L. (1938). The law of effect. *Psychological Review, 45*, 204–205.

Thurstone, L. L. (1947). *Multiple factor analysis*. Chicago: University of Chicago Press.

Van Riper, C. (1982). *The nature of stuttering*. Englewood Cliffs, NJ: Prentice-Hall.

Van Wagenen, R. K. (1991). *Writing a thesis: Sub-*

stance and style. Englewood Cliffs, NJ: Prentice-Hall.

Wallace, I. F., Gravel, J. S., McCarton, C. M., & Rubin, R. J. (1988). Otitis media and language development at one year of age. *Journal of Speech and Hearing Disorders*, *53*, 245–251.

Watson, J. B. (1924). *Behaviorism*. New York: Norton.

Wechsler, D. (1991). *Wechsler Intelligence Scale for Children* (3rd ed.). San Antonio, TX: Psychological Corporation.

Weinberg, N. (1968). *Analysis of fluency and interaction of adult, male stutterers and non-stutterers in small problem-solving groups*. Unpublished Master's thesis, Emerson College, Boston.

Weiner, N. (1948). *Cybernetics*. New York: John Wiley & Sons.

Weismer, S. E., Murray-Branch, J., & Miller, J. F. (1993). The influence of prosodic and gestural cues on novel word acquisition by children with specific language impairment. *Journal of Speech and Hearing Research*, *36*, 1037–1050.

Wigg, E., Secord, W., & Semel, E. (1992). *Clinical Evaluation of Language Fundamentals-Preschool*. San Antonio, TX: Psychological Corporation/ Harcourt Brace Jovanovich.

Wischner, G. J. (1950). Stuttering behavior and learning: A preliminary theoretical formulation. *Journal of Speech and Hearing Disorders*, *15*, 324–335.

Wischner, G. J. (1952). An experimental approach to expectancy and anxiety in stuttering behavior. *Journal of Speech and Hearing Disorders*, *17*, 139–154.

Wolf, F. M. (1986). *Meta-analysis. Quantitative methods for research synthesis*. Beverly Hills, CA: Sage.

Woodcock, R. W., & Johnson, M. B. (1989). *Woodcock-Johnson tests of cognitive ability*. DLM Teaching Resources, Allen, TX.

Yarruss, J. S., & Conture, E. G. (1993). F2 transitions during sound/syllable repetitions of children who stutter and predictions of stuttering chronicity. *Journal of Speech and Hearing Research*, *36*, 883–896.

Young, M. A. (1993). Supplementing tests of statistical significance: Variation accounted for. *Journal of Speech and Hearing Research*, *36*, 644–656.

Zebrowski, P. M. (1994). Duration of sound prolongations and sound syllable repetition in children who stutter: Preliminary observations. *Journal of Speech and Hearing Research*, *37*, 254–263.

Figure and Table Credits

Figure 1.1. Larson, G. (1986). Far Side, May 25, Wednesday. Working alone, Professor Dawson stumbles into a bad section of the petri dish. Kansas City, MO: Andrews McMeel & Parker/Universal Press Syndicate.

Figure 3.1. Taylor, G.R. (1979). Data sets: (a) Cubic; (b) two facing faces; and (c) a puzzle picture with a new principle of concealment. In G.R. Taylor (Ed.), *The Natural History of the Mind* (pp. 198, 199, 201). New York, NY: Penguin Books.

Figure 3.4. Kerlinger, F.N. (1964). Group variances. In F.N. Kerlinger (Ed.), *Foundations of Behavioral Research* (p. 104). Austin, Texas: Holt, Rhinehart and Winston, Inc., Div. Of Harcourt Brace & Co.

Figure 4.1. Jessen, J.K. (1991). Scholarly publications alive and well in ASHA. *Asha, 33,* p.42.

Figure 4.2. Carver, R. (1993). The case against statistical significance testing. In P. Hauser-Cram & F. Martin (Eds.), *Essays on educational research* (p. 24). Danvers, MA: Harvard Educational Review.

Figure 5.1. Schweiger, T.W. (1994). Two possible outcomes of a multiple time-series design. *Research methods in statistics and psychology* (p. 308). Pacific Grove, CA: Brooks/Cole Publishing Company.

Figure 5.3. Weismer, S.E., Murray-Branch, J., & Miller, J.F. (1993). Comparison of two methods for promoting productive vocabulary in late talkers. *Journal of Speech and Hearing Research, 36,* p. 1043.

Figure 5.5. Kazdin, A.E. (1982). Multiple-baseline designs. *Single-case research designs: Methods for clinical and applied settings* (p. 127). New York: Oxford University Press.

Figure 5.6. Pratt, S.R., Heintzelman, A.T., & Deming, S.E. (1993). The efficacy of using the IBM speech viewer vowel accuracy module to treat young children with hearing impairment. *Journal of Speech and Hearing Research, 36,* p. 1067.

Figure 5.8. Kiang, N.Y.S. (1975). Stimulus representation in the discharge patterns of auditory neurons. In D.B. Tower (Ed.), *The nervous system: Vol. 3: Human communication and its disorders.* New York: Raven Press.

Figure 5.9. Kent, R., Read, C. (1992). *The acoustic analysis of speech* (p. 172). San Diego, CA: Singular Publishing Group.

Figure 5.10. Stromsta, C. (1986). *Elements of stuttering* (p. 74). Oshtemo, MI: Atsmorts Publishing.

Figure 5.11. Jerger, J., Hayes, D. (1993). Latency of the acoustic reflex in eighth-nerve tumor. In B.R. Alford, & S. Jerger (Eds.), *Clinical Audiology: The Jerger Perspective* (p. 357). San Diego, CA: Singular Publishing Group.

Figure 6.1. Van Vliet, D., Berkey, D., Marion, M., Robinson, M. (1992). Professional education in audiology. *Asha 34,* p. 51.

Figure 6.2. Lass, N.J., Ruscello, D.M., Pannbacker, M.D., Middleton, G.F., Schmitt, J.F., Scheuerle, J.F. (1995). Career selection and satisfaction in the professions. *Asha 37,* p. 50.

Figure 6.3. Shriberg, L.D., Kwiatkowski, J., Gruber, F.A. (1994). Developmental phonological disorders II: Short-term speech-sound normalization. *Asha 37,* p. 1139.

Figure 6.8. Dunn, L., & Dunn, L. (1981). *Peabody Picture Vocabulary Test-Revised (PPVT-R)* (p. 21). Circle Pines, MN. American Guidance Service.

Figure 7.1. Leaverton, P.E. (1991). *A review of biostatistics: A program for self-instruction,* (4th ed.). Boston: Little, Brown and Company.

Figure 8.5. Oneway ANOVA (1990). SPSS *reference guide, 1990* (p. 846). Chicago: SPSS, Inc.

Figure 9.1. *Guidelines for Research in which Human or Animal Subjects Are Used* (1996). Rockville, MD: American Speech-Language-Hearing Association.

Table 5.6. Bales, R. (1950). Category system for assessment. *Interaction process analysis* (p. 9). Chicago: University of Chicago Press.

Table 7.1. Bell, F. (1995). *Basic biostatistics* (p. 77). Dubuque, IA.: Wm. C. Brown.

Table 8.8. Wechsler, D. (1991). *Wechsler Intelligence Scale for Children.* (3rd ed.) (p. 39). San Antonio: Harcourt, Brace, Jovanovich, Inc.

Table 8.9. Wechsler, D. (1991). *Wechsler Intelligence Scale for Children.* (3rd ed.) (p. 192). San Antonio: Harcourt, Brace, Jovanovich, Inc.

Table A.1. Johnson, J.R., Miller, J.F., Curtis, S., & Tallal, P. (1993). Conversations with children who are language impaired: Asking questions. *Journal of Speech and Hearing Research, 36,* p. 975.

Table A.4. Wallace, I.F., Gravel, J.S., McCarton, C.M., & Rubin, R.J. (1988). Otitis media and language development at one year of age. *Journal of Speech and Hearing Disorders, 53,* p. 246.

Table A.9. Schiff-Myers, N.B. (1983). Pronoun reversals to correct pronoun usage: Aa case study of a normally developing child. *Journal of Speech and Hearing Disorders, 48,* p. 396.

Table A.10. Yaruss, J.S., & Conture, E.G. (1993). F2 transitions during sound/syllable repetitions of children who stutter and predictions of stuttering chronicity. *Journal of Speech and Hearing Research, 36,* p. 891.

Table A.12. Hammen, V.L., Yorkston, K.M., & Minifie, F.D. (1974). Effects of temporal alterations on speech intelligibility in Parkinson's dysarthria. *Journal of Speech and Hearing Research, 37,* p. 250.

Table A.14. Zebrowski, P.M. (1994). Duration of sound prolongations and sound syllable repetition in children who stutter: preliminary observations. *Journal of Speech and Hearing Research, 37,* p. 258–259.

Table A.21. Moore, J.C., & Holbrook, A. (1971). The operant manipulation of vocal pitch in normal speakers. *Journal of Speech and Hearing Research, 14,* p. 287.

Tables C.1–C.6. Chase, W., & Brown, F. (1986). General statistics, (2nd ed.) (pp. A-14–A-21, A-23–A-25). New York, John Wiley & Sons.

Index

Page numbers followed by t or f indicate tables and figures, respectively.